PUBLIC & COMMUNITY HEALTH NURSING PRACTICE

PUBLIC & COMMUNITY HEALTH NURSING PRACTICE

A Population-Based Approach

Demetrius James Porche
Louisiana State University Health Sciences Center

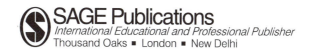
SAGE Publications
International Educational and Professional Publisher
Thousand Oaks ▪ London ▪ New Delhi

For information:

 Sage Publications, Inc.
2455 Teller Road
Thousand Oaks, California 91320
E-mail: order@sagepub.com

Sage Publications Ltd.
6 Bonhill Street
London EC2A 4PU
United Kingdom

Sage Publications India Pvt. Ltd.
B-42, Panchsheel Enclave
Post Box 4109
New Delhi 110 017 India

Printed in the United States of America

Library of Congress Cataloging-in-Publication data

Porche, Demetrius James.
Public and community health nursing practice : a population-based approach / Demetrius James Porche.
    p. cm.
Includes bibliographical references and index.
ISBN 0-7619-2483-3 (cloth)
    1. Public health nursing. 2. Community health nursing. I. Title.
RT97.P67 2004
610.73′4--dc22

                                        2003016654

03   04   05   06   07   10   9   8   7   6   5   4   3   2   1

Acquiring Editor:	Jim Brace-Thompson
Editorial Assistant:	Karen Ehrmann
Production Editor:	Sanford Robinson
Typesetter:	C&M Digitals (P) Ltd.
Copy Editor:	Catherine M. Chilton
Proofreader:	Katherine Pollock
Indexer:	Pilar Wyman
Cover Designer:	Michelle Lee

Contents

Preface

Public health practice focuses on the prevention of disease and disability as a means of promoting the health of communities and the individual constituent members who reside within those respective communities. Our goals for Healthy People 2010 are to increase the quality and quantity of years of healthy life and to eliminate health disparities. The achievement of these goals is dependent on public health nurses' ability to implement the core functions of public health practice: assessment, assurance, and policy development through population-based practice.

Population-based public health practice is the cornerstone to ensuring the health of our nation and the achievement of the Healthy People 2010 objectives. Population-based public health practice uses a defined population or community as the organizing principle for preventive action targeting the broad distribution of diseases and health determinants. Population-based public health practice is consistent with community-level interventions in that both have a widespread intervention scope. A key tenet of population-based public health practice is that a large number of people exposed to a small risk may generate more health alterations than a small number exposed to a high risk. Therefore, the proposition is to target interventions at the larger population group to maximize the public health benefits.

Part I: A Population-Based Framework for Public Health Practice provides the public health underpinnings for population-based public health practice (chapter 1). The public health system (chapter 2) is described from an infrastructure perspective. Basic public health practice content in epidemiological investigations (chapter 3) and behavioral science theories (chapter 4) are presented as foundations to public health nursing practice.

Part II: Public Health–Community Health Assessment Framework focuses on the core function of assessment. The public health nurse practicing at an advanced level is expected to have the skill set to conduct assessments at multiple levels. This section includes assessment strategies for behavioral assessments (chapter 5), public health organizational assessments (chapter 6), environmental health assessments (chapter 7), and a comprehensive community assessment (chapter 8). Assessment methods generating both primary and secondary data are expected to provide supporting data for program planning and the development of community-level interventions.

The content on the assurance core function spans Parts III, IV, and V. Part III emphasizes public health and community health interventions and strategies for program planning. Cultural competence (chapter 9), community development (chapter 10), and community-level interventions (chapter 11) are presented as essential skills needed to conduct public health and community health program planning for populations (chapter 12).

Public health nurses are increasingly held accountable for the effective implementation of population-based public health practice. Communities expect effective use of scarce public health resources. Part IV: Public Health Monitoring, Evaluation, Quality Improvement, Outcome Measures, and Evidence-Based Practice promotes the use of data for public health decision making. This section presents models and methods for program monitoring and evaluation (chapter 13), performance measurement and improvement (chapter 14), and public health research (chapter 15) and concludes with evidence-based public health practice (chapter 16).

The public health infrastructure is dependent on a sufficient number and competency level of public health practitioners to deliver population-based public health services. Part V: Public Health–Community Health Leadership and Administration focuses on the administrative skills necessary for managing and leading public health organizations and professionals. This section covers information about leadership (chapter 17); communication, collaboration, negotiation, and conflict resolution (chapter 18); causal analysis (chapter 19); fiscal and human resource management (chapter 20); and informatics (chapter 21) as public health nursing administrative functions.

The text concludes with content on the core function of policy development, described in Part VI: Public Health Policy, Law, and Ethics. This section familiarizes the public health nurse with health policy and politics (chapter 22); the process of public health policy development (chapter 23); public health policy formulation, implementation, and modification (chapter 24); public health policy analysis and evaluation (chapter 25); review of public health law and the legal system (chapter 26); and the scope of public health law (chapter 27), concluding with an examination of ethical practice in public health (chapter 28). Eight appendixes provide supplemental information that supports the text's chapters.

Acknowledgments

This book has been made possible through the support of my family, friends, and colleagues. First and foremost, I would like to thank my wonderful parents, Hayes and Diane Porche, for providing me with the love and support necessary to achieve an education and successful nursing career. Thanks go also to Anastasia Arceneaux and Chelsealea Lovell, my sisters, as well as their husbands, who always support my professional endeavors and provide me with continual enjoyment, and to Seth and Sebastian Porche, Janson Arceneaux, Jr., and Madeline Lovell, my nephews and niece, who are our family's future.

I extend my appreciation to the Reverend Dr. James A. Ertl, my best friend, for providing me with daily encouragement, support, and guidance to achieve my professional and personal goals and aspirations, and to Lynette Little, who always knows the right encouraging words to keep me focused and motivated and who provides me with numerous laughs.

My graduate community and public health nursing and public health students have encouraged the development and provided the direction for this text. I would also like to thank my mentors, Dr. Myrtis Snowden, Dr. Elizabeth Humphrey, Dr. Grace Guyden, Dr. Velma Sue Westbrook, and Dr. Richard Sowell, for having an impact on my professional career. In addition, I would like to thank my colleagues at Louisiana State University Health Sciences Center and Tulane School of Public Health for their professional affiliation.

Sage Publications acquisitions editor Jim Brace-Thompson and editorial assistant Karen Ehrmann warrant special recognition for their guidance and assistance in bringing this manuscript to fulfillment. My copy editor, Catherine M. Chilton, and production editor, Sanford Robinson, for the hours of talented work and feedback and encouragement, are greatly appreciated.

Thanks,

Demetrius James Porche

Part I

A Population-Based Framework for Public Health Practice

Population-Based Public Health Practice

The health of individuals and our nation are dependent on public health practice. Population-based public health practice provides one paradigm that can influence the health of multiple communities within our nation. This chapter focuses on defining public health practice; describes a population-based approach; differentiates conceptually aggregate, community-based approaches and community-based care; defines community and community health practice; differentiates community and public health nursing practice; provides public health competencies; and concludes with a review of the levels of prevention.

Introduction

Public health practice focuses on the prevention of disease and disability as a means of promoting the health of communities and their constituent members. The Healthy People 2010 agenda is a strategic public health plan that strives to promote the health of communities and community members (Department of Health and Human Services [DHHS], 2000). The national objectives proposed in Healthy People 2010 come at a pivotal point, a point of crisis, in public health practice. A landmark report by the Institute of Medicine (IOM) in 1988 stated that the public health system was in disarray, resulting from uncoordinated public health efforts, a weak public health infrastructure, and inconsistent goals and functions within the public health system. The report also notes that in addition to these problems, Americans continue to take the public health system for granted. Americans appear to take for granted public health issues such as communicable disease control, workplace safety, and environmental protection.

Some of the issues the public health system faces are changing population demographics, cultural tensions, resurgence of infectious diseases, emergence of new infections, and continued environmental hazards. The present state of the public health system and the national Healthy People

2010 objectives require a new paradigm for public health practice. In addition, multiple vulnerable populations exist that would benefit from a new public health practice paradigm of population-based practice. Population-based public health practice will be presented here as the public health practice paradigm for the next century.

Public Health Practice

Public health activity, the public health workforce, and the entire public health system provide the defining framework for public health practice (chapter 2 provides a further description of the public health workforce and public health system). Public health activities are implemented to prevent disease and disability, and this further defines public health practice (Table 1.1). Public health practice focuses on the health of aggregates or groups, family, or community. A key feature of public health practice is the acknowledgment that health is greater than the biological determinants of individual health; public health practice also embraces a host of behavioral, social, economic, and environmental factors that affect the health of a community.

Historically, Winslow (1923) defined public health as

the science and art of preventing disease, prolonging life, and promoting physical health and efficiency through organized community efforts for the sanitation of the environment, the control of community infections, the education of the individual in principles of personal hygiene, the organization of medical and nursing services for the early diagnosis and preventive treatment of disease, and the development of social machinery which will ensure to every individual in the community a standard of living adequate for the maintenance of health. (p. 1)

Winslow's definition of public health continues to remain valid today. A recent definition of public health was provided in the landmark 1988 IOM report on our nation's public health. The IOM defines public health as "organized community efforts aimed at the prevention of disease and promotion of health" (p. 41). In this same report, the IOM describes public health as "what we, as a society, do collectively to assure the conditions in which people can be healthy" (p. 41).

Based on these historical and reputable definitions, public health practice will be defined in this book as those organized public health activities, provided by an educated and trained workforce, that are based on the integration of scientific evidence from biological, behavioral, social, environmental, and epidemiological sciences and are designed to promote health, prevent disease, and improve the quality of life of a population within an

Table 1.1 Public Health Activities

Surveillance and monitoring of the population's health status
Prevention and control of epidemics
Environmental and occupational protection: food, water, and workplace safety practices
Assurance of quality and accessibility of services
Disaster preparation and response
Public health research to develop innovative solutions
Community mobilization and development
Public health policy development

SOURCE: Department of Health and Human Services (1994b).

existing community (Figure 1.1). Public health practice is grounded in public health activities (Table 1.1) that are provided within an organized health-care system comprising multiple types of institutions, both public and private, that promote the health of a community.

The Population-Based Approach

The distinguishing attribute of community and public health practice when compared to medical practice is public health's central focus on the health of a population. The population-based approach uses a defined population (community) as the organizing principle for preventive action targeting the broad distribution of diseases and health determinants. Population-based principles use population-based data as the scientific basis for community level interventions (Novick, 2001; Thomas, 1999). Five principles that characterize the population-based approach are (a) a community perspective, (b) a clinical epidemiology perspective (using population-based data), (c) evidence-based practice, (d) an emphasis on effective outcomes, and (e) an emphasis on primary prevention (Ibrahim, Savitz, Carey, & Wagner, 2001; Novick, 2001). Another term, *population-focused care*, refers to a process that uses the population-based approach. Population-focused care is defined as interventions *aimed* at disease prevention and health promotion that shape a community's overall profile (DHHS, 1994a). For the purposes of this textbook, population-based care will be defined as *community-level interventions* that focus on health promotion and disease prevention activities that *influence the community's overall health profile*.

Community level interventions that affect the determinants of disease within an entire community rather than simply those of a single, high-risk individual are considered population-based interventions. Population-based and individual interventions are not exclusive but complementary strategies (Novick, 2001). The DHHS (1994a) described population-based public health services as interventions aimed at disease prevention and health promotion that shape a community's overall health status profile.

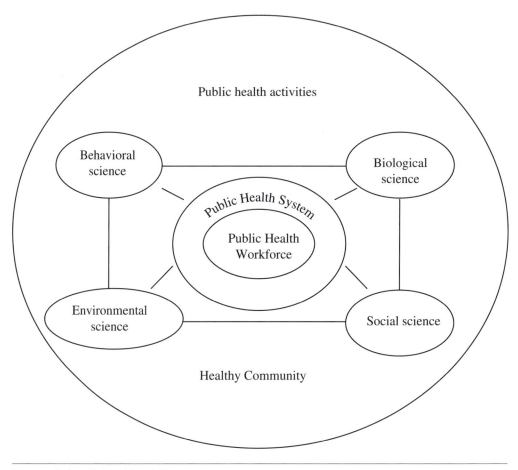

Figure 1.1   Public Health Practice

Clearly, the population-based approach transcends the individual level. The population-based approach does not limit itself to the biological, environmental, and agent determinants of illness but includes as well lifestyle factors and health care organizations (as determinants), as well as other factors that contribute to health determinants. This is consistent with Rose's (1992) philosophy that a widespread problem must have a corresponding widespread intervention. The population-based approach is consistent with Rose's preventive medicine axiom: "A large number of people exposed to a small risk may generate many more cases than a small number exposed to a high risk" (p. 24). Therefore, a preventive strategy targeting only high-risk individuals may benefit these individuals—with little resultant effect on the total burden of a disease within a community.

The Aggregate and Community-Based Approaches and Community-Based Care: Conceptual Differences

The focus of community or public health practice is the health of an entire community. To affect the health of an entire community, the public health nurse targets specific groups and designs interventions at multiple levels (individual, aggregate or group, family, and community). The manner in which the public health nurse identifies the target population, based on population-based data, determines the public health approach to the community: aggregate or community-based care.

An *aggregate* is a subgroup of the community population and is also referred to as a subpopulation. Any community consists of multiple aggregates. The manner in which the aggregate is identified determines the type of aggregate and, eventually, the type of community interventions planned. Community members can be grouped into simple aggregates based on demographic or geographic location; this is the least common type of aggregate used in community health practice. The most common aggregate type is the high-risk aggregate. A *high-risk aggregate* is a subgroup or subpopulation of the community that has a high-risk commonality among its members, such as risky lifestyle behaviors or high-risk health conditions (e.g., adolescent pregnancy). The aggregate concept is used in public health practice to target interventions to specific aggregates or subpopulations within a community.

The concepts of aggregate and community-based approaches and community-based care are different in their intended focus. An *aggregate approach* targets a specific subpopulation within the community. The *community-based approach* focuses the interventions on the entire community, using population-based data. In the community-based approach, interventions are designed to affect the health of an entire community at one time, such as fluoridation of an entire community's water supply. *Community-based care* is often confused with the community-based approach. Community-based care (also referred to as community-based practice) is the delivery of health-care services outside the typical institutional setting, but these services do not necessarily focus on the entire community (American Nurses Association [ANA], 1995). Community-based care is the delivery of health-care services within the community environment, services that target individuals and families. For example, an ambulatory clinic that provides acute episodic care to individuals strategically located within a geographical community is delivering community-based care. The services planned in this clinic may be based on the assessed health needs of individual community members, but they do not strive to affect the health of the community using community-level interventions; rather, these services provide individual-level care. The differentiating factor is the implementation of interventions that affect (a) the individual or family (community-based care) or (b) the community's health (community-based approach). It is possible to deliver community-based care using a community-based approach, provided the public health interventions are community level, delivered in the community, and based on population data.

Community and Community Health Practice

Community and *community health practice* are considered very elusive concepts. The focus of public heath and community health practice is the health of a defined population, which is frequently described as a community. A community can be defined in terms of (a) common interest or characteristics, (b) geographical boundaries, or (c) a system (Helvie, 1998). An individual within a given population can be a member of several different communities at the same time, depending on the defining characteristics of the community. Additionally, depending on the type of community, community members may never have personal contact with each other.

Communities defined by common interest or characteristics may possess similar demographic variables such as age, race, gender, social class, or cultural identity. Communities defined by common interest or characteristics are frequently referred to as associative communities (Turnock, 2001). A geographical community is defined by physical geographic boundaries such as mountains, rivers, or interstates. Other geographical community boundaries are political in nature, such as a census tract or political region. A smaller subsystem or community sector that exists within the larger societal system can be the defining characteristic of a community. Systems that may be considered a community are transportation, emergency response (fire and police), health care, and education.

Community health practice focuses on a defined community and on the capacity of that community to achieve its health goals through effective use of community assets (Turnock, 2001). Community health practices recognize the importance of health determinants that are behavioral, social, and environmental in nature, in addition to the biological determinants of health. Community and public health nurses use community mobilization efforts, such as community engagement, community collaboration, and partnerships, to organize a community to work collectively for community health. Community health practice focuses on population-based problems (identified from population-based data), thereby using a population-based approach to influence the health of a community.

Community Health and
Public Health Nursing Practice

The Quad Council consists of four organizational constituents: the American Nurses Association (ANA), the Association of Community

Health Nurse Educators (ACHNE), the American Public Health Association (APHA), and the Association of State and Territorial District Nurses (ASTDN). The Quad Council defines the scope and standards of practice for each nursing specialty. Table 1.2 presents the respective definitions and standards for community health and public health nursing practice. The scope of practice and standards of practice for community health and public health nursing complement the definition of public health practice given earlier. ACHNE's Task Force on Community Health Nursing Education supports the title and definition of public health nursing by the Quad Council (ACHNE, 2000). Public health nursing practice is considered to include the core functions of public health: assessment, policy development, and assurance activities.

In addition to the Quad Council's definitions, the APHA Ad Hoc Committee on Public Health Nursing (1981) defined public health nursing as

the synthesis of the body of knowledge from the public health sciences and professional nursing theories for the purpose of improving the health of the entire community. This goal lies at the heart of primary prevention and health promotion and is the foundation of public health nursing practice. . . . Identifying subgroups (aggregates) within the population which are at high risk of illness, disability, or premature death, and directing resources toward these groups, is the most effective approach for accomplishing the goal of [public health nursing]. (p. 10)

Public health nursing has specific characteristics (e.g., a focus on public health activities), but it is viewed as a part of the broad area of community health nursing practice. Common characteristics of community and public health nursing are (a) provision of services to an entire population, (b) a focus on the promotion and preservation of health, and (c) care directed to community-level problems.

Public Health Competencies

Public health practice is dependent upon an educated, trained, and competent workforce. The public health workforce is composed of individuals from multiple disciplines and professions associated with health-care delivery. Each discipline and profession brings a specialized combination of knowledge, skill, abilities, perspectives, and competencies to public health practice. The diversity within the public health workforce adds to the richness of public health practice. However, there must be a clear correlation between these diverse sets of competencies in the public health workforce and the community needs. The 1988 IOM report calls for improvements in the training of public health professionals and an improvement of the linkage between academe and public health practice.

Table 1.2   Quad Council Definitions and Standards

Public Health Nursing
DEFINITION

Public health nursing is the practice of promoting and protecting the health of populations using knowledge from nursing, social, and public health sciences (American Public Health Association, Public Health Nursing Section, 1996). Public health nursing is population-focused, community-oriented nursing practice. The goal of public health nursing is the prevention of disease and disability for all people through the creation of conditions in which people can be healthy (American Nurses Association, 1999).

STANDARDS OF CARE

The public health nurse standards of care focus on

1. Assessment of the population's health status using data, community resources identification, input from the population, and professional judgment.

2. Analysis of the assessment data collected in collaboration with community partners to attach meaning to that data and determine opportunities and needs.

3. Participation with community partners to identify expected outcomes in the populations and their health status.

4. Promotion and support of public health program development, policy development, and provision of services that include interventions that improve the health status of populations.

5. Assuring the population access and availability of programs, policies, resources, and services.

6. Evaluation of the population's health status.

STANDARDS OF PROFESSIONAL PERFORMANCE

According to the standards of professional performance, the public health nurse

1. Systematically evaluates the availability, accessibility, acceptability, quality, and effectiveness of nursing practice for the population.

2. Evaluates his or her own nursing practice in relation to professional practice standards and relevant statutes and regulations.

3. Acquires and maintains current knowledge and competence in public health nursing practice.

4. Establishes collegial partnerships when interacting with health-care practitioners and others and contributes to the professional development of peers, colleagues, and others.

5. Applies ethical standards in advocating for health and social policy and in delivery of public health programs to promote and preserve the health of the population.

6. Collaborates with the representatives of the population and other health and human service professionals and organizations in providing for and promoting the health of the population.

7. Uses research findings in practice.

8. Considers safety, effectiveness, and cost in the planning and delivery of public health services when using available resources, to ensure the maximum possible health benefit to the population.

(Continued)

Table 1.2   (Continued)

Community Health Nursing
DEFINITION

Community health nursing is a synthesis of nursing practice and public health practice, applied to promoting and preserving the health of populations. Health promotion, health maintenance, health education and management, coordination, and continuity of care are used in a holistic approach to the management of the health care of individuals, families, and groups in a community (American Nurses Association, 1986).

STANDARDS

Community health nurse standards of care focus on

1. The application of theoretical concepts as a basis for practice decisions.

2. The systematic collection of comprehensive and accurate data.

3. The analysis of community, family, and individual level data to determine diagnoses.

4. The development of plans to specify nursing actions unique to individual client needs based on the level of prevention.

5. Nursing plans developed to guide interventions that promote, maintain, or restore health; prevent illness; and effect rehabilitation.

6. Evaluation of community, family, and individuals' responses to interventions as a means of determining progress toward goal achievement and revising the database, diagnoses, and plan.

7. Participation in peer review and other means of evaluation to assure quality of nursing practice. The responsibility for professional development and professional growth of others is a responsibility of the nurse.

8. Collaboration with other health-care providers, professionals, and community representatives in the assessment, planning, implementation, and evaluation of community health programs.

9. Use of research as a means of contributing to theory and practice development in community health nursing.

SOURCE: American Nurses Association (1986, 1999), American Public Health Association, Public Health Nursing Section (1996).

As a measure to meet both of these objectives—improving public health workforce training and linking academic research and knowledge to public health—the Council on Linkages Between Academia and Public Health Practice was formed. The council comprises leaders from national organizations representing both public health practice and academic communities. The council's mission is "to improve public health practice and education by defining and implementing recommendations of the Public Health/ Faculty/Agency Forum, establishing links between academia and the agencies of the public health community, and creating a process for continuing public health education throughout one's career" (Council on Linkages Between Academia and Public Health Practice, 2001). This mission is consistent with the U.S. Public Health Service's efforts to implement certain components of *The Public Health Workforce: An Agenda for the 21st Century* report (Public Health Functions Project, 1997) pertaining to public health competencies.

The Council on Linkages adopted core competencies on April 11, 2001, for a 3-year period. These core competencies represent a set of skills, knowledge, and attitudes designed to transcend the boundaries of a specific discipline and ensure the delivery of essential public health services. The competencies are divided into eight domains:

- Analytic assessment skills
- Basic public health science skills
- Cultural competency skills
- Communication skills
- Community dimensions of practice skills
- Financial planning and management skills
- Leadership and system thinking skills
- Policy development and program planning skills

The skill or knowledge level (ranging from aware to knowledgeable to proficient) required for each competency is defined for frontline staff, senior-level staff, and supervisory and management staff. Appendix A presents the Council on Linkages Between Academia and Public Health Practice competencies for each domain. It is expected that all public health professionals should be aware of these core competencies, including public health nurses. Additionally, public health professionals should be educated and trained to ensure that they have the appropriate level of knowledge and skills that corresponds to their respective public health duties for each core competency (Council on Linkages Between Academia and Public Health Practice, 2001).

Prevention Levels: Primary Prevention and Health Promotion—A Public Health Focus

Public health practice focuses on altering the interaction of biologic, behavioral, social, cultural, and environmental determinants that would result in disease. Alterations in the interaction of these health determinants are based on planned public health interventions from population-based data. These public health interventions can be characterized as three levels—primary, secondary, and tertiary prevention. A major emphasis of public health practice that is aligned with public health goals is primary prevention. Primary prevention involves individual, aggregate or group, or community-level

Table 1.3 Primary, Secondary and Tertiary Prevention Strategies

Primary Prevention Strategies
- Health education and counseling—healthy lifestyle behaviors, exercise, stress management, nutrition, genetic, family
- Immunizations
- Adequate housing and employment opportunities
- Educational and recreational opportunities
- Environmental modifications and regulations—clean air and water, environmental sanitation
- Occupational hazard protection
- Injury prevention

Secondary Prevention Strategies
- Screening test and surveys
- Community assessments
- Case-finding activities
- Routine physical and mental exams
- Early medical treatment

Tertiary Prevention Strategies
- Effective and complete medical treatment
- Work therapy and workforce retraining and reeducation

interventions, based on population data, to promote and protect health (health promotion) and prevent disease (disease prevention). Health promotion and disease prevention are two different concepts. Health promotion consists of lifestyle-related activities designed to improve or maintain health. Disease prevention consists of those activities designed to prevent the development of disease or its related consequences (Thomas, 1999). Secondary prevention involves individual, aggregate or group, or community-level interventions, based on population data, to promote early detection and treatment of disease. After a disease state exists, tertiary interventions are directed at preventing disability through restoration of optimal functioning. Table 1.3 presents primary, secondary, and tertiary prevention strategies.

Each prevention level has a different impact on the status of diseases within a population. Primary prevention interventions prevent disease occurrence; therefore, the incidence rates of diseases within a population are reduced. Screening, testing, and treatment are secondary prevention strategies that result in earlier identification of cases of the disease and promote early treatment of disease; therefore, the prevalence rates of a disease within a population are reduced. Secondary prevention strategies strive to decrease a population's burden of a disease. Tertiary prevention strategies reduce the long-term complications and disabilities that result from a disease and also affect prevalence rates of disease within a population. Tertiary prevention strategies that promote quality of life but do not end the disease state can increase the prevalence rate of a disease within a population. Although tertiary prevention strategies do affect the individual's disease burden, if they increase the disease burden within the community, more population-based services will be required.

Public health levels of prevention can also be related to medical practice. *Medical practice* is defined as the services provided under the direct supervision of a health-care provider, which can be divided into four service levels: population-based public health services, primary medical care, secondary medical care, and tertiary medical care. These levels of medical practice were developed independently from the levels of prevention, but they correlate with the levels of prevention (Turnock, 2001).

Population-based public health services consist of health promotion and disease prevention interventions that affect the health of an entire community. Population-based public health and medical practice are not mutually exclusive concepts. Population-based public health practice uses medical interventions to affect the health of an entire community. Primary prevention correlates with population-based public health practice. Primary medical care consists of medical services delivered at the first point of contact that includes clinical preventive services and ongoing care for common medical conditions. Primary medical care frequently encompasses primary, secondary, and tertiary levels of prevention. Secondary medical care consists of medical services requiring specialized treatment and ongoing management of common and less common medical conditions. Secondary medical care is correlated with secondary prevention (routine examinations or screenings and treatment of health conditions). Tertiary medical care consists of medical services that require highly specialized and technologically sophisticated medical and surgical care for unusual and complex medical conditions. Secondary and tertiary medical care are correlated with tertiary prevention (DHHS, 2000; Turnock, 2001).

Summary

Key issues in population-based public health practice are as follows.

- Public health practice focuses on the prevention of disease and disability as a means of promoting the health of communities and their constituent members.
- A key feature of public health practice is the acknowledgment that health is greater than the biological determinants of individual health. Public health practice also embraces a host of behavioral, social, economic, and environmental factors that affect the health of a community.
- Public health practice is defined as the organized public health activities that are (a) provided by an educated and trained workforce; (b) based on the integration of scientific evidence from biological,

behavioral, social, environmental, and epidemiological sciences; and (c) designed to promote health, prevent disease, and improve the quality of life of a population within an existing community.

- The population-based approach uses a defined population (community) as the organizing principle for preventive action that targets the broad distribution of diseases and health determinants.
- Five principles that characterize the population-based approach are (a) a community perspective, (b) a clinical epidemiology perspective (population-based data), (c) evidence-based practice, (d) emphasis on effective outcomes, and (e) emphasis on primary prevention.
- Community-level interventions that affect the determinants of disease within an entire community rather than those of a single high-risk individual are considered population-based interventions.
- An aggregate, also referred to as a subpopulation, is a subgroup of the community population.
- A high-risk aggregate is a subgroup of the community population that has a high-risk commonality among its members.
- The community-based approach focuses interventions on the entire community, using population-based data.
- Community-based care is the delivery of health-care services outside the typical institutional setting. These services do not necessarily focus on the entire community.
- A community can be defined in terms of (a) common interest or characteristics, (b) geographical boundaries, or (c) a system.
- Community health practice focuses on the capacity of a community to achieve its health goals through effective use of community assets.
- Common characteristics of community and public health nursing are (a) provision of services to an entire population, (b) a focus on the promotion and preservation of health, and (c) care directed to community-level problems.
- Public health competencies are divided into eight domains: (a) analytic assessment skills, (b) basic public health science skills, (c) cultural competency skills, (d) communication skills, (e) community dimensions of practice skills, (f) financial planning and management skills, (g) leadership and system thinking skills, and (h) policy development and program planning skills. The skill or knowledge level (aware, knowledgeable, proficient) required for each competency is defined for frontline staff, senior-level staff, and supervisory and management staff.
- Public health levels of prevention are primary, secondary, and tertiary.
- Medical practice has four service levels—population-based public health services, primary medical care, secondary medical care, and tertiary medical care—that are different from but relate to the levels of prevention.

References

American Nurses Association. (1986). *Standards of community health nursing practice.* Washington, DC: Author.

American Nurses Association. (1995). *Scope and standards of population-focused and community-based nursing practice.* Washington, DC: Author.

American Nurses Association. (1999). *Scope and standards of public health nursing practice.* Washington, DC: Author.

American Public Health Association. (1981). *The definition and role of public health nursing practice in the delivery of health care: A statement of the public health nursing section.* Washington, DC: Author.

American Public Health Association, Public Health Nursing Section. (1996). *Definition and role of public health nursing.* Washington, DC: Author.

Association of Community Health Nurse Educators, Task Force on Community/Public Health Masters Level Preparation. (2000). *Graduate education for advanced practice in community/public health nursing.* Louisville, KY: Author.

Association of Community Health Nurse Educators, Task Force on Basic Community Health Nursing Education. (1990). *Essentials of baccalaureate nursing education for entry level community health nursing practice.* Louisville, KY: Author.

Council on Linkages Between Academia and Public Health Practice. (2001). *Competencies project.* Retrieved June 5, 2003, from http://www.trainingfinder.org/competencies/background.htm

Department of Health and Human Services. (1994a). *Consensus conference on the essentials of public health nursing practice and education: Report of the conference.* Rockville, MD: Author.

Department of Health and Human Services, Public Health Services. (1994b). *For a healthy nation: Returns on investments in public health.* Washington, DC: Author.

Department of Health and Human Services. (2000). *Healthy people 2010: Understanding and improving health.* Washington, DC: Author.

Helvie, C. (1998). *Advanced practice nursing in the community.* Thousand Oaks, CA: Sage.

Ibrahim, M., Savitz, L., Carey, T., & Wagner, E. (2001). Population-based health principles in medical and public health practice. *Journal of Public Health Management, 7*(3), 75-81.

Institute of Medicine. (1988). *The future of public health.* Washington, DC: National Academy Press.

Novick, L. (2001). Defining public health. In L. Novick & G. Mays (Eds.), *Public health administration: Principles for population-based management* (pp. 3-33). Gaithersburg, MD: Aspen.

Public Health Functions Project. (1997). The public health workforce: An agenda for the 21st century. Washington, DC: U.S. Department of Health and Human Services.

Rose, G. (1992). *The strategy of preventive medicine.* New York: Oxford University Press.

Thomas, S. (1999). Caring in community health nursing. In J. Hitchcock, P. Schubert, & S. Thomas (Eds.), *Community health nursing: Caring in action* (pp. 3-16). Boston, MA: Delmar.

Turnock, B. (2001). *Public health: What it is and how it works.* Gaithersburg, MD: Aspen.

Winslow, C.-E. A. (1923). *The evolution and significance of the modern public health campaign.* New Haven, CT: Yale University Press.

2

The Public
Heath System

The public health system is an intricate component of the nation's health-care delivery systems. The public health infrastructure supports the delivery of public health services to the community's populations. This chapter focuses on the IOM public health report, public health infrastructure, public health's core functions and essential services, the nation's Healthy People 2010 plan, and privatization of public health services.

Introduction

The defining characteristics of public health are dependent upon the services provided through the public health system and the professional disciplines represented within the public health system. Chapter 1 provides various definitions of public health and Figure 1-1 provides a model of the components of public health practice. Even with these definitions, there has been a growing impression that public health, as a profession, governmental agency, or integrated health-care system is not clearly defined, adequately supported, or completely understood (IOM, 1988). This chapter proposes to expand and further clarify the meaning of public health and public health systems.

Institute of Medicine Public Health Report

An IOM committee examined the mission, current state, and barriers to improvement in public health. "The public health system is in disarray" is a frequently quoted statement from this report, which provides further direction for the development of the public health system. The committee reported, "effective public health activities are essential to the health and well-being of the American people, now and in the future" (IOM, 1988,

p. 6). Additionally, based on the committee's study of the public health system, recommendations were provided in three areas: the mission of public health, the government's role in fulfilling the mission, and the unique responsibilities of each level of government.

According to the IOM committee (IOM, 1988), the mission of public health is very expansive and comprehensive, with a central focus on maintaining a healthy population. The IOM committee defined the mission of public health as "fulfilling society's interest in assuring conditions in which people can be healthy" (p. 7). The public health system that addresses this broad mission is expected to encompass public and community-based agencies, individuals, and private organizations within the broader health-care delivery system. However, governmental public health agencies are expected to maintain the vital elements of the public health infrastructure to achieve this mission.

Core functions of public health—assessment, policy development, and assurance—are recommended as essential to achieving the mission of public health. These core functions of public health are common to the federal, state, and local governments, with each level of government maintaining unique responsibilities. States are considered the central force in public health, with direct responsibility for the public sector's health. States are expected to define the basic authority and responsibility entrusted to public health agencies, boards, and officials at the state and local levels and establish the relationships between such entities (IOM, 1988). Table 2.1 outlines the governmental levels of responsibility as identified in the 1988 IOM report.

Public Health System

The view that public health exists as an isolated entity is eroding as a result of the 1988 Institute of Medicine (IOM) committee report on the disarray within public health. Public health has historically solved and continues to solve population-based problems through scientific and technical information, with an eye to society's values. Public health knowledge and societal values remain the primary decisive elements that shape public health practice and, ultimately, the public health system. Public health's vision is "healthy people in healthy communities" with an articulated mission to "promote physical and mental health and prevent disease, injury and disability" (Centers for Disease Control and Prevention [CDC], 2001).

The public health system is composed of a complex network of people, systems, and organizations that are working together at local, state, and national levels to improve the health of populations (CDC, 2001). The public health-care system is only one component of the national health-care system. A distinguishing aspect of the public health system is its primary

Table 2.1 Public Health Duties at Each Governmental Level

Federal

- Support of knowledge development and dissemination through data gathering, research, and information exchange
- Establishment of nationwide health objectives and priorities
- Stimulation of debate on interstate and national public health issues
- Provision of technical assistance to help states and localities determine their own objectives and carry out action on national and regional objectives
- Provision of funds to states to strengthen states' capacity to deliver services, especially services that will achieve national objectives
- Assurance of actions and services that are in the public interest of the entire nation

State

- Assessment of health needs in the state, based on statewide data collection
- Assurance of an adequate statutory base for health activities
- Establishment of statewide health objectives: Power is delegated to localities for this purpose as appropriate, and the state holds them accountable
- Assurance of appropriate, organized, statewide effort to develop and maintain essential personal, educational, and environmental services; provision of necessary services; and solution of those problems that are inimical to health
- Guarantee of at least a minimum of essential health services

Local

- Assessment, monitoring, and surveillance of local health problems and needs
- Policy development and leadership that fosters local involvement and a sense of ownership of specific, emphasized, local needs, with an equitable distribution of resources commensurate with community need
- Assurance of high-quality services that are available and accessible; assurance that the community receives proper consideration for allocation of federal and state resources; assurance that the community is kept informed

emphasis on preventing disease and disability and its focus on the health of an entire population at the community level, rather than at the individual level. As a system, public health consists of governmental and nongovernmental agencies. Figure 2.1 provides the U.S. Department of Health and Human Services organizational chart.

Relationships exist in the public health system between governmental and nongovernmental agencies to accomplish the core functions of public health. There are at least five types of relationship that exist between (a) different health agencies at various governmental levels, (b) public health agencies and other health-related agencies (community-based organizations), (c) public health agencies and private sector agencies, (d) private sector and voluntary agencies, and (e) various combinations of these relationships (Novick, 2001). Both private and public agencies have key roles and responsibilities in maintaining an intact public health system. An intact public health system is dependent on a strong infrastructure that provides the foundation for public health practice.

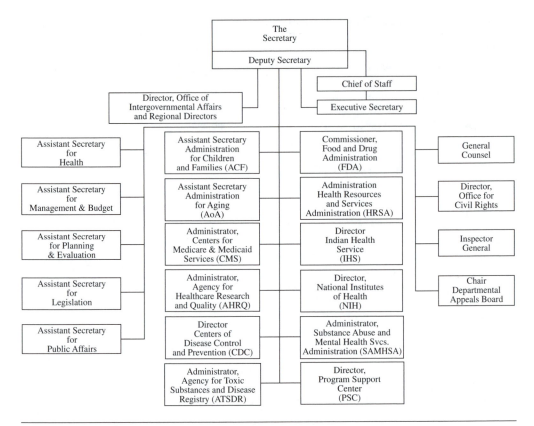

Figure 2.1 U.S. Department of Health and Human Services Public Health Services Organizational Chart

SOURCE: DHHS (2001).

Public Health Infrastructure

Public health infrastructure is the underlying foundation that supports the planning, delivery, and evaluation of public health practice (CDC, 2001). A solid public health infrastructure depends on sustained, coordinated, and effective activities at the local, state, and federal levels. Turnock (2001) describes the public health infrastructure as "the nerve center of the public health system, representing the capacity necessary to carry out public health's core functions" (p. 208). Public health core functions, assessment, assurance, and health policy will be referenced throughout this book. The infrastructure relies on the accessibility of sufficient human, financial, and organizational resources.

Novick (2001) identifies five components of the public health infrastructure: (a) a skilled public health workforce, (b) integrated electronic information systems, (c) public health organizations, (d) resources, and (e) research. The CDC (2001) identifies three essential components of the public health infrastructure that are similar to Novick's description of public health infrastructure: (a) workforce capacity and competency, (b) information

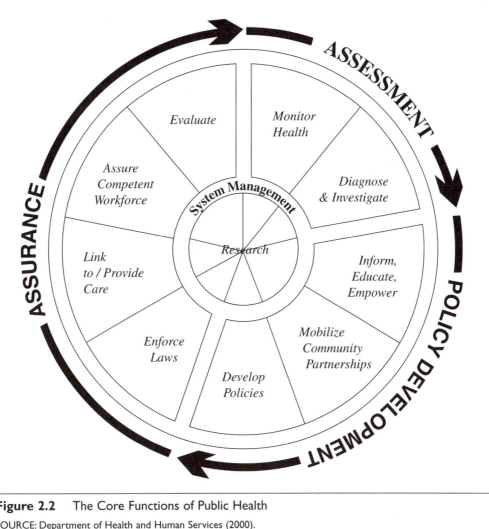

Figure 2.2   The Core Functions of Public Health

SOURCE: Department of Health and Human Services (2000).

and data systems, and (c) organizational capacity. The CDC states that these three essential components provide for a prepared public health system, which can then provide for and protect the nation's health.

Core Functions of Public Health

The IOM's dismal portrait of the public health system was a major impetus for the establishment of core public health functions. These core public health functions are designed to target the public health problems encountered today within the existing public health infrastructure. Public health practices are based in the core public health functions of assessment, policy development, and assurance (IOM, 1988). Figure 2.2 provides a model for the core functions of public health with their defining activities.

Assessment calls for regular and systematic collection, assembling, analysis, and dissemination of information on the health status of specific populations within the community. Two processes of assessment are (a) monitoring a population's health status to identify population-based community problems and (b) diagnosing and investigating health problems and health hazards in the community. The assessment function provides the foundation for the policy development and assurance functions. Policy development consists of activities that promote the development of comprehensive public health policies through the use of scientific knowledge and assessment data. The policy development function informs, educates, and empowers communities to mobilize community groups, promote community partnership, and develop policies that affect the nation's health. The assurance function means that public health agencies will provide what is necessary to achieve agreed-on community health goals, either through encouraging actions by other entities (public or private), by regulatory requirements, or by the direct provision of services (IOM). As part of the assurance function, laws and other public health regulations are enforced, community members are linked to health-care services or receive health-care services, a competent public health workforce is assured, and the effectiveness of public health functions are evaluated. Table 2.2 provides a broader perspective of the defining activities for each core public health function (Turnock, 2001).

Essential Services of Public Health

Essential public health services are important processes that further develop and operationalize the core public health functions. The essential public health services are a formulation of processes used in public health to prevent epidemics and injuries, protect against environmental hazards, promote healthy behaviors, respond to disasters, and ensure the quality and accessibility of health-care services (Turnock, 2001). Table 2.3 lists the 10 essential public health services.

Essential public health services provide a framework that can be applied to each area of public health practice. These essential public health services are used by public health agencies to explain what constitutes public health practice and define the services that are provided in the public health system (Novick, 2001).

Healthy People 2010

The Healthy People initiative was begun by the United States Department of Health and Human Services (DHHS) in 1979 with *Healthy People: The Surgeon General's Report on Health Promotion and Disease Prevention.* The focus in the 1979 initiative was on reducing premature deaths and

Table 2.2 Core Functions of Public Health Activities

Assessment

- Community assessment—identify community needs, resources, and assets
- Identification of health threats and hazards
- Determination of health-care services—service utilization and service needs

Policy Development

- Community development
- Development and mobilization of community partnerships
- Coalition building
- Leadership development in the community
- Systematic program planning at various levels—local, regional, state, and national
- Development of measurable health objectives and indicators
- Development of public health policy and legislation

Assurance

- Enforcement of laws and regulations
- Linking health-care providers together and to community members
- Assurance of a competent workforce
- Evaluation of effectiveness, accessibility, and quality of individual and population-based care
- Population-based public health research

SOURCE: Turnock (2001).

Table 2.3 Essential Public Health Services

- Monitor health status to identify community health problems
- Diagnose and investigate health problems and health hazards in the community
- Inform, educate, and empower people regarding health issues
- Mobilize community partnerships to identify and solve health problems
- Develop policies and plans that support individual and community health efforts
- Enforce laws and regulations that protect health and ensure safety
- Link people to needed personal health services and assure the provision of health care when otherwise unavailable
- Assure a competent public health and personal health-care workforce
- Evaluate effectiveness, accessibility, and quality of personal and population-based health services
- Conduct research to gain new insights and innovative solutions to health problems

preserving the independence of older adults. This initiative was followed in 1990 by the Healthy People 2000 initiative. The Healthy People 2000 goals were increasing the span of a healthy life, reducing health disparities, and securing access to preventive health services.

A progress review of the Healthy People 2000 objectives in 1998 and 1999 determined that 15% of the objectives had been met or had surpassed the 2000 targets (Office of Disease Prevention and Health Promotion [ODPHP], 2000). Progress toward targeted objectives was achieved for another 44% of the objectives. Eighteen percent of the objectives had data reporting movement away from the targeted projections (i.e., things were worse). Mixed results were reported for 6%, and 2% had no change from baseline data. Three percent had no baselines established at the time the fact sheet was put together, and 11% had baseline data but no current data to evaluate progress toward the Healthy People 2000 objectives. Overall, there was some indication that the nation's health had improved in relation to the Healthy People 2000 objectives.

For the third time in history, the DHHS has developed a strategic initiative to improve the nation's health. The health objectives in the Healthy People 2010 document address the nation's health concerns for the 21st century. The Healthy People 2010 initiative presents a comprehensive, nationwide agenda for health promotion and disease prevention.

The overarching purpose of the Healthy People 2010 initiative is to promote health and prevent illness, disability, and premature death. Healthy People 2010 is expected to serve as the instrument to address the nation's health problems, confront emerging health issues, reverse unfavorable health trends, and expand the previous achievements in health seen with the 1979 and 2000 initiatives. The two goals of Healthy People 2010 are to (a) increase the quality and years of healthy life and (b) eliminate health disparities. These two goals are divided into specific objectives in 28 focus areas. Table 2.4 lists the Healthy People 2010 focus areas (Department of Health and Human Services, 2000). Appendix B provides a detailed list of the 467 Healthy People 2010 objectives.

The Healthy People 2010 initiative has four key elements to facilitate systematic improvement in health. The two goals provide the initiative's overall focus and direction, as well as the guiding framework for the development of the objectives that will be measured to evaluate the nation's progress. Leading health indicators are identified in Table 2.5; these will be used to measure the nation's progress in meeting the Healthy People 2010 objectives.

The objectives were developed to focus on the determinants of health that consist of the combined effects of the individual and community physical and social environments, the policies and interventions used to promote health, and access to quality health care. Figure 2.3 displays a diagram of the systematic approach to healthy improvements. These determinants of heath affect the nation's health status, which is the ultimate measure of success in Healthy People 2010 goals and objectives. The individual is considered to consist of a biological and a behavioral component. The biological component consists of the individual's genetic makeup and his or her physical and mental health states. Individuals' reactions to internal or external stimuli and personal lifestyle choices compose their behavioral component. Individuals exist within and interact with a physical and social environment. The social environment consists of family, friends,

Table 2.4   Healthy People 2010 Focus Areas

 1. Access to quality health services

 2. Arthritis, osteoporosis, and chronic back conditions

 3. Cancer

 4. Chronic kidney disease

 5. Diabetes

 6. Disability and secondary conditions

 7. Educational and community-based programs

 8. Environmental health

 9. Family planning

10. Food safety

11. Health communication

12. Heart disease and stroke

13. Human immunodeficiency virus

14. Immunization and infectious diseases

15. Injury and violence prevention

16. Maternal, infant, and child health

17. Medical product safety

18. Mental health and mental disorders

19. Nutrition and overweight

20. Occupational safety and health

21. Oral health

22. Physical activity and fitness

23. Public health infrastructure

24. Respiratory diseases

25. Sexually transmitted diseases

26. Substance abuse

27. Tobacco use

28. Vision and hearing

SOURCE: U. S. Department of Health and Human Services (2000).

coworkers, community members, and other social institutions, such as schools, churches, and businesses. The physical environment consists of tangible elements such as the weather and toxic substances in the environment.

Table 2.5   Leading Health Indicators

1. Physical Activity

2. Overweight and obesity

3. Tobacco use

4. Substance abuse

5. Responsible sexual behavior

6. Mental health

7. Injury and violence

8. Environmental quality

9. Immunizations

10. Access to health care

SOURCE: Department of Health and Human Services (2000).

Policies and interventions are those public health or governmental strategies that attempt to affect certain health determinants. The accomplishment of improved health status is dependent on access to health-care services. This model illustrates the Healthy People 2010 systematic approach to developing national goals and objectives derived from determinants of health that are associated with the nation's health status. Population-based public health interventions directed toward affecting these determinants of health are expected to improve the nation's health status.

Changes for the Future:
A Population-Based Approach

In the past, public health practice remained separate from the traditional health-care practice delivered in the private sector. Advancements in technology, the current state of the public health system, community-based mobilization initiatives, and the growth of managed care have blurred distinctions between traditional public health systems and health-related practice settings. Core functions of public health are redefining public health practice to a population-based approach. Public health practice is moving away from the provision of individually focused care. At the same time, managed care organizations are assuming more health-care responsibilities for population-based health (Roper & Mays, 1998) but continuing to provide individual-level care (Bibeau, Lovelace, & Stephenson, 2001).

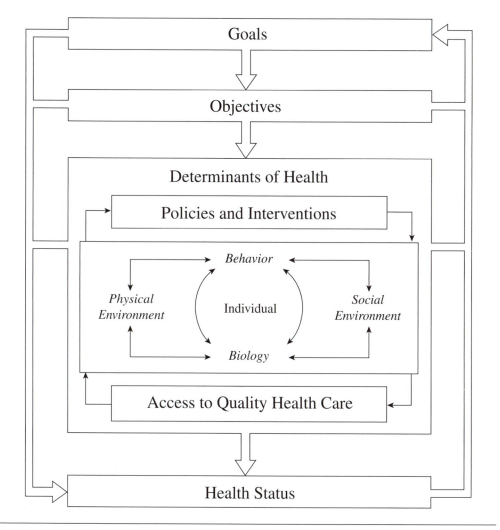

Figure 2.3   A Systematic Approach to Public Health Improvements

These changes in the health-care delivery system are occurring at a time when the functions of public health are changing and the public health infrastructure is being reconceptualized and redefined into a system for the 21st century. In this redefined and expansive public health infrastructure, collaborative partnerships between public health agencies and health-related agencies, such as community-based organizations (CBOs), are developing managed care agreements that include consumers of the traditional public health system in managed care plans. These managed care agreements are the foundation of an integrated community health system. These integrated community health systems will provide information exchange networks and community interventions targeting population-based health problems and will deliver individual-level care services. The delivery of individual-level-care services, along with other public health services, is being outsourced to medical practice settings so public health agencies may focus on the core functions of public health at a population-based level. The outsourcing of public health services into the private sector is frequently referred to as the privatization of public health practice.

Privatization of Public Health

Public health agencies are contracting out (outsourcing) or delegating services that were traditionally provided by public health agencies to nongovernmental community-based agencies and other health-care institutions (Keane, Marx, & Ricci, 2001). A major emphasis in the 1988 IOM report is the elimination of the provision of individual-level care services to focus on the core functions of assessment, policy development, and assurance. Bibeau, Lovelace, & Stephenson (2001) examined the privatization of public health services in 83 local public health departments in North Carolina that employed health educators. These researchers determined that these local health departments were more likely to provide infectious disease and sexually transmitted disease clinics (97%), family planning clinics (96%), and environmental services (96%). The local health departments were least likely to provide nonclinical chronic disease services (39%), school health clinics (48%), and home health services (49%). The most frequently privatized public health services were laboratory services (20%), prenatal care clinics (16%), and home health services (14%).

Examination of local health department directors determined that almost three quarters (73%) of these public health departments had privatized public health services (Keane et al., 2001). More than half of the local health departments (57%) reported delegating the direct performance of at least one service. The likelihood of the local health department's having privatized public health services increased as the department's sphere of influence approached jurisdictions with a population of 100,000 people. Keane, Marx, and Ricci (2001) identified individual-level services as the most frequently privatized public health services, along with environmental heath services, health education, community outreach, and data processing. Common reasons cited by local health department directors for privatization were the lack of capacity or expertise, desire to develop partnerships or collaborate with community agencies, and compliance with state mandates for privatization. Bibeau, Lovelace, and Stephenson (2001) noted that the privatization of services did free up the public health educator's time to focus on the core functions of public health practice. A remaining tension with the privatization of public health services is the need for the appropriation of funds to support public health agencies' implementation of core public health functions (Keane et al., 2001).

Summary

Key issues in the public health system are as follows.

- The defining characteristics of public health are dependent on the services provided through the public health system and the professional disciplines represented within the public health system.
- Core functions of public health are assessment, policy development, and assurance.
- The vision for public health is "healthy people in healthy communities" (CDC, 2001).
- The mission of public health is to "promote physical and mental health and prevent disease, injury and disability" (CDC, 2001).
- Private and public agencies have key roles and responsibilities in maintaining an intact public health system.
- The public health infrastructure is described as "the nerve center of the public health system, representing the capacity necessary to carry out public health's core functions" (Turnock, 2001).
- The five components of the public health infrastructure are (a) a skilled public health workforce, (b) integrated electronic information systems, (c) public health organizations, (d) resources, and (e) research.
- The three essential components of the public health infrastructure are (a) workforce capacity and competency, (b) information and data systems, and (c) organizational capacity.
- Public health practices occur within the core public health functions of assessment, policy development, and assurance.
- The essential public health services are a formulation of processes used in public health to prevent epidemics and injuries, protect against environmental hazards, promote healthy behaviors, respond to disasters, and ensure the quality and accessibility of health-care services.
- The two goals of Healthy People 2010 are to (a) increase the quality and years of healthy life and (b) eliminate health disparities.
- Leading health indicators are used to measure the nation's progress in relation to Healthy People 2010 objectives.
- Core functions of public health are redefining public health practice so that it now uses a population-based approach.
- Public health agencies are contracting out (outsourcing) or delegating services that were traditionally provided by public health agencies to nongovernmental, community-based agencies and other health-care institutions.

References

Bibeau, D., Lovelace, K., & Stephenson, J. (2001). Privatization of local health department services: Effects on the practice of health education. *Health Education & Behavior, 28*(2), 217-230.

Centers for Disease Control and Prevention. (2001). Public health's infrastructure: A status report. Retrieved June 7, 2003, from http://www.phppo.cdc.gov/documents/phireport2_16.pdf

Department of Health and Human Services. (2000). *Healthy People 2010: Understanding and improving health* (2nd ed.). Washington, DC: U.S. Government Printing Office.

Institute of Medicine. (1988). *The future of public health*. Washington, DC: National Academy Press.

Keane, C., Marx, J., & Ricci, E. (2001). Privatization and the scope of public health: A national survey of local health department directors. *American Journal of Public Health, 91*(4), 611-617.

Novick, L. (2001). A framework for public health administration and practice. In L. Novick & G. Mays (Eds.), *Public health administration: Principles for population-based management* (pp. 34-62). Gaithersburg, MD: Aspen.

Office of Disease Prevention and Health Promotion, U.S. Department of Health and Human Services. (2000). *Healthy People 2000 fact sheet*. Retrieved June 7, 2003, from http://odphp.osophs.dhhs.gov/pubs/HP2000/hp2kfact.htm

Roper, W., & Mays, G. (1998). The changing managed care–public health interface. *Journal of the American Medical Association, 280*(20), 1739-1740.

Turnock, B. (2001). *Public health: What it is and how it works*. Gaithersburg, MD: Aspen.

3

Epidemiology: Population-Based Data

Epidemiological investigations yield population-based data. Epidemiology is frequently cited as a basic science for public health practice. Epidemiology can be described as the investigation of illness or health-related data in relation to variables of person, place, and time. This chapter focuses on defining epidemiology, describing surveillance, discussing morbidity and mortality measures, introducing screening measures, reviewing epidemiological study designs, presenting the epidemiological approach to investigation, and differentiating causation from association.

Introduction

Population-based practice is based on population-based data derived from epidemiological research. The core public health competency of analytical assessment skills is based in principles of epidemiology. Epidemiology is a basic science of public health practice that affects all facets of population-based public health practice—interventions, program development, social and legal actions, and public health policy. Public health nurses should be versed in epidemiology and epidemiological terminology. Appendix C provides a brief glossary of essential terms that should be in the public health nurse's epidemiological knowledge base and vocabulary.

Epidemiology

The term *epidemiology* is derived from the Greek words *epi* (upon), *demos* (people), and *logos* (science; literally, reason or wisdom; Valanis, 1999). Thus epidemiology is a science that studies a group or population of people. This supports epidemiology as a core component of population-based practice. Epidemiology is typically defined as the study of the distribution and determinants of health-related states or events in specified populations and the application of this study to the control of health problems (Last, 1988). Valanis (1999) defined epidemiology as the study of the distribution of health states and the determinants of health deviations in human populations. For the purpose of this text, epidemiology is defined as the methods used to study the determinants and distribution of health-related events in a population.

The basic objectives of epidemiology are to (a) identify the etiology and risk factors for disease or unhealthy conditions, (b) determine the extent of disease or unhealthy conditions in a population, (c) study the natural history and prognosis of diseases, (d) evaluate public health interventions and health-care delivery, and (e) provide data that support the development of public health policy and regulations related to population-based health. (Gordis, 2000).

The term epidemiology is frequently used to refer both to a particular method applied in the study of the determinants and distribution of health-related events and to the body of knowledge derived from epidemiological investigations. Epidemiology can be divided into three different classifications, depending on the methods and purpose of the investigation: substantive, descriptive, or analytical. Substantive epidemiology refers to the cumulative collection of epidemiological knowledge generated through epidemiological research in a defined population. Substantive epidemiology consists of descriptions of the natural history of an illness, known patterns of occurrence, factors associated with the risk of illness, and basic descriptors of various states of health. Some epidemiologists use the terms substantive and descriptive interchangeably. Descriptive epidemiology consists of descriptions of the patterns of diseases according to variables of person, place, and time. Epidemiologists generate research hypotheses based on descriptive epidemiology. Analytical epidemiology is the use of epidemiological methods to investigate these research hypotheses (Last, 1988; Moon & Gould, 2000; Valanis, 1999). For example, analytical epidemiology can compare populations exposed and not exposed to risk factors known to cause lung cancer in relation to the occurrence of cancer based on person, place, and time variables.

Epidemiology can further be defined by its focus on illness or health in relation to the population investigated, and can be classified by its primary focus (clinical, social, communicable disease, chronic disease, community, or occupational). Clinical epidemiology focuses on individual patterns of disease with an etiological orientation. Social epidemiology emphasizes the determinants and distribution of health and illness in society, based on a societal paradigm. A focus on diseases that are transmitted through direct or indirect contact forms the basis of communicable disease epidemiology. Diseases such as diabetes mellitus and heart disease, which have a chronic orientation, formulate chronic disease epidemiology. Community epidemiology focuses on the application of epidemiological methods to a defined community in real-world settings. Occupational epidemiology focuses on workplace and workforce issues related to disease determinants and distribution (Moon & Gould, 2000).

Surveillance

Population-based data is derived through an integrated network of surveillance systems. The CDC and the Agency for Toxic Substances and Disease Registry (ATSDR) define surveillance as the "ongoing systematic collection, analysis, and interpretation of outcome-specific data for use in the planning, implementation, and evaluation of public health practice (Thacker & Berkelman, 1988). Today, surveillance is frequently used in the broadest sense to collect data on public health problems other than communicable diseases. In this manner, surveillance is frequently referred to as epidemiologic surveillance. The application of epidmiologic surveillance to the public as a whole denotes what is referred to as public health surveillance. Public health surveillance also indicates the contextual environment in which surveillance activities or the surveillance system is structured.

Surveillance is a vital activity for the public health nurse. Public health surveillance activities are used to assess the health status of a population, determine public health problems and priority areas, evaluate public health programs, and conduct research (Thacker, 2000). Surveillance activities provide the public health nurse with data that answer the questions What is the problem? Who is affected by the problem? Where is the problem occurring? How should public health interventions be focused? and To what extent will public health interventions be effective?

Primarily, public health surveillance data are used to

- Identify, characterize, and monitor patterns and trends in health status within a population
- Identify, characterize, and monitor the patterns and trends in the determinants of health status within a population
- Determine public health strategies to prevent or treat health problems using evidence- or research-based data
- Implement health promotion and disease prevention and control programs
- Identify public health problems to support health promotion and disease prevention and control programs
- Monitor a public health organization or community-based agency's capacity to implement the public health program
- Evaluate the effectiveness of the public health program (Parrish & McDonnel, 2000)

Table 3.1 summarizes the multiple uses of public health surveillance data (Thacker, 2000).

Table 3.1   Use of Public Health Surveillance Data

- Estimate the magnitude of a health problem
- Describe the natural history of disease
- Determine incidence or prevalence of disease
- Document the distribution of a disease in a population
- Facilitate research efforts
- Evaluate public health programs
- Monitor changes in disease states over time
- Monitor effectiveness of isolation measures
- Detect changes in public health practice
- Facilitate program planning

Due to the limited resources available in public health practice, public health nurses have to prioritize what will be subjected to surveillance activities. Public health surveillance activities provide the continuous monitoring that is needed to detect insidious, rare, or "sentinel" events. Teutsch (2000) proposed criteria to determine which high priority health events should be subjected to surveillance activities. These criteria are (a) frequency of disease occurrence (incidence and prevalence), (b) severity of disease (mortality data, years of productive life lost, disability rate), (c) surveillance cost, (d) preventability or potential treatment or control of disease, (e) communicability, and (f) public interest. Once priority areas for public health surveillance are determined, a surveillance system must be established. This is the process for establishing a surveillance system:

1. Establish the purpose, goals, and objectives of the system.

2. Develop case definitions and criteria for noting incidences of disease occurrence.

3. Determine data sources and data collection procedures.

4. Develop data collection instruments.

5. Establish the public health informatics structure to support data collection and transfer.

6. Pilot test and revise methods.

7. Develop and test analytic approaches to the collected surveillance data.

8. Develop a timely method for disseminating surveillance data.

9. Assess the use of surveillance data.

10. Continually evaluate the effectiveness of the surveillance system in relation to the originally stated purpose, goals, and objectives.

An effective public health surveillance system is dependent on accurate and timely collection of surveillance data. There are four basic types of surveillance processes with which to collect population-based surveillance data: active, passive, mixed, and sentinel. Active surveillance denotes a system in which the public health professional conducts periodic field visits to health-care agencies to collect surveillance data (also known as active case finding). Active surveillance is consistent with the concept of, for example, active partner notification used with sexually transmitted infections (STIs). Passive surveillance denotes a system in which the responsibility for the generation and reporting of surveillance data is primarily dependent on the health-care provider. In a passive surveillance system, the public health professional in the surveillance system depends on the health-care provider to report the required surveillance data. Passive surveillance is consistent with the concept of partner or client-center partner notification for illnesses such as STIs. A mixed surveillance system is a combination of active and passive surveillance. In a mixed system, the public health surveillance professional may routinely depend on the health-care provider to generate reportable surveillance data, but in certain situations, the public health surveillance professional may actively visit the health-care agency to gather data on specific health problems (Gordis, 2000). Sentinel surveillance is conducted by a designated group of public health providers for specifically targeted health problems. The term sentinel surveillance also has two other types of applications. Sentinel surveillance can refer to surveillance that occurs in special "sentinel groups" that have a particular risk profile for the occurrence of a particular disease. For example, sentinel surveillance is conducted for human immunodeficiency virus (HIV) infection in blood donors, pregnant women, and military applicants. Secondly, sentinel surveillance is conducted to identify "sentinel health events." Sentinel health events refer to conditions or events for which even one case serves as a warning signal for public health nurses that quality improvement measures are needed to prevent health problems. Sentinel health events are typically considered unusual or avoidable events (Hatzell, Aldrich, Cates, & Shin, 2001).

Active, passive, mixed, and sentinel surveillance systems consist of multiple networks of data sources. Table 3.2 lists sources of surveillance data. The CDC and the World Health Organization (WHO) have several surveillance programs in place that generate data for public health surveillance purposes. These programs, in collaboration with state and local public health agencies, have mandatory reporting systems, primarily for communicable diseases. The APHA defined five classifications of reportable diseases: universally mandatory, regularly reportable, selectively reportable, obligatory report of epidemic—no case report required, and official report not ordinarily justifiable (Valanis, 1999).

Universally mandatory reportable diseases require international health regulations and quarantine of a defined population to prevent or control disease transmission. Plague, cholera, yellow fever, and smallpox are

Table 3.2   Selected Sources of Surveillance Data

Vital Statistics
- United States Census
- National Vital Statistics Program
- Birth certificates
- Death certificates
- Fetal death certificates

Registries
- The National Cancer Institute's Surveillance, Epidemiology and End Results Program
- State disease registries

Health Surveys
- National Health and Nutrition Examination Survey (NHANES)
- National Health Provider Inventory
- National Home and Hospice Care Survey
- National Ambulatory Medical Care Survey
- AIDS surveillance
- Hospital discharge survey
- National Health Interview Survey
- National Traumatic Occupational Fatalities Surveillance System
- National Household Surveys on Drug Abuse
- Drug Abuse Warning Network (DAWN)
- Behavioral Risk Factor Surveillance Survey

Notifiable and Reportable Diseases
- National Notifiable Diseases Surveillance System

Surveillance Systems Within Regulatory and Governmental Agencies
- Healthy People 2000 and 2010
- Healthy Communities 2000 and 2010
- National Health expenditures
- Medicare Statistical System
- Medicaid Data System
- Physician Supply Projections—Health Resources and Services Administration (HRSA)
- Nurse Supply Estimates—HRSA
- National Geographic Information System—Environmental Protection Agency (EPA)
- Hazardous Substance Release/Health Effects Database (HazDat)—Agency for Toxic Substances and Disease Registry (ATSDR)

diseases under surveillance by WHO that are universally mandatory reportable diseases. The WHO also requires reporting of louse-borne typhus fever, relapsing fever, paralytic poliomyelitis, malaria, and viral influenza as universally mandatory reportable diseases. There are two sub-classifications of regularly reportable diseases: diseases requiring rapid reporting to the local public health agency, such as typhoid and diphtheria, and those that require routine weekly reports to the local public health agency, such as brucellosis and leprosy. Selectively reportable diseases occur in endemic areas. Examples of selectively reportable diseases are tularemia, bartonellosis, coccidioidomycosis and clonorchiasis. Obligatory reports of an epidemic, or outbreak report, must be made for food poisoning, infectious keratoconjunctivitis, and other unidentified syndromes. The last classification, "official report not ordinarily justifiable," consists of diseases that are usually sporadic in nature and uncommon. These are often not directly transmissible from person to person, or they occur where the reporting of such information is of little public health value (Benson, 1990; Valanis,1999). Each state defines the list of reportable diseases through legislative processes. Public health nurses must be familiar with the list of reportable diseases in their respective states.

Morbidity and Mortality Measures

Morbidity and mortality data provide the public health nurse with data on the number of individuals within a defined population who are experiencing illness or other types of health alterations. Morbidity and mortality data are used in the development and planning of public health programs to promote health, prevent and control disease, and develop treatments. It is beyond the scope of this text to fully examine all measures of disease morbidity and mortality. This text will limit the discussion of morbidity and mortality data to the most common measures used by public health nurses.

A common measure for both morbidity and mortality data is the rate. A rate is a measure of the frequency of occurrence of an event. All rates are ratios. This simply means that they consist of one number (a numerator of events) divided by another number (a denominator or population at risk). Tables 3.3 and 3.4 provide lists of frequently used rates and ratios in epidemiology and the formulas for morbidity and mortality rates, respectively. The typical equation for a rate is

$$\frac{\text{Number of events in a specified time period}}{\text{At-risk population during specified time period}}$$

Rates can be presented as crude, specific, or standardized. A crude rate presents all cases for an entire population. A specific rate presents the cases for a defined characteristic of a population. For example, specific rates present a measure of a disease in a subpopulation based on the defining characteristic, such as age (age-specific rate) or gender (sex-specific rate). An age-specific mortality rate is the mortality rate only for a defined age group within a population. A standardized rate is used to compare two or more populations, controlling for the effects of other variables by adjusting the risk population.

Table 3.3   Frequently Used Rates and Ratios in Epidemiology

Mortality Statistics

Rate or Ratio	Common Expression (multiplier)
Crude mortality or death rate	per 1000
Age-specific mortality or death rate	per 1000 persons
Cause-specific mortality or death rate	per 100,000 persons
Maternal mortality rate	per 100,000 live births
Infant mortality rate	per 1000 live births
Neonatal mortality rate	per 1000 live births
Fetal mortality rate	per 1000 live births and fetal deaths
Birth-death ratio	per 100
Case fatality ratio	per 100

Morbidity Statistics

Incidence	per 1000 persons
Prevalence	per 1000 persons

Vital Statistics

Crude birth rate	per 1000 persons
General fertility rate	per 1000 females from 15-44 years old
General marriage rate	per 1000 persons 15 years old or older
General divorce rate	per 1000 persons 15 years old or older
Dependency ratio	per 100

Morbidity Measures

Incidence and prevalence are the most common morbidity measures. Incidence is a measure of the occurrence of new diseases within a defined population in a specified period of time. Incidence measures that use the population size at the midpoint of a specified period of time for a large population are measuring what is frequently referred to as cumulative incidence. Incidence is used to present a measure of risk in a population. Another significant type of incidence measure is incidence density. Incidence density is a modification of the cumulative incidence that is often used with cohort studies over time. Incidence density measures account for those individuals who are lost during a specific period of time due to death, who are lost to follow-up, or who have contracted the disease and are no longer considered at risk for the entire study period, using a measure called person-years as the denominator. A person-year is one person who is at risk for one year. The incidence density is a measure of the total number of new cases accumulated during a study period divided by the person-years accumulated by the study subjects and multiplied by a constant.

Prevalence is a measure of all cases of an event, new cases and old cases, in a defined population within a specific period of time. Prevalence provides public health nurses with data to assess the burden of illness on public

Table 3.4   Morbidity, Mortality, and Screening Formulas

Morbidity Measures

$$\text{Incidence} = \frac{\text{New cases of disease in time period}}{\text{Population at risk in time period}}$$

$$\text{Prevalence} = \frac{\text{Total number of existing cases in time period}}{\text{Population at risk in time period}}$$

Mortality Measures

$$\text{Crude death rate} = \frac{\text{Number of deaths in a year}}{\text{Average (midyear) population}}$$

$$\text{Cause-specific death rate} = \frac{\text{Number of deaths in a year due to a specific cause}}{\text{Average (midyear) population}}$$

$$\text{Age-specific death rate} = \frac{\text{Number of deaths among persons in given age group in a year}}{\text{Average (midyear) population in specific age group}}$$

$$\text{Proportional mortality rate} = \frac{\text{Number of deaths from specific cause in specific time period}}{\text{Total deaths in the same time period}}$$

$$\text{Case fatality rate} = \frac{\text{Number of deaths due to a specific disease}}{\text{Number of cases of specific disease}}$$

$$\text{Survival rate} = \frac{\text{Number of cases alive at the end of a specific time period}}{\text{Number of cases at start of period}}$$

$$\text{Maternal (puerperal) mortality rate} = \frac{\text{Number of deaths from puerperal cases in a year}}{\text{Number of live births in the same year}}$$

$$\text{Infant mortality rate} = \frac{\text{Number of infant deaths during year}}{\text{Number of live births in same year}}$$

$$\text{Neonatal mortality rate} = \frac{\text{Number of deaths in a year of children younger than 28 days}}{\text{Number of live births in same year}}$$

$$\text{Fetal death rate} = \frac{\text{Number of fetal deaths during a year}}{\text{Number of live births and fetal deaths in same year}}$$

$$\text{Perinatal mortality rate} = \frac{\text{Number of fetal deaths 28 weeks or more and infant deaths younger than 7 days of age during year}}{\text{Number of live births and fetal deaths 28 weeks or more gestation in same year}}$$

(Continued)

Table 3.4   (Continued)

Validity Measures

$$\text{Sensitivity} = \frac{\text{True positives}}{\text{True positives} + \text{false negatives}} \times 100$$

$$\text{Specificity} = \frac{\text{True negatives}}{\text{True negatives} + \text{false positives}} \times 100$$

Predictive Measures

$$\text{Predictive value positive} = \frac{\text{True positives}}{\text{True positives} + \text{false positives}} \times 100$$

$$\text{Predictive value negative} = \frac{\text{True negatives}}{\text{True negatives} + \text{false negatives}} \times 100$$

health resources. Two types of prevalence measure are frequently used: point and period prevalence. Point prevalence measures the total amount of an event, new and old cases, in a population at one point in time. For example, point prevalence may measure all individuals with influenza on January 1. Period prevalence measures the total amount of an event, new and old cases, in a population during a specified period of time. For example, period prevalence would measure all individuals with influenza during the entire month of January.

Incidence and prevalence measures are intricately related. Prevalence is a product of the incidence rates of a disease in a population and the duration of the disease in the population (Prevalence = Incidence × Duration of illness). The prevalence of a disease in a population is dependent on the incidence of disease occurrence (incidence) and the rate at which people in the population recover or die from the disease (duration) (Unwin, Carr, Leeson, & Pless-Mulloni, 1997). If the incidence rate of a disease continues to increase in a population but the mortality or cure rates remain constant, the prevalence of the disease will increase in the defined population. In a population in which the incidence rate remains stable and the mortality or cure rates increase, the prevalence of the disease will decrease in the population. A situation could occur in a population in which the incidence rates and mortality or cure rates remain constant for a period of time, resulting in a stable prevalence rate. These explanations exemplify the intricate relationship between the incidence and prevalence of a disease in a population.

Mortality Measures

Mortality rates are a measure of the amount of death from an event within a defined population. Mortality rates describe the incidence of death.

The most common mortality measures are crude and specific: disease and age, case fatality, standardized mortality ratio. The crude mortality rate is total number of deaths from all causes within a defined population in a specific time period. Specific mortality rates can be calculated with regard to subpopulations according to disease or age. A disease-specific or cause-specific mortality rate is the total number of deaths associated with the specific disease in a defined population in a specific time period. For example, a disease-specific mortality rate can be cancer-related deaths from January 1 to December 31 in a given year. Age-specific mortality rates are the total number of deaths in a population defined by age within a specific time period. An age-specific mortality rate could consist of all individuals who died from January 1 to December 31 who were 20 to 39 years old. Case fatality rates provide public health nurses with a measure of the effectiveness of an intervention. A case fatality rate uses the number of cases of a disease as the denominator or population at risk, and the numerator is the number of persons who die from the disease. The case fatality rate is calculated as a percentage and demonstrates disease severity. The standardized mortality ratio (SMR) adjusts the population statistics according to age groups.

Screening Measures

Screening is a systematic process used to identify the presence of an illness or condition within an individual or population. Screening is defined as the presumptive identification of unrecognized disease or defects through the application of tests, examinations, or other procedures that are systematically applied to an individual or population (Last, 1988). Effective screening programs are developed based on the following criteria: (a) an identified need; (b) a problem of significant frequency and magnitude (significant incidence, mortality, disability, discomfort, or financial cost); (c) the test meets standards of simplicity and safety; (d) measures exist to identify at-risk individuals; (e) the test is acceptable to the at-risk population; (f) an intervention to correct the identified problem exists, or the test identifies disease at an early enough stage to prevent or delay disease presentation; (g) the benefits of screening outweigh the costs (cost-benefit ratio); and (h) the screening test is reliable and valid, with high sensitivity and specificity (Unwin et al., 1997; Valanis, 1999).

The reliability of a screening test is determined when the test repeatedly provides the same results in the same person. The validity of a test is its ability to measure what it is intended to measure. Validity is determined by sensitivity and specificity measures. Sensitivity is the ability of a test to correctly identify those individuals who have a disease. Specificity is the ability of a test to correctly identify those individuals who do not have a disease (Gordis, 2000; Unwin et al., 1997). Table 3.4 provides formulas for the calculation of these characteristics.

Screening tests are assessed within a population by calculating predictive values. The predictive value is a measure of the frequency with which test results correctly identify a disease in the population screened. Predictive values are dependent on the prevalence of a disease within a population. The predictive value of a positive test is the proportion of those individuals testing positive who actually have the disease. The predictive value of a negative test is the proportion of those individuals in a population who test negative and who do not have the disease. These are expressed as the percentage of positives or negatives in a population who are correctly identified.

Epidemiological Study Designs

The study of the determinants and distribution of diseases within a population relies on the systematic collection of data through epidemiological investigations using multiple epidemiological and research methods. Chapter 15 further delineates the public health research process. This section is limited to frequently used epidemiological study designs. Epidemiological study designs are typically descriptive, analytical, or experimental in nature.

Descriptive studies provide information on the frequency of a disease in a defined population according to the variables of person, place, and time. A commonly used descriptive design is the cross-sectional study or prevalence survey. Cross-sectional studies measure the occurrence of a disease or the health status of individuals within a defined period of time.

The association between a determinant of a disease and the occurrence of the disease is examined through analytical study designs. Common case-analytical study designs are cohort and case-control studies.

Cohort study involves a group of individuals who are investigated over time according to a cohort variable such as age. Cohort studies are generally prospective in nature, examining the effects of exposures in groups of individuals. In a cohort study, the public health nurse examines groups of exposed and nonexposed individuals over time to compare the incidence of disease in the two groups (Figure 3.1). In a case-control study, two groups of individuals are identified: those with the disease (cases) and those without the disease (controls). Then the proportions of individuals in the case and control groups that were or were not exposed are compared (Figure 3.2).

Experimental designs measure the effectiveness of a public health intervention in a population. The gold standard for intervention studies is experimental designs. True experimental designs have three essential components: a control group, randomization, and manipulation of an intervention under the researcher's control. The common experimental design is a randomized clinical trial. Public health professionals use experimental methods to conduct randomized community trials.

Randomized clinical trials randomly assign individuals to treatment and control groups in which one group receives the treatment or intervention

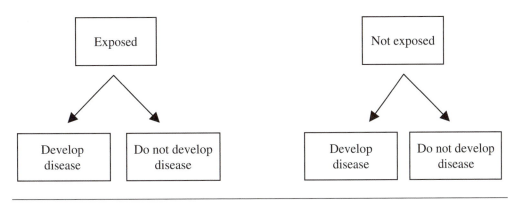

Figure 3.1 Cohort Designs

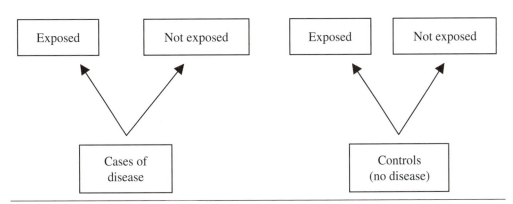

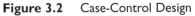

Figure 3.2 Case-Control Design

under investigation (experimental group) and one group does not (control group). Randomized clinical trials are frequently double blind, with neither the investigator nor the subject knowing who is assigned to which group. Public health professionals have modified the randomized clinical trial design into a randomized community trial design. The subject that is investigated and randomized in this design is the community. Communities are identified and randomized to either a treatment or control group. Randomized community trials are being proposed as a method to measure the effectiveness of population-based public health interventions.

Epidemiological Approach

Fundamental to the principles of epidemiology and guiding the epidemiological approach are the concepts that are frequently known as the epidedmiological triad: agent, host, and environment. Figure 3.3 illustrates the interrelationship among these variables.

The agent is a factor whose presence or absence is identified as a determinant of the disease. There are several types of agents: physical, chemical,

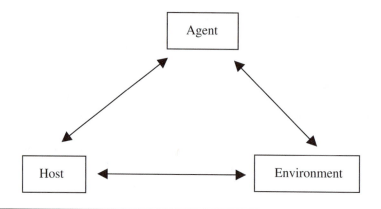

Figure 3.3   Epidemiological Triad: Agent, Host, and Environment

nutrient, genetic, psychological, and biological. Physical agents include mechanical forces or atmospheric conditions that have the potential to produce injury. Chemical agents are substances that have the potential to affect human physiological processes. Nutrient agents are chemical in nature and specific to the consumption of dietary products. Genetic agents are predetermined through a host's DNA. Psychological agents are factors that affect the psychosocial well-being of a host, such as stress. Biological agents consist of all living organisms (bacteria, viruses, fungus, parasites, etc.) that affect the host (Valanis, 1999).

The individual in whom an agent produces disease is known as the host. A host possesses immunity that will influence whether an agent contributes to the occurrence of a disease process. Immunity is the resistance that a host presents against specific infectious agents. Immunity can be derived actively, passively, or naturally. A host develops active immunity after experiencing exposure to an agent, resulting in the presence of antibodies. Passive immunity is derived through the transmission of maternal antibodies to an infant or through the artificial administration of immunoglobulins. Natural immunity is a host's inherent resistance to a disease agent (Valanis, 1999).

The environment consists of all conditions external to the host that influence the interaction of the agent and the host and influence the impact of an agent on the host. Three essential components of the environment that are typically examined in the epidemiological approach are physical, socioeconomic, and biologic environments. The physical environment consists of geographical structures external to the host such as water sources, mountains, and reservoirs. The socioeconomic environment consists of broad social and economic conditions that may directly or indirectly affect the host, such as unemployment, poor city finances affecting garbage disposal and removal, or lack of access to medical care. All living organisms external to the host, such as plants, animals, and vector-type organisms, make up a host's biological environment (Valanis, 1999).

Table 3.5   The Epidemiological Approach to an Investigation

1. Define the epidemic
   a. Define the cases (numerator data)
      i. Case definition
      ii. Clinical features
      iii. Laboratory evidence
   b. Define the population at risk (denominator data)

2. Case distribution is examined
   a. Data according to place
   b. Data according to time

3. Examine data for interactions and correlations—assess for relationships that exist between agent, host, and environmental conditions

4. Develop preliminary hypothesis
   a. Use existing data to generate hypothesis
   b. Establish a priori hypothesis based on literature and previous disease occurrence patterns
   c. Examine plausibility of hypothesis

5. Test hypothesis, if applicable. Analyze existing data using case-control design

6. Recommend prevention and control measures
   a. Write narrative report of investigation
   b. Develop prevention and control interventions
   c. Develop recommendations to guide future disease investigations

Agent, host, and environment are the primary variables that guide an epidemiological investigation using the epidemiological approach, in addition to the variables of person, place, and time. The epidemiological approach is used to examine the distribution and determinants of suspected disease occurrences. Table 3.5 outlines the epidemiological approach for disease investigation (Gordis, 2000).

Causation Versus Association

Most public health problems are the result of multiple causes or associated factors. Public health professionals typically rely on measures of association to determine causation. The criteria used to evaluate causation are as follows:

- Temporal association (cause precedes event)
- Strength of association, measured through relative risk or odds ratios
- Dose-response relationship (increased exposure associated with increased disease occurrence)
- Consistency of causal relationship (findings are replicable)
- A biologically plausible explanation
- Cessation of exposure prevents disease occurrence
- Confounding explanations are not plausible (Gordis, 2000; Valanis, 1999)

An association entails a simple relationship between a disease and some illness determinant (risk factor). Due to the multiple criteria necessary to prove causation, public health professionals infrequently identify sole causes of a disease; more usually, they will identify associative factors and describe the amount of association between the disease determinant and occurrence of the disease.

Summary

Key issues of population-based epidemiology are as follows.

- Epidemiology is a science basic to public health practice that affects all facets of population-based public health practice.
- Epidemiology can be described as the investigation of illness- or health-related data in relation to variables of person, place, and time.
- Epidemiology is defined as the methods used to study the determinants and distribution of health-related events in a population.
- The objectives of epidemiology are to (a) identify the etiology and risk factors of disease or unhealthy conditions, (b) determine the extent of disease or unhealthy conditions in a population, (c) study the natural history and prognosis of diseases, (d) evaluate public health interventions and health-care delivery, and (e) provide data that support the development of public health policy and regulations related to population-based health.
- Epidemiology can be divided into several different types, depending on the methods and purpose of the investigation.
- Epidemiology can be classified by focus: clinical, social, communicable disease, chronic disease, community, and occupational.
- Public health surveillance data is primarily used to (a) identify, characterize, and monitor patterns and trends in health status within a population; (b) identify, characterize, and monitor patterns and trends in the determinants of health status within a population; (c) determine public health strategies to prevent or treat health problems, using evidence- and research-based data; (d) implement health promotion and disease prevention and control programs; (e) identify public health problems to support health promotion and disease prevention and control programs; (f) monitor a public health or community-based agency's capacity to implement public health programs; and (g) evaluate the effectiveness of public health programs.
- Criteria to determine what illness or conditions will be under surveillance are (a) frequency of disease occurrence, (b) severity of disease, (c) surveillance cost, (d) preventability or potential treatment or control of disease, (e) communicability, and (f) public interest.
- The process for establishing a surveillance system is to (a) establish the purpose, goals, and objectives of the system; (b) develop case definitions

and criteria for noting incidences of disease occurrence; (c) determine data sources and data collection procedures; (d) develop data collection instruments; (e) establish a public health informatics structure to support data collection and transfer; (f) pilot test and revise methods; (g) develop and test analytic approaches to the collected surveillance data; (h) develop a method of timely dissemination of surveillance data; (i) assess the use of surveillance data; and (j) continually evaluate the effectiveness of the surveillance system in relation to the original purpose, goals, and objectives.

- The APHA has five classifications of reportable diseases: universally mandatory, regularly reportable, selectively reportable, obligatory report of epidemic—no case report required, and official report not ordinarily justifiable.
- A rate is a measure of the frequency of occurrence of an event.
- Rates can be presented as crude, specific, or standardized.
- Incidence is a measure of the occurrence of new diseases within a defined population in a specified period of time.
- Incidence density measures account for those individuals who are lost during a specific period of time due to death, who are lost to follow-up, or who have contracted the disease and are no longer considered at risk for the entire study period. A measure called person-years is used as the denominator in the equation.
- Prevalence is a measure of all cases of an event, new cases and old cases, in a defined population within a specific period of time.
- Prevalence is a product of the incidence rates of a disease in a population and the duration of the disease in the population (Prevalence = Incidence × Duration of illness).
- Mortality rates are a measure of the amount of death from an event within a defined population.
- Screening is a systematic process used to identify the presence of an illness or condition within an individual or population.
- Screening is the presumptive identification of unrecognized disease or defects through the application of tests, examinations, or other procedures that are systematically applied to an individual or population.
- The reliability of a screening test is determined when the test repeatedly provides the same results in the same person.
- The validity of a test is its ability to measure what it is intended to measure.
- Sensitivity is the ability of a test to correctly identify those individuals who have a disease.
- Specificity is the ability of a test to correctly identify those individuals who do not have a disease.
- Predictive value is a measure of the frequency with which a test correctly identifies a disease in the population screened.
- The predictive value of a positive test is the proportion of those individuals testing positive who actually have the disease.

- The predictive value of a negative test is the proportion of those individuals testing negative who do not have the disease.
- Descriptive studies provide information on the frequency of a disease in a defined population according to the variables of person, place, and time.
- True experimental designs have three essential components: a control group, randomization, and manipulation of an intervention under the researcher's control.
- The epidedmiological triad consists of agent, host, and environment.
- Agent, host, and environment are the primary variables that guide an epidemiological investigation.
- The criteria used to evaluate the presence of causation are (a) temporal association, (b) strength of association, (c) dose-response relationship, (d) consistency of causal relationship, (e) biological plausibility, (f) cessation of exposure prevents disease occurrence, and (g) confounding explanations are not plausible.

References

Benson, A. (1990). *Control of communicable diseases in man* (15th ed.). Washington, DC: American Public Health Association.

Gordis, L. (2000). *Epidemiology* (2nd ed.). Philadelphia, PA: W. B. Saunders.

Hatzell, T., Aldrich, T., Cates, W., & Shin, E. (2001). Public health surveillance. In L. Novick & G. Mays (Eds.), *Public health administration: Principles for population-based management* (pp. 202-221). Gaithersburg, MD: Aspen.

Last, J. (1988). *Dictionary of epidemiology* (2nd ed.). New York: Oxford University Press.

Moon, G., & Gould, M. (2000). *Epidemiology: An introduction.* Philadelphia, PA: Open University Press.

Parrish, R., & McDonnel, S. (2000). Sources of health-related information. In S. Teutsch & R. Churchill (Eds.), *Principles and practice of public health surveillance* (2nd ed., pp. 30-75). New York: Oxford University Press.

Teutsch, S. (2000). Considerations in planning a surveillance system. In S. Teutsch & R. Churchill (Eds.), *Principles and practice of public health surveillance* (2nd ed., pp. 17-29). New York: Oxford University Press.

Thacker, S. (2000). Historical development. In S. Teutsch & R. Churchill (Eds.), *Principles and practice of public health surveillance* (2nd ed., pp. 1-16). New York: Oxford University Press.

Thacker, S., & Berkelman, R. (1988). Public health surveillance in the United States. *Epidemiological Reviews, 10,* 164-190.

Unwin, N., Carr, S., Leeson, J., & Pless-Mulloni, T. (1997). *An introductory study guide to public health and epidemiology.* Philadelphia, PA: Open University Press.

Valanis, B. (1999). *Epidemiology in health care* (3rd ed.). Stamford, CT: Appleton & Lange.

4

Behavioral Health Theories

Behavioral choices are cited as a predominant precursor to disease. Behavioral theories provide the foundational concepts from which to understand and predict human behavior. Public health nursing interventions directed at behavior modification should be guided by sound behavioral theories. This chapter defines certain behavioral theories; describes the linkage between theory, research, and practice; and summarizes several behavioral theories used in public health.

Introduction

Lifestyle and personal behaviors are the predominant causes of disease within a community. The determinants of a disease and its contributing factors are often directly related to personal behavior. Public health practice focuses on the prevention of risky lifestyle or personal behaviors that cause or facilitate the occurrence of a disease. Public health nurses must plan interventions that modify an individual's risky behaviors as a measure to improve health, reduce risk factors, and improve the quality of life for individuals within a community. Successful public health behavior modification programs are more likely to succeed if they are based on a clear understanding of the target population's health behaviors and the environmental context within which such behaviors exist. Behavioral health theories and models provide the theoretical perspective that guides the assessment of risky behaviors and the development and refinement of interventions to target a population's risky health behaviors.

Health behavior theories are so intricately linked to healthy behavior that the American Psychological Association has declared 2000 to 2010 as the "Decade of Behavior." During the Decade of Behavior, attention will be focused on the many contributions of the behavioral and social sciences in addressing society's health challenges. This initiative is designed to increase awareness and understanding of the contributions of behavioral and social sciences in solving our nation's problems from a practice and theoretical perspective (Tyler, 1999).

Theory

A theory is a set of concepts, constructs, and/or variables that are interrelated through propositional statements that provide a specific view of events or situations. Theories seek to explain or predict events, situations, or behaviors. Some theories are specifically constructed to develop behavior changes.

The various behavioral theories to be considered have common structural elements. The concepts within a theory are the basic building blocks of that theory. Concepts are abstract ideas that provide meaning to one's perceptions and permit generalizations (King, 1997). A concept is also referred to as a linguistic label that is given to describe a phenomenon or class of phenomena (Kim, 1997). Concepts in a theory provide the basis for the theoretical constructs. A construct is less abstract than a concept. Concepts that have been developed or adopted for use in a particular theory are referred to as constructs. Variables are referred to as the empirical (measurable) or operational forms of constructs (Glanz, Rimer, & Lewis, 2002). Propositions are statements that describe the relationship of one concept to another concept within the specific theory. Depending on the level of theoretical development in the theory, these essential components are typically evident and form the basis for explaining or predicting human behavior.

The two basic levels of theory development are grand and midrange theories. Grand theories are those theories that have the broadest scope. Middle-range theories are narrower in scope and encompass a limited number of concepts (Fawcett, 1997). These levels of theory exert various amounts of influence on human behavior.

Theories may also be classified, according to their level of influence on health-related behaviors, as intrapersonal (individual), interpersonal, institutional or organizational, community, or public policy. A theory's developmental level and level of influence affects which theory is used in the linking of public health research and practice to a particular theoretical perspective.

Linkage of Theory, Research, and Practice

Historically, the distinction between *theoria* and *praxis* dates back to the time of Aristotle, who differentiated between the two concepts. *Theoria* meant those sciences and activities that were concerned with ways of knowing or inquiry. *Praxis* was concerned with the way or manner in which people performed or acted (Glanz et al., 2002). The ways of knowing formulate the bases for the mode of research inquiry. There are four universally accepted ways of knowing: empirical, ethical, personal, and aesthetic.

The linkage between theory, research, and practice begins with the philosophical ways of knowing. Empirical knowing uses verifiable, factual descriptions, explanations, or predictions that are based on the collection of subjective or objective data. Empiricism correlates with empirical research, which uses measurable methods of data collection. Ethical knowing uses moral obligations and values as a means of inquiry that focuses on the identification and analysis of beliefs and values held by individuals and the relationship of these beliefs and values to human behavior. Matters of obligation and what ought to be done are related to ethical knowing. Ethical knowing correlates with values clarification and qualitative methods of data collection. Personal knowing is being knowledgeable regarding one's own personal lifestyle and the inner experience of becoming whole and self-aware. The quality and authenticity of interpersonal relationships formulate personal knowing. An individual must be open and centered on ways of being authentic to develop personal knowing. Personal knowing correlates with autobiographical case studies and reflective data. Aesthetic knowing relates to what is considered important and significant in a person's behavior. Aesthetic knowing permits an individual to sense the meaning of the moment and to envision what may be possible but not yet real. Aesthetic knowing relates to aesthetic criticism (Chinn & Kramer, 1995; Fawcett, Watson, Neuman, Walker, & Fitzpatrick, 2001).

These ways of knowing shape the research questions posed and the research methods selected. The ways of knowing define an approach to scientific inquiry. The theories provide the conceptual basis that assists in defining what will be measured to answer the research question posed about public health practice and provide a framework to explain or predict the research findings.

The interrelationship between theory, research, and practice is multifaceted. First, public health practice provides the area from which research questions are generated (practice generates questions). Second, the approach to answering specific research questions is defined by the public health practitioner's way of knowing and theoretical perspective with respect to the research question and the methodology to answer the research question. Third, the answers to public health practice questions generated through research further develop or verify the theoretical explanations of human behavior (research develops theories). Fourth, the body of knowledge that forms the domain of public health practice is representative of multiple theories based on ways of knowing and research (research builds the discipline's body of knowledge). Finally, public health research provides the data to answer practice questions grounded in public health and behavioral theories; this research data provides the scientific evidence that supports public health practice (theory and research provide the scientific evidence to support public health practice). Research-based and evidence-based public health practice will be discussed later in the text.

Health Belief Model

The health belief model (HBM) is one of the most widely used theoretical perspectives in health behavior. The HBM is widely used to explain behavior change and maintenance and guides the selection and development of behavioral interventions. The U.S. Public Health Service initially developed the HBM in the 1950s to explain the failure of people to participate in preventive health programs.

The HBM is a value expectancy theory that explains intrapersonal behavior. The major components of the HBM are perceived susceptibility, perceived severity, perceived benefits, perceived barriers, cues to action, and self-efficacy. These major components account for an individual's "readiness to act" (Glanz & Rimer, 1997; Glanz et al., 2002).

Perceived susceptibility is an individual's opinion regarding his or her personal chances of developing a condition. Perceived susceptibility measures the individual's subjective perception of risks. An individual's opinion about the seriousness of a specific condition and its consequences is referred to as perceived severity. These two concepts—perceived susceptibility and perceived severity—form the individual's perception of the threat of a condition. The hope is that emphasis on the perceived threat along with recommended health-related behaviors will lead to healthy behavior. The course of action or health-related behavior that an individual selects depends on his or her perceived benefit of the recommended health behavior. The perceived benefit is an individual's perception of the efficacy of the recommended health-related behavior in reducing his or her personal risk of contracting the condition (perceived threat). Individuals who do not believe the recommended health-related behavior will reduce their risk are less likely to adopt the recommended health-related behavior. Any impediments to adopting a recommended health-related behavior are the individual's perceived barriers. Perceived barriers negatively influence the adoption of health-related behavior. Thus individuals decide to adopt specific health-related behaviors based on their perception of their susceptibility and of the severity (perceived threat) of a condition, plus the perceived benefits from adopting the health-related behavior, and minus the perceived barriers to adopting the health-related behavior. Public health nurses can influence individuals' decisions through cues to action. Cues to action are strategies that activate "readiness." Cues to action could be postal reminders for health checks, posters with educational messages, or counseling. To adopt a health-related behavior, an individual must possess self-efficacy in relation to the behavior. Self-efficacy is the belief that an individual is capable of carrying out the recommended behavior. In addition to these major components, an individuals' demographic, sociopsychological, and structural variables affect their perceptions and influence their health-related behaviors (Glanz & Rimer, 1997; Janz, Champion, & Strecher, 2002).

For example, according to the HBM, an individual is likely to engage in the safe-sex practice of wearing a condom if the following conditions are present: the individual perceives that he or she can "get" human immunodeficiency virus (HIV) from his or her sexual behavior and considers HIV infection to be a severe or deadly illness. These two beliefs create a perceived health threat of HIV in an individual. An individual with these perceptions will decide to use a condom based on the perceived benefits of using a condom (decreased risk of HIV exposure) in relation to the perceived barriers of adopting condom use, such as cost and having to alter sexual practices. For an individual to adopt condom use, that individual has to be self-efficacious about condom use (he or she has to be able to use a condom correctly). To assist the individual in making a decision, public health nurses can implement cues to action such as placing safe-sex posters in community settings and having condoms readily available for use.

The Transtheoretical Stages of Change Model

Prochaska introduced the stages of change model as a framework to identify an individual's readiness to change behavior. The basic premise of the stages of change model is that human behavior change is a process, with individuals at varying levels of motivation or readiness for change (Glanz & Rimer, 1997). This model is a circular, not linear, model of human behavior. It accepts that individuals relapse in their behavior and recycle through previous stages of change. Public health interventions are matched to the individual's identified stage of change. There are six distinct stages of change in this model that are associated with a temporal dimension: precontemplation, contemplation, preparation and decision or determination, action, maintenance, and termination (see Figure 4.1; Prochaska, Redding, & Evers, 2002; Zimmerman, Olsen, & Bosworth, 2000).

An individual who is unaware of a health problem or risk and has no intention to change behavior within the next 6 months is in the precontemplation stage of change. Individuals who are aware of the "pros" of behavior change and intend to change their behavior within the next 6 months are in the contemplation stage. In the preparation stage, individuals have a plan of action for behavior change and intend to take action in the next month. Once overt behavior modifications have taken place, the individual is considered to be in the action stage. The maintenance stage of behavior change is not achieved until the individual has modified his or her behavior for from 6 months to 5 years. Relapse prevention is the goal in the maintenance stage. Termination is the last stage of change: in it, an individual has no temptation to repeat the previous, unhealthy behavior. Persons in the termination stage are typically self-efficacious. Termination of unhealthy behaviors is not appropriate for all types of behavior modification (Glanz & Rimer, 1997; Prochaska, Norcross, & DiClemente, 1994; Prochaska et al., 2002).

As an individual makes progress through these stages of change, a decisional balance occurs. The decisional balance is the individual's personal

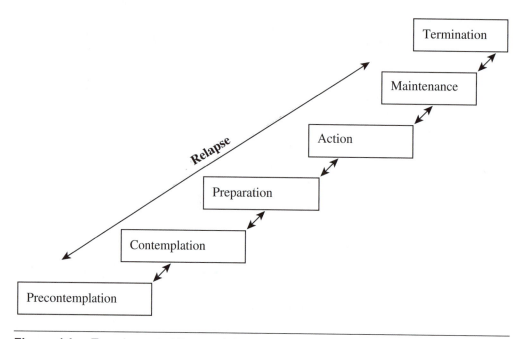

Figure 4.1   Transtheoretical Stages of Change

weighing of the pros and cons of behavior change. The four categories of pros are instrumental gains to self, instrumental gains for others, approval of self, and approval from others. The four categories of cons are instrumental cost to self, instrumental cost to others, disapproval from self, and disapproval from others (Prochaska et al., 2002; Zimmerman et al., 2000).

The processes of change are the covert and overt actions or interventions used to assist an individual in progressing through the six stages of change to achieve behavior modification. The 10 processes of change are consciousness raising, dramatic relief, self-reevaluation, environmental reevaluation, self-liberation, helping relationships, counterconditioning, contingency management, stimulus control, and social liberation. Table 4.1 presents the definition of each process of change, with examples.

Precaution Adoption Process Model

The precaution adoption process model (PAPM) is a stage theory similar to but different from the transtheoretical stages of change. In the PAPM, the adoption of a new precaution (healthy behavior) or the reduction or elimination of a risky behavior requires deliberate human action. This model focuses on the psychological process that occurs within an individual during behavior modification consideration. There are seven stages: unaware,

Table 4.1   Processes of Change: Definitions and Examples of Interventions

Process of Change	Definition	Examples of Interventions
Consciousness raising	Increasing awareness through facts and ideas that support behavior change	Feedback, confrontations, interpretations, bibliotherapy, media campaigns
Dramatic relief	Experiencing of negative emotions associated with unhealthy behavioral risks	Psychodrama, role-playing, grieving, personal testimonials, media campaigns
Self-reevaluation	Cognitive or affective assessment of one's self-image	Values clarification, role modeling, mental imagery
Environmental reevaluation	Cognitive or affective assessment of how one's social environment affect one's health	Empathy training, documentaries, family interventions
Self-liberation	Belief that one can change and the commitment to act on that belief	New Year's resolutions, public testimonials
Helping relationships	Social support for healthy behaviors	Rapport building, therapeutic alliances, buddy systems, counselors
Counterconditioning	Learn healthy behaviors that substitute for unhealthy behaviors	Relaxation, assertion, desensitization, positive self-talk
Contingency management	Increase rewards for healthy behavior and decrease rewards for unhealthy behavior	Contingency contracts, reinforcements, group recognition
Stimulus control	Remove reminders or cues to engage in unhealthy behavior and add cues that remind of healthy behavior	Avoidance, environmental reengineering, self-help groups
Social liberation	Realization of social norms that support healthy behaviors	Advocacy, empowerment

unengaged, deciding to act, decision not to act, decision to act, acting, and maintenance (see Figure 4.2; Weinstein & Sandman, 2002a, 2002b).

In stage 1, an individual is not aware of the health issue. Once the individual learns about the health issue, he or she is no long unaware and moves into the second stage but is still unengaged by the health issue. In stage 3 are individuals who are in the decision-making stage: They are engaged by the health issue and are planning their response. If an individual decides not to act (stage 4), the precaution adoption process ends with the individual aware and engaged but not acting. If the individual decides to act (stage 5), he or she progresses to the next step, acting (stage 6), and initiates behavior

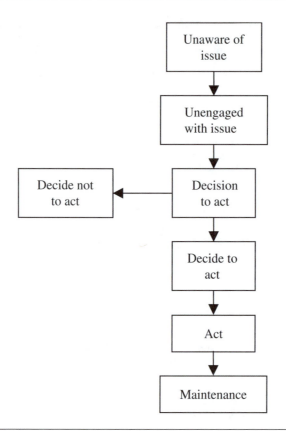

Figure 4.2   Precaution Adoption Process Model

changes. Stage 7 is the final stage. This stage is characterized by behavioral maintenance over time (Weinstein & Sandman, 2002a, 2002b).

PAPM is a stage-sequential model. Individuals are considered to move through each stage sequentially but at different rates of time. They may move back to earlier stages as well as forward as they attempt to modify their behaviors.

Theory of Reasoned Action and Theory of Planned Behavior

Motivational factors are considered the immediate determinants of behavior change in the theory of reasoned action (TRA) and the theory of planned behavior (TPB). Fishbein first introduced the TRA in 1967. The TPB is an extension of the TRA. Both theories assume that such factors such as demographics and environment operate through the models' constructs and do not independently contribute to the explanation of an individual's likelihood

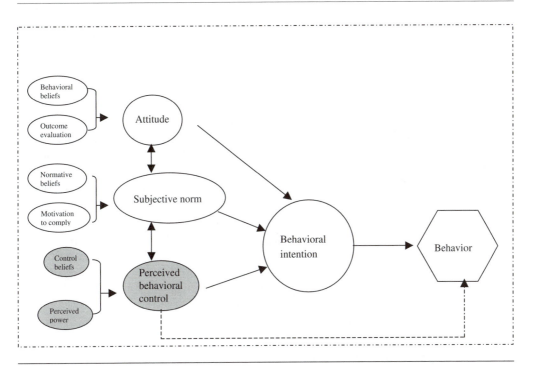

Figure 4.3   The Theories of Reasoned Action and of Planned Behavior

Note: White areas indicate the original theory of reasoned action. Gray areas denote those constructs added with the theory of planned behavior. Solid lines indicate direct relationship.

of behavior change (Ajzen, 1991; Fishbein, 1967; Montano & Kasprzyk, 2002; Sheeran, Conner, & Norman, 2001).

The TRA asserts that behavioral intention is the most important determinant of human behavior. The direct determinants of individuals' behavioral intentions are their attitude toward performing the behavior and their subjective norm associated with the behavior. An individual's attitude toward the behavior is determined by that individual's beliefs about the outcomes or attributes of performing the behavior (behavioral beliefs) and his or her evaluation of the outcomes or attributes of performing the behavior. The subjective norm is determined by the normative beliefs of the individual's peer group and his or her motivation to comply with those normative beliefs. An assumption of TRA is that individuals are rational actors who process information and are motivated to act on the information. TRA asserts that the likelihood of an individual performing a behavior results from his or her behavioral intention, which is determined by the individual's combined attitude toward the behavior and his or her subjective norms in relation to the behavior (see Figure 4.3; Montano & Kasprzyk, 2002).

The TPB is an expansion of the TRA; the construct of perceived behavioral control has been added. Perceived behavioral control was added to this theory to account for factors outside the individual's volitional control. According to the TPB, beliefs about perceived behavioral control are determined by control beliefs regarding the resources needed to carry out the behavior and the impediments to performing a behavior. TPB asserts that individuals' beliefs about behavioral control are weighed by their perceived power and result in their perception of behavioral control. Perceived power is the individual's belief about the ability of the resources or impediments to promote or inhibit a behavior (Ajzen, 1991; Sheeran et al., 2001).

For example, a woman's intention to receive a mammogram is dependent on her attitude toward mammograms, her subjective norms, and her perceived behavioral control. Her attitude is influenced by her beliefs about receiving mammograms to detect cancer (behavioral beliefs) and beliefs about the benefits of receiving a mammogram (outcome evaluation). Her subjective norm is created by her referent peers, such as family members or friends who encourage her to seek a mammogram, and her motivation to comply with their recommendations. Her perceived behavioral control is dependent on her perception of how much the mammogram is within her control and how much power she has to receive a mammogram.

Social Cognitive Theory

Social cognitive theory (SCT) is an interpersonal theory of human behavior. SCT explains human behavior in terms of a triadic, dynamic, and reciprocal model in which behavior, personal factors, and environment influence each other in what is termed reciprocal determinism (Bandura, 1986). Reciprocal determinism proposes that the environment maintains and affects behavior and that people in turn maintain and affect their environment. A central concept of SCT is behavioral capability.

Behavioral capability asserts that an individual must have the knowledge and ability to perform the expected behavior. Bandura (1986) considers self-efficacy as the most important aspect that determines behavior change. Self-efficacy is an individual's confidence in his or her ability to enact and continue with the health behavior. SCT embraces the idea that antecedent determinants of behavior are influenced by outcome expectations.

Outcome expectations are the anticipatory aspects of behavior. Outcome expectations are learned in four ways: (a) performance attainment—previous experience with behavior, (b) vicarious experience—observing others in similar behavior situations, (c) verbal persuasion—hearing about similar situations from others, and (d) physiological arousal—emotional or physical ability to conduct the behavior or the response to behavior (Baranowski, Perry, & Parcel, 2002). Outcome expectations affect an individual's self-efficacy. Additionally, three strategies for increasing self efficacy are (a) setting small, incremental, and attainable goals, (b) behavioral contracting—establishing goals and specific rewards, and (c) monitoring and reinforcement (Cervonne, 2000; Glanz & Rimer, 1997).

Table 4.2 Diffusion of Innovation: Attributes to Speed and Extend Adoption

Relative advantage	Innovation is better than what it replaces
Compatibility	Innovation matches intended audience
Complexity	Innovation is easy to use
Trialability	Innovation can be subjected to a trial
Observability	Innovation outcome is observable and measurable
Impact on social relations	Does innovation affect social environment?
Reversibility	Innovation can be reversed or discontinued
Communicability	Innovation is easily and clearly understood
Time required	Innovation can be adopted with minimal time investment
Risk and uncertainty	Innovation can be adopted with minimal risk and uncertainty
Commitment required	Innovation can be used with modest commitment
Modifiability	Innovation can be updated and modified over time

Diffusion of Innovation

Diffusion of innovation is considered an organizational or community-level theory. Diffusion of innovation focuses on the dissemination of innovations within an organization or community to affect human behavior. Rogers (1983) defines an innovation as "an idea, practice, or object that is perceived as new by an individual or other unit of adoption" (p. 11). Diffusion is defined as the process by which the innovation is communicated through appropriate channels over time to members of a social system or community. The diffusion process involves the channels used to communicate a message (communication channel) and the environmental system in which the communication occurs (diffusion context). Communication is considered a two-way process in which the communicator affects the community's behavior and the community's behavior affects the mediator's message. A critical element in this diffusion theory is the communicator's ability to communicate with individuals at various levels of adoption.

In addition to the communication channels and diffusion context, a focus on the characteristics of an innovation can improve the chances that the innovation will be adopted. Table 4.2 presents the key determinants of the speed and extent of innovation diffusion that must be addressed in planning an innovation for community diffusion (Oldenburg & Parcel, 2002).

Five mutually exclusive adopter categories—innovators, early adopters, early majority adopters, late majority adopters, and laggards—were identified that affect the level of diffusion of an innovation. Innovators are risk takers who are excited by the adoption of new behaviors. Early adopters are frequently respected members of a community or social system and may serve as role models. These individuals require a high degree of opinion leadership. Early majority adopters require a long time of deliberation before adopting a new behavior. Late majority adopters are frequently skeptical and change behavior because of increased pressure from others or a change in the social norms of a group. Laggards are the last members of a social system to adopt an intervention. Laggards are traditionally conservative and suspicious of innovations. Green, Gottlieb, and Parcel (1987) suggest that interventions to be diffused into a community should be targeted based on the type of adopters involved. Cognitively oriented interventions should target early adopters, a motivational emphasis may reach majority adopters, and measures to eliminate barriers are best for late adopters.

Learning Theories

Learning theories reinforce the idea that behavior change is complex. Changing behavior requires learning new and different patterns of complex behaviors, requiring the modification of many smaller behaviors that compose the overall complex behavior (Skinner, 1953). Behavior modification includes the belief that reducing complex behaviors into smaller segments improves behavior-change learning. The attainment of smaller changes in behavior reinforces the belief that achievement of the final goal, changing the complex behavior, is reachable. Reinforcement can be defined as the consequences that motivate an individual to continue or discontinue a behavior (Bandura, 1986; Skinner, 1953). Classical learning theory is an individual-level theory in which the key concepts are shaping behavior, providing behavioral cues, and behavioral reinforcement. It is beyond the scope of this text to provide a thorough explanation of classical learning theory.

The PRECEDE-PROCEED Planning Model

PRECEDE-PROCEED is a systematic planning model for the development of health education and health promotion programs. Green and Kreuter (1991) developed the PRECEDE component of this model in the 1970s and extended the model in 1991 to include the PROCEED component. The model begins at the end by focusing on the outcome of interest and works backwards to determine how best to achieve the desired outcome. This model consists of nine phases that assert that human behavior is complex, multidimensional, and influenced by a variety of factors that must be assessed and diagnosed.

The first five (diagnostic) phases are (a) social diagnosis—individuals' perceptions of needs, wants, resources, barriers, and quality of life; (b) epidemiological diagnosis—vital statistics and morbidity and mortality data; (c) behavioral and environmental diagnosis—behavioral and environmental risk factors; (d) educational and organizational diagnosis—predisposing, reinforcing, and enabling factors that affect behavior; and (e) administration and policy diagnosis—policies and procedures, regulations, or organizational conditions that may facilitate or block a program's implementation. In the educational and organizational diagnosis, predisposing factors include knowledge, attitudes, beliefs, personal preferences, existing skills, and self-efficacy beliefs about a behavior. Reinforcing factors are elements that serve as incentives or rewards for a behavior. Enabling factors affect the behavior directly or indirectly through environmental factors. Each diagnostic phase identifies objectives and strategies to achieve the community-level goal of meeting the community's self-determined health education and health program needs and wants (Green & Kreuter, 1991).

The PRECEDE-PROCEED model's final four phases focus on implementation and evaluation. Implementation involves health behavior change strategies targeting health education, policy, regulations, or organizational resources. Process evaluation consists of assessing the health behavior intervention's impact on predisposing, reinforcing, and enabling factors; impact evaluation assesses the intervention's impact on behavior, lifestyle, and environment. The final phase is outcome evaluation, which focuses on health status and quality of life measures (Gielen & McDonald, 2002; Green & Kreuter, 1991).

The Social Marketing Model

Social marketing is a consumer-oriented process that tailors interventions and programs to serve a defined target population using marketing theory. Andreasen (1995) describes social marketing as the application of commercial marketing technologies to the analysis, planning, execution, and evaluation of programs designed to influence the voluntary behavior of target populations as a measure to improve healthy behaviors. The basic principles of marketing—product, price, place, and promotion—are integrated into the social marketing model. The product is the intervention being marketed. Price is what it will cost the person to adapt a health behavior. The place corresponds to the environmental and contextual barriers to selling the intervention. Promotion is the advertising and communication of the intervention through identified channels. Social marketing is a valuable process of promoting health behavior change (see Figure 4.4).

Social marketing is considered to be most valuable when implemented in a systematic, continuous manner, with each step of the process based on market research. The major concepts of the social marketing model are consumer orientation, audience segmentation, channel analysis, strategy, and process tracking. Each concept is evident in the six phases of the social marketing model:

- *Phase 1: Planning and strategy.* The organization's overall mandates and goals are analyzed, there is an economic analysis, and the geographical market, distribution outlets, market trends and projections, and target population are analyzed.

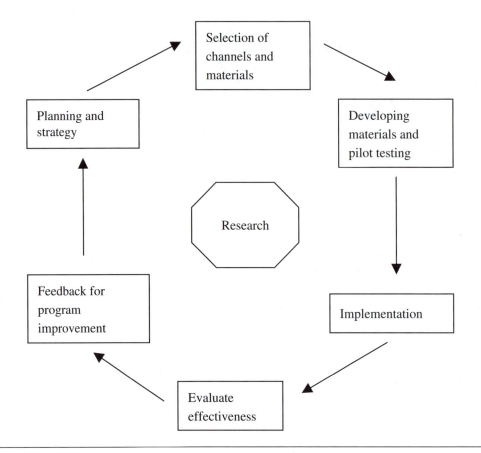

Figure 4.4   Social Marketing Model

- *Phase 2: Selecting channels and materials.* The program's structure and organization are established, program objectives are developed, the target population is segmented, the strategy for market entry is selected, and marketing mix is defined (product, price, and promotion).
- *Phase 3: Developing materials and pretesting.* Materials are developed and pilot tested. This is the hallmark of the social marketing model.
- *Phase 4: Implementation.* The program is completely implemented.
- *Phase 5: Assessing effectiveness.* A systematic evaluation of program objectives and goals is conducted.
- *Phase 6: Feedback to refine program.* Evaluation data provides continuous feedback to revise the program as the target population (market) evolves over time (Andreasen, 1995; Glanz & Rimer, 1997).

The Structural Model of Health Behavior

The structural model of health behavior builds on ecological theory by specifying structural mechanisms by which population-level factors effect behavior change. A key factor in ecological theory is that environmental or structural factors are critical determinants of individual health behavior. Ecological theories propose that public health interventions should manipulate or adjust the conditions in which people live to influence individual health behavior (Cohen & Scribner, 2000; Cohen, Scribner, & Farley, 2000; McLeroy, Bibeau, Steckler, & Glanz, 1988). The structural model of health behavior changes the environment's structural context in which a behavior exists; therefore, it is considered a population-level health behavior theory.

The goal of structural interventions, based on the structural model of health behavior, is to change the behavior of an entire population. Four factors that constitute a structural model of health behavior affecting a population are (a) the availability and accessibility of consumer products, (b) physical structures, (c) social structures and policies, and (d) media and cultural messages (Cohen & Scribner, 2000; Cohen et al., 2000). Cohen and Scribner define availability as the accessibility of consumer products that are associated with health behavior outcomes. Availability of products can change behavior without directly affecting an individual's attitudes, beliefs, or cognitions. Public health economic policy interventions can negatively affect the availability of harmful products that contribute to risky behaviors. Physical structures refer to the physical characteristics or products that either reduce or increase an individual's opportunities for healthy behaviors and outcomes. Manufacturing requirements, safety laws, and zoning regulations are examples of public health interventions directed at physical structures. Physical structures can change health outcomes without changing an individual's attitudes, beliefs, cognitions, or behavior. Laws or policies that require or prohibit certain behaviors are social structures. Social structures influence health behavior directly without changing attitudes or beliefs but also work indirectly through changing social norms and expectations. Cultural practices and messages seen and heard frequently form cultural and medial messages. Media is considered a structural intervention when it influences social norms (Cohen & Scribner, 2000; Cohen et al., 2000).

Summary

Key issues in behavioral health theories are as follows.

- A theory is a set of concepts, constructs, and/or variables that are interrelated through propositional statements that provide a specific view of events or situations.
- Concepts are abstract ideas that provide meaning to one's perceptions and permit generalizations.
- Propositions are statements that describe the relationship of one concept to another within the specific theory.

- Empirical knowing uses verifiable, factual descriptions, explanations, or predictions that are based on the collection of subjective or objective data.
- Ethical knowing uses moral obligations and values as a means of inquiry that focuses on the identification and analysis of beliefs and values held by individuals and the relationship of these beliefs and values to human behavior.
- Personal knowing is being knowledgeable regarding one's own personal style of being with another person and the inner experience of becoming whole and self-aware.
- Aesthetic knowing relates to what is considered important and significant in a person's behavior.
- The major components of the health belief model are perceived susceptibility, perceived severity, perceived benefits, perceived barriers, cues to action, and self-efficacy.
- The transtheoretical stages of change include six distinct stages that are associated with a temporal dimension: precontemplation, contemplation, preparation and decision or determination, action, maintenance, and termination.
- Ten processes of change, according to the transtheoretical stages of change, are consciousness raising, dramatic relief, self-reevaluation, environmental reevaluation, self-liberation, helping relationships, counterconditioning, contingency management, stimulus control, and social liberation.
- The precaution adoption process model has seven stages: unaware, unengaged, deciding to act, decision not to act, decision to act, acting, and maintenance.
- The theory of reasoned action asserts that behavioral intention is the most important determinant of human behavior.
- The direct determinants of individuals' behavioral intention are their attitude toward performing the behavior and their subjective norm associated with the behavior.
- The theory of planned behavior is an expansion of the TRA; the construct of perceived behavioral control has been added.
- Beliefs about perceived behavioral control are determined by control beliefs regarding the resources needed to carry out the behavior and the impediments to performing a behavior.
- Reciprocal determinism proposes that the environment maintains and affects behavior and people in turn maintain and affect their environment.
- A central concept of social cognitive theory is behavioral capability.
- Self-efficacy is an individual's confidence in his or her ability to enact and continue with the health behavior.
- Outcome expectations are learned in four ways: (a) performance attainment, (b) vicarious experience, (c) verbal persuasion, and (d) physiological arousal.

- Three strategies for increasing self efficacy are (a) setting small, incremental and attainable goals; (b) behavioral contracting; and (c) monitoring and reinforcement.

- The diffusion process involves the channels used to communicate a message (communication channel) and the environmental system in which the communication occurs (diffusion context).

- The speed of diffusion is affected by five mutually exclusive adopter categories: innovators, early adopters, early majority adopters, late majority adopters, and laggards.

- PRECEDE-PROCEED is a systematic planning model for the development of health education and health promotion programs.

- The first five diagnostic phases are (a) social diagnosis, (b) epidemiological diagnosis, (c) behavioral and environmental diagnosis, (d) educational and organizational diagnosis, and (e) administration and policy diagnosis.

- The PRECEDE-PROCEED model's final four phases focus on implementation and evaluation.

- Social marketing is a consumer-oriented process that tailors interventions and programs to serve a defined target population, using marketing theory.

- The six phases of the social marketing model are planning and strategy, selecting channels and materials, developing materials and pretesting, implementation, assessing effectiveness, and feedback.

- Ecological theories propose that public health interventions should manipulate or adjust the conditions in which people live to influence individual health behavior.

References

Ajzen, I. (1991). The theory of planned behavior. *Organizational Behavior and Human Decision Processes*, *50*, 179-211.

Andreasen, A. (1995). *Marketing social change: Changing behavior to promote health, social development, and the environment*. San Francisco: Jossey-Bass.

Bandura, A. (1986). *Social foundations of thought and action*. Englewood Cliffs, NJ: Prentice-Hall.

Baranowski, T., Perry, C., & Parcel, G. (2002). How individuals, environments, and health behavior interact: Social cognitive theory. In K. Glanz, B. Rimer, & F. Lewis (Eds.), *Health behavior and health education: Theory, research, and practice* (pp. 165-184). San Francisco: Jossey-Bass.

Cervonne, D. (2000). Thinking about self-efficacy. *Behavior Modification*, *24*(1), 30-51.

Chinn, P., & Kramer, M. (1995). *Theory and nursing: A systematic approach* (4th ed.). St. Louis, MO: Mosby.

Cohen, D., & Scribner, R. (2000). An STD/HIV prevention intervention framework. *AIDS Patient Care and STDs*, *14*(1), 37-45.

Cohen, D., Scribner, R., & Farley, T. (2000). A structural model of health behavior: A pragmatic approach to explain and influence health behaviors at the population level. *Preventive Medicine, 30,* 146-154.

Fawcett, J. (1997). The structural hierarchy of nursing knowledge: Components and their definitions. In I. King & J. Fawcett (Eds.), *The language of nursing theory and metatheory* (pp. 11-17). Indianapolis, IN: Sigma Theta Tau International.

Fawcett, J., Watson, J., Neuman, B., Walker, P., & Fitzpatrick, J. (2001). On nursing theories and evidence. *Journal of Nursing Scholarship, 32*(2), 115-119.

Fishbein, M. (1967). *Readings in attitude theory and measurement.* New York: Wiley.

Gielen, A., & McDonald, E. (2002). Using the PRECEDE-PROCEED planning model to apply health behavior theories. In K. Glanz, B. Rimer, & F. Lewis (Eds.), *Health behavior and health education: Theory, research, and practice* (pp. 409-436). San Francisco: Jossey-Bass.

Glanz, K., & Rimer, B. (1997). *Theory at a glance: A guide for health promotion practice.* Washington, DC: National Cancer Institute.

Glanz, K., Rimer, B., & Lewis, F. (2002). Theory, research and practice in health behavior and health education. In K. Glanz, B. Rimer, & F. Lewis (Eds.), *Health behavior and health education: Theory, research, and practice* (pp. 22-44). San Francisco: Jossey-Bass.

Green, L., Gottlieb, N., & Parcel, G. (1987). Diffusion theory extended and applied. In W. Ward (Ed.), *Advances in health education and promotion.* Greenwich, CT: JAI.

Green, L., & Kreuter, M. (1991). *Health promotion planning: An educational and environmental approach* (2nd ed.). Mountain View, CA: Mayfield.

Janz, N., Champion, V., & Strecher, V. (2002). The health belief model. In K. Glanz, B. Rimer, & F. Lewis (Eds.), *Health behavior and health education: Theory, research, and practice* (pp. 45-66). San Francisco: Jossey-Bass.

Kim, H. (1997). Terminology in structuring and developing nursing knowledge. In I. King & J. Fawcett (Eds.), *The language of nursing theory and metatheory* (pp. 27-36). Indianapolis, IN: Sigma Theta Tau International.

King, I. (1997). Knowledge development for nursing: A process. In I. King & J. Fawcett (Eds.), *The language of nursing theory and metatheory* (pp. 19-25). Indianapolis, IN: Sigma Theta Tau International.

McLeroy, K., Bibeau, D., Steckler, A., & Glanz, K. (1988). An ecological perspective on health promotion programs. *Health Education Quarterly, 15,* 351-377.

Montano, D., & Kasprzyk, D. (2002). The theory of reasoned action and the theory of planned behavior. In K. Glanz, B. Rimer, & F. Lewis (Eds.), *Health behavior and health education: Theory, research, and practice* (pp. 67-98). San Francisco: Jossey-Bass.

Oldenburg, B., & Parcel, G. (2002). Diffusion of innovation. In K. Glanz, B. Rimer, & F. Lewis (Eds.), *Health behavior and health education: Theory, research, and practice* (pp. 312-334). San Francisco: Jossey-Bass.

Prochaska, J., Norcross, J., & DiClemente, C. (1994). *Changing for good: A revolutionary six-stage program for overcoming bad habits and moving your life positively forward.* New York: Avon.

Prochaska, J., Redding, C., & Evers, C. (2002). The transtheoretical model and stages of change. In K. Glanz, B. Rimer, & F. Lewis (Eds.), *Health behavior and health education: Theory, research, and practice* (pp. 99-120). San Francisco: Jossey-Bass.

Rogers, E. (1983). *Diffusion of innovation* (3rd ed.). New York: Free Press.

Sheeran, P., Conner, M., & Norman, P. (2001). Can the theory of planned behavior explain patterns of health behavior change? *Health Psychology, 20*(1), 12-19.

Skinner, B. (1953). *Science and human behavior*. New York: Macmillan.

Tyler, J. (1999). The decade of behavior 2000-2010. *Society for Public Health Education: News & Views, 25*(6), 1.

Weinstein, N., & Sandman, P. (2002a). The precaution adoption process model and its application. In R. DiClemente, R. Crosby, & M. Kegler (Eds), *Emerging theories in health promotion practice and research: Strategies for improving public health* (pp. 16-39). San Francisco: Jossey-Bass.

Weinstein, N., & Sandman, P. (2002b). The precaution adoption process model. In K. Glanz, B. Rimer, & F. Lewis (Eds.), *Health behavior and health education: Theory, research, and practice* (pp. 121-143). San Francisco: Jossey-Bass.

Zimmerman, G., Olsen, C., & Bosworth, M. (2000). A "stages of change" approach to helping patients change behavior. *American Family Physician, 61*, 1409-1416.

Part II

Public Health—Community Health Assessment Framework

5

Behavioral Assessment

Behavioral theories provide the theoretical framework for understanding human behavior and identify the behavioral concepts that should be assessed in a behavioral assessment. Behavioral assessments provide the population data on risky behaviors and risk factors for illness and related health conditions. A comprehensive, population-based, community assessment should include a component of a behavioral assessment. This chapter focuses on identifying the determinants of health and leading health indicators for the United States, describes behavioral assessments, and summarizes the Youth Risk Behavior Surveillance System.

Introduction

Public health professionals are continually challenged to use behavioral science theories to modify or change individuals' risk-related behaviors. Behavioral science theories provide the concepts that can be used to assess and predict an individual's behavior. Understanding individual behaviors as a component of the community assessment process is a public health strategy that can affect population-based morbidity and mortality through behavior modification interventions.

In the United States, 70% of all premature deaths are related to individual behaviors and environmental factors. The leading causes of death in the United States have changed from causes that are primarily infectious in origin to those that originate in behavior. Deaths from these causes are a direct result of risky behaviors such as injury, violence, environmental factors, unavailability or inaccessibility of quality health-care services, and unhealthy lifestyle choices. The nation's progress in achieving the Healthy People 2010 goals and objectives is dependent on the integration of behavioral assessments as a component of public health, environmental, and community assessment processes (Department of Health and Human

Services [DHHS], 2000, 2001). Individual behavioral assessments are often neglected as a component of the population-level community assessment. Public health professionals conducting behavioral assessments should be knowledgeable and integrate into the assessment and planning processes the determinants of health and leading health indicators as outlined in Healthy People 2010.

Determinants of Health

The determinants of health identified in Healthy People 2010 are individual biology, individual behaviors, physical environment, social environment, policies and interventions, and access to quality health care (see Figure 2.3; DHHS, 2000). These determinants of health are defined in chapter 2.

Behaviors are defined as individual responses or reactions to internal stimuli and external conditions. Behaviors are generally classified as healthy, health-seeking, or risk behaviors. Healthy or health-seeking behaviors are actions taken by the individual that increase his or her chances of experiencing positive health-related outcomes. In contrast, risk behaviors are those actions that increase the chance or likelihood that the individual will be exposed to some untoward health-related outcome.

Neither healthy nor risky individual human behaviors exist in isolation. There is a reciprocal relationship between an individual's biological makeup and his or her behavioral choices. Additionally, an individual's physical and social environment are considered to directly influence that individual's behavior, in the same reciprocal manner. Policies and interventions are considered to have a powerful impact on an individual's health and the community. Lastly, access to quality health care directly affects the health of individuals and the community. Through behavioral, public health, environmental, and community assessments, the reciprocal relationship of these determinants of health is better understood. An understanding of the behavioral determinants of health assists the public health professional with the identification of public health interventions that can modify individuals' risky behaviors. Behavioral assessment is an important public health measure that can improve the health of individuals, communities, and the nation. Behavioral assessments are generally conducted through survey research.

Leading Health Indicators

Leading health indicators were identified from the Healthy People 2010 determinants of health. These leading health indicators identify individual behaviors, physical and social environmental factors, and health-care system policies and access to care issues that affect the health of individuals and communities. The nation's leading health indicators communicate to the public the importance of health promotion and disease prevention activities in the next decade.

The major public health concerns of the United States are reflected in the leading health indicators. The Healthy People 2010 specific objectives (Appendix B) were derived from these leading health indicators. The leading health indicators are

- Physical activity
- Overweight and obesity
- Tobacco use
- Substance use
- Responsible sexual behavior
- Mental behavior
- Injury and violence
- Environmental quality
- Immunization
- Access to health care (DHHS, 2000).

The Healthy People 2010 initiative proposes that strategies and action plans developed to address one or more of these indicators that are consistent with the specific Healthy People 2010 objectives can have a significant effect on reaching the nation's goals and creating healthy people in healthy communities. These leading health indicators form the basis for 10 public health priority areas that are consistent with the Healthy People 2010 objectives (Table 5.1). Behavioral assessment and interventions are an essential component in affecting the leading health indicators. All of the leading health indicators are directly or indirectly related to human behavior choices, health seeking or risky. Population-based surveys should be conducted by public health nurses to identify risky behaviors that need modification to achieve the Healthy People 2010 objectives. The leading health indicators can be used as a framework to understand which behavioral areas to assess as a component of the comprehensive population-based community assessment.

Behavioral Assessment

Behavior as an essential determinant of health has produced a plethora of health-related surveys as a method of determining what patterns of health or risk behaviors exist within defined populations. Behavioral surveys are conducted at the national, regional, state, and local levels using various methods (e.g., self-administered questionnaires and surveys, interviews, focus groups). The primary purposes of a behavior assessment are to determine which behaviors should be routinely under surveillance and to

Table 5.1   Healthy People 2010 Public Health Priorities

- Promote daily physical activity
- Promote good nutrition and healthier weights
- Prevent and reduce tobacco use
- Prevent and reduce substance abuse
- Promote responsible sexual behavior, including abstinence
- Promote mental health and well-being
- Promote safety and reduce violence
- Promote healthy environments
- Prevent infectious disease through immunizations
- Increase access to quality health care

determine which behaviors should be targeted in public health behavioral intervention programs.

Green and Kreuter (1999) identified a five-step behavioral assessment process:

1. Delineating the behavioral and nonbehavioral causes of a defined health problem

2. Developing a classification of behaviors (the leading health indicators can be used to frame the classification categories)

3. Rating the importance level of the behaviors

4. Rating the behavior's changeability

5. Selecting behavioral targets or baseline measurements

The first step in a behavioral assessment is the delineation of an extensive list of behavioral and nonbehavioral causes of a defined health problem. These causative behaviors are typically based on epidemiological data. Epidemiological studies identify the behavioral risk factors associated with specific diseases. These behaviors are the ones that are the focus of the behavioral assessment for the specified diseases. After the behavioral causes are identified, these behavioral factors are classified as preventive behaviors or treatment procedures. Behavioral causes are classified as primary, secondary, or tertiary preventive behaviors to identify potential actions that can be implemented to prevent or alter the disease. In addition, the causal behaviors are targeted as the behaviors to be prevented, reduced, or eliminated in prevention and treatment programs (Green & Kreuter, 1999).

Once the behavioral causes are classified as preventive or treatment behavioral activities, the extensive list of behaviors is reduced into a manageable list. Rating the importance of behaviors narrows the list. Two criteria used to narrow the list of behaviors to be assessed are frequency of occurrence and strength of the relationship between the behavior and the health problem (relative risk assessments or odds ratios may be used for this). The fourth step in the behavioral assessment is rating the behavior's changeability. The basic question at this point is "How susceptible to change are the behaviors that have been selected?" The attribute method is frequently used to assess the changeability of a behavior. The attribute method uses the "adoption of innovations" criteria of relevance, social approval, advantages, complexity, compatibility with values, experiences and needs, divisibility or trialability, and observability to rate the changeability of each behavior listed. Rating the changeability of behaviors assists the public health nurse in deciding what behaviors are to be measured under surveillance and recommended for behavior modification interventions. The last step in the behavioral assessment process is the determination of baseline behavioral measurements or targets (Green & Kreuter, 1999). Two approaches to determining baseline behavioral measurements are the baseline measurement approach and the importance and changeability dimensional approach.

Baseline Measurement Approach

A behavioral assessment provides a baseline measurement of the health- or risk-related actions of constituents within a defined population. The behavioral assessment baseline is the standard against which the accomplishment of goals and objectives is measured. The purposes of developing a behavioral baseline measure are to (a) determine the effectiveness of a behavioral modification intervention, (b) clarify the understanding of behavioral trends in the assessment data, (c) determine the appropriate time to initiate an intervention, (d) verify the necessity for a behavioral intervention, and (e) identify health- or risk-related actions in comparison to some standard on the national, regional, or local population level (Martin & Pear, 1992).

Public health professionals responsible for conducting behavioral assessments identify baseline behavioral measures specific to the population under investigation. Baseline behavioral measurements are developed by identifying an indicator or indicators that best reflect the behaviors that are most important and determining the measurements for each behavioral indicator. To identify the importance of the behavior, the following questions can be posed:

- Is this what is most important and pertinent to the community?
- Is the measure a valid measure?
- Can this measure be used comparatively with another community?

The behavioral indicators for the respective behaviors can be identified through the following questions:

- What characteristics of the behavior should be measured (frequency, rate of behavior, or duration of behavior)?
- Will the data be collected through a sampling, continuously, or at specified intervals? What will be the intervals of data collection?

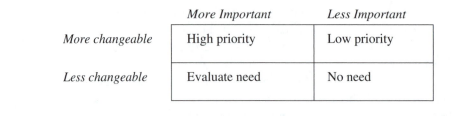

	More Important	*Less Important*
More changeable	High priority	Low priority
Less changeable	Evaluate need	No need

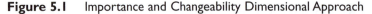

Figure 5.1   Importance and Changeability Dimensional Approach

Importance and Changeability Dimensional Approach

The importance and changeability dimensional approach classifies each behavior according to two dimensions: changeability and importance. Changeability refers to the degree to which the behavior can be changed. Importance refers to the level of significance of the behavior as related to health outcomes. Figure 5.1 demonstrates how each behavior may be placed into one of four dimensional quadrants: more changeable and more important, more changeable and less important, less changeable and more important, or less changeable and less important.

In summary, completion of the five-step behavioral assessment identifies which behaviors should be measured for specific health problems in a defined population. The behavioral assessment identifies and prioritizes the behaviors that should be targeted in public health interventions as a means to affect the population-based morbidity and mortality statistics of a defined health problem. Inherent in the behavioral assessment process is not only the determination of which behaviors should be assessed but which behaviors are highly changeable and important for behavior modification.

Behavioral theories provide the framework to guide the behavioral assessment. For example, the theory of reasoned action can be integrated into the five steps of the behavioral assessment for HIV infection. First the behavioral and nonbehavioral causes of HIV infection can be identified using the major concepts in this theory (attitudes toward the behavior and subjective norms). Next the behaviors or behavior-related beliefs associated with each of the noted concepts are classified according to the theory— behavioral beliefs and outcome beliefs, normative beliefs, and motivation, respectively. Each behavior in each category is rated according to level of importance and changeability. The major concepts of the theory are used to identify and measure behavioral targets and conduct baseline measurements (attitude toward HIV prevention and subjective norms related to HIV prevention). In addition, the concepts provide guidance on what types of interventions should be implemented to modify risky behaviors.

Youth Risk Behavior Surveillance System

The Youth Risk Behavior Surveillance System (YRBSS, 2003) is an example of a population-level behavioral assessment. This assessment survey is conducted every 2 years by the CDC to assess a number of youth behaviors that contribute to the nation's leading causes of death. The YRBSS is conducted on youths because healthy or risky behaviors are established during this developmental period. The purposes of the YRBSS are fivefold: (a) determine the prevalence and age of initiation of health-risk behaviors; (b) assess whether health risk behaviors increase, decrease, or remain the same over time; (c) examine the cooccurrence of health-risk behaviors among youth; (d) provide comparable national, state, and local data; and (e) monitor the nation's progress toward achieving the Healthy People 2010 goals and objectives. Data from the YRBSS are used to (a) implement or modify programs to address the behaviors of young people in a specific area, (b) set program goals and objectives and monitor progress toward these goals and objectives, (c) create an awareness of the extent of risk behaviors among young people, (d) promote state-level changes that support specific education curricula and coordinated school health programs, and (e) provide data to support the need for federal, state, and private funding (Centers for Disease Control and Prevention, 2001a).

The YRBSS has been conducted since 1991 as a behavioral assessment to identify trends in youth behaviors that pose health-related threats. This surveillance system uses some of the behavioral assessment techniques discussed earlier to discern which behaviors should be monitored. The CDC (2001b) notes that from 1991 to 1999, the following behaviors have continued to improve: never or rarely wearing a seat belt, never or rarely wearing a bicycle helmet, riding with a drunk driver, carrying a gun, carrying a weapon on school property, involvement in physical activity, involvement in physical fights on school property, consideration of suicide, using smokeless tobacco, ever engaging in sexual intercourse, having four or more sexual partners, using a condom at last intercourse, HIV/AIDS education in school, and participating in strengthening exercises. Behaviors that have worsened from 1991 to 1999 are cigarette use, episodic heavy drinking, lifetime marijuana use, current cocaine use, lifetime illegal steroid use, using birth control, and attending physical education classes daily. These trends in the youth data that were examined over time provide support for the usefulness of behavioral assessment data to conduct population-based behavioral interventions in this youth population. The development of behavioral assessment and surveillance systems such as the YRBSS strengthens the ability of public health infrastructures to appropriately conduct public health program planning.

Summary

Key issues in behavioral assessment are as follows.

- Individual behavioral assessments are a component of the community assessment process that can affect population-based morbidity and mortality through the identification of behaviors that need modification.
- The determinants of health identified in the Healthy People 2010 document are individual biology, individual behaviors, physical environment, social environment, policies and interventions, and access to quality health care.
- Behaviors are defined as individual responses or reactions to internal stimuli and external conditions.
- Healthy or health-seeking behaviors are those actions that increase an individual's chances of experiencing positive health-related outcomes.
- Risk behaviors are those actions that increase an individual's chance or likelihood of exposure to some untoward health-related outcome.
- The leading health indicators are physical activity, overweight and obesity, tobacco use, substance use, responsible sexual behavior, mental behavior, injury and violence, environmental quality, immunization, and access to health care.
- Behavioral assessments are a method of determining what patterns of health or risk behaviors exist within defined populations.
- The five-step behavioral assessment process consists of (a) delineating the behavioral and nonbehavioral causes of a defined health problem, (b) developing a classification of behaviors, (c) rating the importance level of the behaviors, (d) rating the behavior's changeability, and (e) selecting behavioral targets or baseline measurements.
- The behavioral assessment baseline is the standard against which the accomplishment of goals and objectives is measured.
- The purposes of developing a behavioral baseline measure are to (a) determine the effectiveness of a behavioral modification intervention, (b) clarify the understanding of behavioral trends in the assessment data, (c) determine the appropriate time to initiate an intervention, (d) verify the necessity for a behavioral intervention, and (e) identify health- or risk-related actions in comparison to some standard on the national, regional, or local population level.
- The importance and changeability dimensional approach classifies each behavior according to two dimensions: changeability and importance.
- The Youth Risk Behavior Surveillance System is an example of a population-level behavioral assessment.

References

Centers for Disease Control and Prevention. (2001a). *Assessing health risk behaviors among young people: Youth risk behavior surveillance system.* Retrieved June 10, 2003, from http://www.cdc.gov/nccdphp/dash/yrbs/yrbsaag.htm

Centers for Disease Control and Prevention. (2001b). *Fact Sheet: Youth risk behavior trends.* Retrieved February 19, 2002, from http://www.cdc.gov/nccdphp/dash/yrbs/trend.htm

Department of Health and Human Services. (2000). *Healthy People 2010: Understanding and improving health* (2nd ed.). Washington, DC: U.S. Government Printing Office.

Department of Health and Human Services. (2001). *Healthy people in healthy communities: A community planning guide using Healthy People 2010.* Washington, DC: U. S. Government Printing Office.

Green, L., & Kreuter, M. (1999). *Health promotion planning: An educational and ecological approach* (3rd ed.). London: Mayfield.

Martin, G., & Pear, J. (1992). *Behavior modification: What it is and how to do it.* Englewood Cliffs, NJ: Prentice-Hall.

Youth Risk Behavior Surveillance System. (2003). Retrieved June 10, 2003, from http://www.cdc.gov/nccdphp/dash/yrbs/index.htm

6

Public Health Organizational Assessment

Public health and community-based organizational assessments analyze the capability of agencies to meet population-based health needs. Conducting a public health or community-based organizational assessment is a first step to planning strategies that improve an agency's organizational capacity. The public health or community-based agency assessment is one component of a comprehensive community assessment. It is essential that the agencies delivering public health services are assessed in relation to their capability in meeting expectations. This chapter focuses on the model standards assessment process and proposes an organizational assessment method for community-based nonprofit organizations.

Introduction

Public health and community-based organizations are the backbone of the public health infrastructure. These agencies are key entities in community organization and mobilization efforts to developing healthy communities. The nation's Healthy People 2010 objectives are dependent on concentrated efforts at the community and population level that direct interventions to meet the established national objectives (appendix B). Achievement of these national objectives requires an appropriate alignment of individual and population-based interventions with the Healthy People 2010 objectives and organizational capacity and assets to deliver public health services. To ensure alignment of organizational capacity and resources with public health interventions, organizations must conduct an organizational assessment as a component of the behavioral, environmental, and community assessment processes. These public health or community-based organizational assessments are a component of agencies' blueprint to move the nation closer to achieving the Healthy People 2010 goals and objectives.

The CDC proposed *Healthy Communities 2000: Model Standards* (APHA, 1991) as a guidebook that offers tools for the assessment and planning of public health services to link the individual community's capacity with the national objectives of the Healthy People 2000 objectives. The *Model Standards* can still be used with the Healthy People 2010 initiative as a philosophical paradigm and process to assess public health organizations' capacity to accomplish the nation's objectives.

The *Model Standards* Assessment Process

The *Model Standards* assist public health and community-based agencies in focusing resources, setting priorities, and mobilizing the community in an organized, rational manner (APHA & CDC, 1993). The *Model Standards* encourage a philosophical perspective that each state should adopt when conducting population-based public health assessments. The philosophical principles of the *Model Standards* are (a) an emphasis on health outcomes, (b) a focus on the entire community, (c) a government presence at the local level, (d) accessibility to services, (e) an emphasis on programs, (f) flexibility, and (g) the importance of negotiation.

The CDC has defined 11 steps that can help state and local health departments to implement the model standards as a means to assess the local community and plan community-level interventions. These standards contain a health assessment function; therefore, the steps of the model standards will be presented as a component of the public health assessment process. The 11 steps to implementing a public health assessment using the *Model Standards* process are presented and explained here:

1. Assess and determine the role of the public health agency.

2. Assess the lead public health agency's organizational capacity.

3. Develop a public health agency plan to build the organization's capacity.

4. Assess the community's organizational and power structures.

5. Organize the community to build a stronger constituency for public health and establish partnerships for public health.

6. Assess health needs and available community resources.

7. Determine local health priorities.

8. Select objectives compatible with the nation's Healthy People goals and objectives and with local health priorities.

9. Develop community-level intervention strategies.

10. Develop and implement a plan of action.

11. Monitor and evaluate community efforts continually (APHA & CDC, 1993).

These 11 steps outline the need for any assessment process—behavioral, environmental, or community—to begin with an assessment of the agency itself. The steps outline an assessment process for the public health or community-based agency. An assessment and determination of the public health agency's role begins with a comparison of the public health agency's mission statement with the community's vision for a healthy community. Public health agencies' organizational capacity assessment focuses on their readiness to exercise leadership and technical assistance throughout the public health assessment and community-level intervention process. Any deficits or weaknesses identified in the organizational capacity assessment process need to be corrected if the public health agency is to serve as the lead agency conducting the assessment. In addition, assets identified need to be expanded to encompass areas of weakness. The agency develops a plan of action that focuses on building its internal strengths, overcoming weaknesses, and enhancing organizational effectiveness (APHA & CDC, 1993; Griffin & Welch, 1995).

Public health agencies are encouraged to work in partnership with other community-based agencies, community leaders, special-interest coalitions and groups, and community members throughout the assessment process. In the public health assessment process, the lead agency must identify formal and informal power structures within the agency and among those entities interacting with the agency through partnerships. This provides the public health agency with a list of key stakeholders to involve in other community-level assessments and interventions. Once these individuals and other organizations are identified, the agency convenes meetings to form partnerships among the public health agencies. Through these meetings, the lead public health agency assesses the health needs and health problems each respective agency has the capacity to target. The lead agency also assesses and coordinates responsibilities among the organizations that partner with public health agencies.

At this point, the model standards move the public health agency to conduct a community assessment to assess the community's health needs and what community resources are available to implement Healthy People 2010 objectives (the community assessment process will be discussed in detail in chapter 8). As a part of the public health assessment and also the community assessment process, local priorities will be determined. From the public health agency assessment vantage point, the focus will be on determining local health priorities that the public health agency has the capacity to target either singularly or in partnership with other agencies. The public health agency assessment and community assessment process will identify objectives and community-level interventions consistent with the Healthy People 2010 goals and objectives. A plan of action is developed to implement these community-level interventions through program planning processes (program planning will be discussed in detail in chapter 12). Monitoring and evaluation of these efforts will be accomplished at the public health agency level. Therefore an essential component of the public health agency assessment is an assessment of the agency's capability to conduct a community health program evaluation (evaluation will be discussed in detail in chapter 13).

The model standards provide the public health agency or community-based agency with a framework for an organizational assessment. Before public health or community-based agencies engage in behavioral, environmental, or community assessments, it is critical that these agencies accurately assess their capability to conduct assessments, implement community-level interventions through program planning, and conduct monitoring and evaluation. The CDC has proposed two planning tools to assist public health agencies in implementing the model standards (APHA & CDC, 1993; Griffin & Welch, 1995). These tools are referred to as the Assessment Protocol for Excellence in Public Health (APEXPH) and the Planned Approach to Community Health (PATCH). APEXPH is primarily a local-based activity; PATCH emphasizes a partnership among national, state, local, and other community-based organizations. Both of these public health agency assessment tools are discussed below.

APEXPH

APEXPH was developed by the CDC and National Association of County and City Health Officials (NACCHO) as a process for public health agencies to use as a self-assessment of their ability to meet their community's needs. APEXPH outlines a process that the public health agency can use to assess and improve its organizational capacity, assess the health status of the community, and involve the community in improving public health. The APEXPH assessment model (NACCHO, 1991) supports enhancing organizational capacity and strengthening the leadership role of the public health agency in the local community. The APEXPH assessment tool has three parts, with parts 1 and 2 each consisting of eight steps.

Part 1 is the "Organizational Capacity Assessment," which studies the agency's authority to operate, involvement in community assessments, policy development, and administrative areas (Figure 6.1). Through the organizational capacity assessment, an organizational action plan should be developed to set priorities for correcting identified organizational weaknesses. This assessment should minimally focus on the following capabilities:

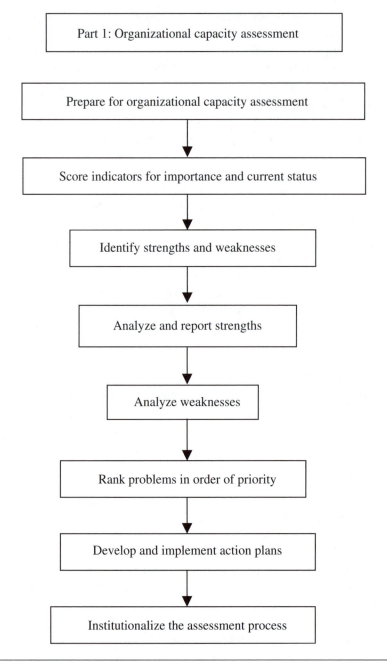

Figure 6.1   Part 1: Steps of APEXPH

- Authority to operate
- Community relations
- Community health assessment
- Public policy development
- Assurance of public health services

- Financial management
- Personnel management
- Program management (NACCHO, 1991).

Part 2 is the "Community Process" (Figure 6.2). The community process is the conducting of a community assessment (community assessment will be further discussed in chapter 8). The assessment process in this model focuses on the collection and analysis of community health data, the community's perception of its health status, and the involvement of a community advisory committee in the community planning process. The public health agency develops a community advisory committee or community assessment team that identifies the priority health problems. From these priority health problem areas, programmatic goals and objectives are developed that are consistent with the Healthy People 2010 initiative (NACCHO, 1991).

Part 3 is known as "Completing the Cycle." It consists of the monitoring and evaluation functions that are necessary to ensure that the organizational action plan rectifies organizational weaknesses and that the community health initiatives are effectively implemented. The APEXPH model has been used to improve public health systems in a community by enhancing the public health agency's capacity to perform core public health functions—assessment, policy development, and assurance.

PATCH

The CDC developed PATCH in 1985 as a standard process that enables public health agencies to conduct community planning and to implement and evaluate programs. PATCH is a model that not only emphasizes assessment and the use of the data but incorporates program planning as an essential component of the process. This model increases a community's capacity to analyze selected health problems, determine their root causes, identify key interventions, and plan effective strategies through the systematic process that focuses on the use of assessment data at an organizational level. PATCH consist of six phases (Figure 6.3) that focus on five key aspects:

- Active participation from community members
- Use of data to determine health priorities, plan programs, and conduct program evaluation
- Development of a comprehensive health promotion strategy based on data from the health priority assessment and community resource assessment
- Evaluation of process and outcome, emphasizing quality improvement
- Skill and resource development within the community (Greene, 1992; NACCHO, 1991).

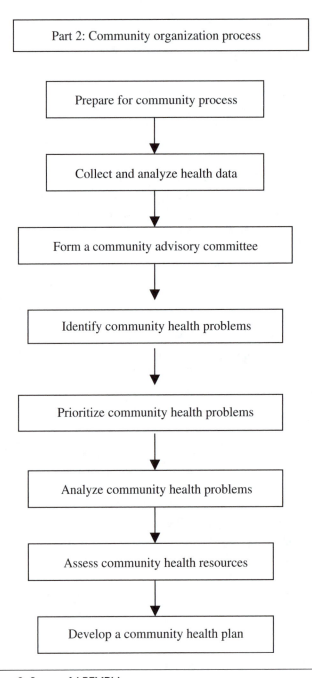

Figure 6.2   Part 2: Steps of APEXPH

Phase 1 is "Community Mobilizing." Community coalitions and partnerships are formed to define the community and increase community members' capability to address health problems. During this phase, community working groups are formed. Phase 2 is "Data Collection and

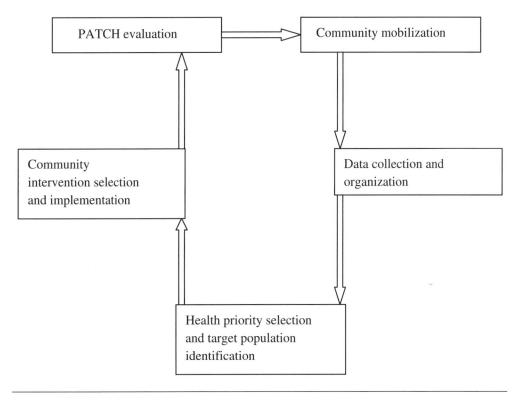

Figure 6.3 PATCH Model

Organization." This phase consists of collecting mortality, morbidity, behavioral, and environmental health data. Phase 3 involves the selection of health priority areas and identification of the respective target populations. Phase 4 consists of selecting and implementing community-level interventions. Phase 5 concludes the PATCH model with process and outcome evaluations of the model and the community interventions (Greene, 1992; NACCHO, 1991).

APEXPH and PATCH are two public health processes and tools used to assess the public health agency and the public health infrastructure's capability to meet the community's needs. The National Public Health Performance Standards Program (NPHPSP) is collaborative effort to build and enhance the nation's public health infrastructure. The NPHPSP developed assessment tools and strategic approaches (such as "mobilizing for action through planning and partnerships," or MAPP) to community health improvement and measurement of public health practice using performance standards. These assessment tools and approaches focus on a quality improvement perspective and will therefore be presented in chapter 14.

Community-Based Organization Assessments

Community-based organizations differ from public health organizations in that they are typically nonprofit organizations that deliver public health–related services to specific health conditions or populations. Organizational assessments of community-based organizations use an assessment format typically used for nonprofit organizations. Community-based organizational assessments can be conducted internally or by an external evaluator.

A community-based organizational assessment tool is used to ascertain essential information regarding the organization's capacity to deliver public health services. Representatives from various levels of the organization typically complete the organizational assessment tool. These individuals are familiar with the organization's functions. The community-based organizational assessment tool collects data in the following areas: (a) organizational infrastructure, (b) strategic development, (c) board functions, (d) financial management, (e) human resources, (f) leadership and management effectiveness, (g) physical and technological resources, (h) outcome measurement and evaluation, and (i) program planning, development, and implementation (Lewis, 2000). Appendix D provides some assessment items for each of the listed areas.

Summary

Key issues in public health organizational assessment are as follows.

- Public health and community-based organizations are the backbone of the public health infrastructure.
- The principles in *Model Standards* are (a) an emphasis on health outcomes, (b) a focus on the entire community, (c) government presence at the local level, (d) accessibility to services, (e) an emphasis on programs, (f) flexibility, and (g) the importance of negotiation.
- The *Model Standards* process proceeds as follows: (a) Assess and determine the role of the public health agency, (b) assess the lead public health agency's organizational capacity, (c) develop a public health agency plan to build the organization's capacity, (d) assess the community's organizational and power structures, (e) organize the community to build a stronger constituency for public health and establish partnerships for public health, (f) assess health needs and available community resources, (g) determine local health priorities, (h) select objectives compatible with the nation's Healthy People goals and objectives and the local health priorities, (i) develop community-level

intervention strategies, (j) develop and implement a plan of action, and (k) monitor and evaluate community efforts continually.

- The APEXPH assessment model supports enhancing organizational capacity and strengthening the leadership role of the public health agency in the local community.

- Organizational capacity assessment studies agencies' authority to operate, involvement in community assessment, policy development, and administrative areas.

- "Community process" is the conducting of a community assessment.

- The "Completing the Cycle" phase consists of the monitoring and evaluation functions that are necessary to ensure that the organizational action plan rectifies organizational weaknesses and that community health initiatives are effectively implemented.

- PATCH is a standard process that enables public health agencies to conduct community planning and to implement and evaluate programs.

- PATCH consist of six phases that focus on five key aspects: (a) active participation from community members; (b) use of data to determine health priorities, plan programs, and conduct program evaluation; (c) development of a comprehensive health promotion strategy based on data from the health priority assessment and community resource assessment; (e) evaluation of process and outcome, emphasizing quality improvement; and (f) skill and resource development within the community.

- Organizational assessments of community-based organizations use an assessment format typically used for nonprofit organizations.

- The community-based organizational assessment tool collects data in the following areas: (a) organizational infrastructure, (b) strategic development, (c) board functions, (d) financial management, (e) human resources, (f) leadership and management effectiveness, (g) physical and technological resources, (h) outcome measurement and evaluation, and (i) program planning, development, and implementation.

References

American Public Health Association. (1991). *Healthy communities 2000: Model standards* (3rd ed.). Washington, DC: Author.

American Public Health Association and Centers for Disease Control and Prevention. (1993). *The guide to implementing model standards: Eleven steps toward a healthy community.* Washington, DC: American Public Health Association. Retrieved June 10, 2003, from http://www.apha.org/ppp/science/theguide.htm

Greene, L. (1992). PATCH: CDC's planned approach to community health, an application of PRECEDE and an inspiration for PROCEED. *Journal of Health Education, 23*(3), 140-147.

Griffin, S., & Welch, P. (1995). Performance-based public health in Texas. *Journal of Public Health Management and Practice, 1*(3), 44-49.

Lewis, A. (2000). Nonprofit organizational assessment tool. Retrieved June 10, 2003, from http://www.uwex.edu/li/learner/assessment.htm

National Association of County and City Health Officials. (1991). *Assessment Protocol for Excellence in Public Health (APEXPH)*. Washington, DC: Author.

7

Environmental Health Assessment

The environment is intricately associated with the health of a population. There is a reciprocal relationship that exists between individuals and their environment. To conduct a comprehensive community assessment on the population's health status, an environmental assessment of the community must be included as a component. This chapter focuses on defining environmental health, identifying environmental hazards, describing an ecological environmental health approach, conducting a risk assessment of the environment, and communicating risk to the community population.

Introduction

Industrialization and globalization have affected the environment and resulted in an ecological impact on the health of individuals and communities. The symbiotic, reciprocal, and dependent relationship between the environment and individuals is considered the associative factor that links environmental hazards to all aspects of human life. With the influential effects of the environment so far reaching, the environment is considered a fundamental factor in determining the health of individuals and populations (Institute of Medicine [IOM], 1995). Thus an environmental assessment must be a component of a community assessment.

Environmental Health Defined

The environment is considered a primary determinant of individual and community health. There is a growing concern regarding the effect of the environment on individual and community-level health. Everything external to an individual is considered environmental in nature. In addition, individuals and communities have their own internal environment, which consists of intrapersonal or intracommunity psychosocial factors that exist within the individual or community's immediate sphere of existence.

A personal health perspective definition of environmental health is freedom from illness or injury related to exposures to toxic agents and other environmental conditions that may pose a detrimental effect to the health of the individual (IOM, 1995). A definition of environmental health from a scientific perspective is the systematic development, promotion, and conduct of measures that modify or otherwise control those external factors in the indoor or outdoor environments that might cause illness, disability, or discomfort (DHHS, 1998). The final determination of whether an environment meets the definition of "healthy" is dependent on the results of evaluations of individuals within the context of their community or the community within the context of the larger society. The interrelationships that exist between an individual, the community, the presence or absence or environmental hazards, and the detrimental effects of such hazards are the ultimate determinants of whether an environment is healthy. This determination is dependent on the environmental assessment and the analysis of environmental health indicators.

Environmental Health Indicators

Environmental health indicators establish measures for key environmental health issues. These environmental health indicators can be used to monitor trends in the environment, identify potential health risks, monitor trends in health status, compare communities in terms of environmental health status, monitor and assess the effectiveness of environmental health policies, and provide data on associative linkages between the environment and health. Good environmental health indicators should be relevant to conditions of interest to the community, scientifically sound, testable, measurable, sensitive to changes, and robust (Corvalan, Briggs, & Kjellstrom, 1996). In addition to the environmental assessment framework provided below, environmental health indicators provide guidance to what data should be measured and collected during the environmental health assessment process. Table 7.1 provides environmental health indicators and measures for some environmental health concerns (World Health Organization [WHO], 1999).

Understanding the environmental health risk that exists in a community is intricately related to understanding the health status of a population; therefore, an environmental assessment is an essential component of any community assessment process. The ability to perform an environmental health assessment is one of the competencies recommended for public health nurses and environmental health practitioners (see Table 7.2; IOM, 1995; National Center for Environmental Health, CDC, and APHA, 2001). Knowledge of the potential environmental health hazards that may exist in a community is

Table 7.1   Key Environmental Health Indicators

Environmental Health Issue	Indicator	Measurement
Sociodemographic	Poverty	Human poverty index
	Population density	Population density
	Rate of population growth	Annual net rate of population growth
	Dependent population	Percentage of people < 16 or > 65 years
	Rate of urbanization	Annual net rate of change in proportion of people residing in urban areas
	Infant mortality	Annual infant death rate
	Life expectancy	Number of years a newborn is expected to live
Air pollution	Ambient air concentrations of pollutants	Mean annual concentrations of ozone, CO, SO_2, NO_2, O_3, and lead
	Sources of indoor air pollution	Percentage of households using coal, wood, or kerosene as primary heating source
	Childhood respiratory illness	Annual mortality rate due to acute respiratory illness
	Capability for air management	
	Availability of lead-free gasoline	Percentage of lead-free gasoline consumption
Sanitation	Access to basic sanitation	Proportion of population with access to excreta disposal and sewer systems
	Childhood diarrhea	Morbidity and mortality rates for diarrhea in children < 5 years old
Shelter	Building regulations	Percentage of population living in informal settlements
	Informal settlement living	Scope and extent of housing regulations
Safe drinking water	Access to safe drinking water	Percentage of population with access to adequate amounts of safe drinking water
	Childhood diarrhea	Incidence of diarrhea in children < 5 years old
	Water-borne illness outbreaks	Incidence of water-borne illness outbreaks
	Intensity of water quality monitoring	Density of water quality monitoring network
	Piped water supply	Percentage of households with piped water
Solid waste management	Municipal waste collection	Percentage of population served by regular waste collection services
Hazardous substances	Blood lead levels	Percentage of children with blood lead levels > 10 $\mu g/dl$
	Mortality due to poisoning	Mortality rate due to poisoning
Food safety	Food-borne illness	Incidence of food-borne illness outbreaks
	Childhood diarrhea	Morbidity and mortality rates of diarrhea in children under 5 years old
Radiation	Cumulative radiation dose	Percent of population receiving radiation doses above 5 mSv/yr
	UV light index	UV light index
Nonoccupational risk	Motor vehicle mortality	Mortality rate due to motor vehicles
	Childhood injuries	Incidence of physical injury to children < 5 years old
	Childhood poisonings	Number of poisonings reported in children < 5 years old

(Continued)

Table 7.1 (Continued)

Environmental Health Issue	Indicator	Measurement
Occupational health risk	Morbidity and mortality due to health hazards	Morbidity and mortality rates due to health hazards
Vector-borne disease	Adequacy of vector control and management Vector-borne disease	Percentage of risk population covered by effective vector control and management programs Morbidity and mortality of vector-borne disease

Note: This list is not comprehensive.

SOURCE: WHO (1999).

necessary to conduct an environmental assessment. These environmental hazards are the primary offenders assessed and analyzed in relation to the health status of individuals and the entire community population.

Environmental Hazards

Environmental hazards identified during the environmental assessment are classified into six categories: physical, biological, chemical and gaseous, mechanical, psychosocial, and organizational. Appendix E presents environmental hazardous agents, common routes of exposure, and symptoms produced.

Each of these environmental hazards is interrelated in a manner or system that can potentially affect an individual's health status (Figure 7.1). Following is a description of the dimensions of each of these environmental hazards.

Physical

Physical environmental hazards consist of radiation, noise, waste disposal, and accidents. Ionizing radiation, from electromagnetic waves such as X-rays, nuclear power, and natural radiation in the soil (radon), and nonionizing radiation, such as electric and magnetic fields, ultraviolet radiation, visible light, and infrared radiation, pose risk to individuals and communities. Exposure to noise over 80 dB can produce hearing loss. Solid waste disposal such as burning and dumping, along with toxic waste disposal such as radiological or chemical, can potentially release hazardous substances into the environment. Motor vehicle accidents, falls, drowning, and fires are common physical accidents.

Table 7.2   Environmental Health Competencies

Fourteen Environmental Health Practitioner Competencies, Grouped in Three Primary Functions

Assessment

- *Information gathering.* The capacity to identify sources and compile relevant and appropriate information, and the knowledge of where to obtain the information.
- *Data analysis and interpretation.* The capacity to analyze data, recognize meaningful test results, interpret results, and present the results in an appropriate manner to various stakeholders.
- *Evaluation.* The capacity to evaluate the effectiveness of procedures, interventions, and programs.

Management

- *Problem solving.* The capacity to identify appropriate solutions to environmental health problems.
- *Economic and political issues.* The capacity to use information about the economic and political implications of decisions.
- *Organizational knowledge and behavior.* The capacity to function effectively as a team player within the culture of the organization.
- *Project management.* The capacity to plan, implement, and maintain fiscally responsible programs and projects.
- *Computer and information technology.* The capacity to use information technology.
- *Reporting, documentation, and record keeping.* The capacity to produce reports to document actions, keep records, and inform appropriate stakeholders.
- *Collaborating.* The capacity to form collaborative partnerships and alliances.

Communication

- *Education.* The capacity to use the environmental health practitioner's frontline role to effectively educate the public about environmental health issues and the public health rationale for public health interventions.
- *Communication.* The capacity to effectively communicate risk to and exchange information with various stakeholders.
- *Conflict resolution.* The capacity to facilitate resolution of conflicts within the agency, in the community, and with regulated parties.
- *Marketing.* The capacity to articulate basic concepts of environmental health and public health and convey an understanding of their value and importance to clients and the public.

Institute of Medicine Environmental Health Nursing Competencies

Basic Knowledge and Concepts

- All nurses should understand the scientific principles and underpinnings of the relationship between individuals or populations and the environment, including the basic mechanisms and pathways of exposure to environmental hazards, basic prevention and control strategies, interdisciplinary nature of effective interventions, and the role of research. *Assessment and Referral*
- All nurses should be able to successfully complete an environmental health history or assessment, recognize potential environmental hazards and sentinel illnesses, and provide referrals for conditions with probable environmental etiologies. Nurses should be able to access and provide information to patients and communities and locate referral sources.

Advocacy, Ethics, and Risk Communication

- All nurses should be able to demonstrate knowledge of the role of advocacy (case and class), ethics, and risk communication in patient care and community intervention with respect to the potential adverse effects of the environment on health.

Legislation and Regulation

- All nurses should understand the policy framework and the legislation and regulations that affect the environment.

SOURCE: National Center for Environmental Heath, CDC, and APHA (2001) and the Institute of Medicine (1995).

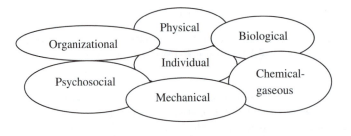

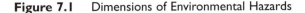

Figure 7.1   Dimensions of Environmental Hazards

Biological

Infectious agents, plants, insects, rodents, and animals are biological hazards. Infectious agents consist of contamination of water, food, or air with pathogenic microorganisms. Plants create allergic responses and can be the initiating agent in accidental poisonings. Insects (mosquitoes, fleas, ticks), rodents, and other animals serve as vectors between the environmental source and humans.

Chemical and Gaseous

Chemical and gaseous agents can leach into the soil or water or concentrate in the air. Metal and metallic compounds that leach into the environment, such as lead, mercury, arsenic, and cadmium, pose harm to humans. Routinely monitored pollutants in the air include carbon monoxide, ozone, sulfur oxides, volatile organic compounds, nitrogen oxides, lead, and particles. Automobiles serve as a source of air pollutants from their emission systems, along with industrial plants. Another source of chemical air pollution is cigarette smoking. Pesticides used for agricultural purposes leach into the soil and create a bioaccumulation effect in the soil, as well as in the plants produced from that soil, which may be consumed by humans or livestock.

Mechanical

Mechanical hazards are prevalent in work environments. Commonly reported mechanical hazards are exposure to continuous vibrations, repetitive motions (carpal tunnel syndrome), lifting, and poor ergonomic workplace designs.

Psychosocial

Psychological and social hazards in the environment consist of socio-economic and cultural differences, societal and intimate partner violence, overcrowded conditions, and traffic. Psychological and social hazards produce intrapersonal and interpersonal conflicts that result in numerous tensions or stressors that adversely affect individuals within a specific community population. Some psychosocial and social hazards, such as overcrowding, can lead to disease outbreaks of an infectious nature.

Organizational

Organizational hazards are those potential threats created in an environment through institutions, organizations, and other systematic social structures. These institutions or organizations may produce policies and procedures or physical, biological, chemical, gaseous, mechanical, or psychosocial hazards that may adversely affect an individual's health status. Common organizational hazards are the political climate, legal and judicial system, economic and employment conditions, health-care systems, educational systems, transportation systems, housing, and recreational facilities.

Ecological Environmental Health Approach

An ecological approach views environmental health as the product of the interrelationships of the individual ecosystem and subsystems of the larger ecosystem, such as family, community, culture, and physical and social environments (Green & Kreuter, 1999). From an ecological perspective, all these aspects of the larger ecosystem and their interrelationships are considered as antecedents that affect environmental health. Sormanti, Pereira, El-Bassel, Witte, and Gilbert (2001) identify four subsystems of the ecological approach: ontogenetic, microsystem, exosystem, and macrocultural.

The ontogenetic subsystem consists of an individual's unique biological and personal factors, such as knowledge level, attitudes, values, beliefs, communication skills, and acculturation. The interactional factors that exist within the immediate environmental context comprise the microsystem; for example, an environment in which an individual may be exposed to environmental toxins. The exosystem consists of factors that act as external stressors or buffers to the likelihood of an environmental exposure, such as employment status, socioeconomic status, and social support and networks. Broad cultural values and beliefs comprise the macrocultural level of an ecological approach. Macrocultural factors consist of the larger social norms existing within a community (Sormanti et al., 2001). The ecological approach as a whole may be expressed as the cumulative interaction and interrelationships that exist between factors that exist in the environment at each level.

The ecological approach assumes complex interdependencies within the environmental health ecological web. This approach lends itself to the application of multilevel and multisectoral environmental health interventions.

One environmental framework that can be used for developing multilevel or multisectoral environmental interventions is the "DPSEEA" (*d*riving forces, *p*ressures, *s*tate of the environment, *e*xposure, health *e*ffects, *a*ctions taken to reduce exposure to hazards) framework. This framework has also been used to develop the environmental health indicators noted above. I recommend the use of this framework to focus environmental health interventions on the ecological relationships that exist with environmental exposures. If this framework is used in this manner, the interventions will simultaneously be directed at the environmental health indicators.

DPSEEA Framework

The DPSEEA framework proves a perspective from which to understand ecological environmental interrelationships (Figure 7.2). The driving forces (D) refer to the factors that motivate and push the environmental processes. Driving forces consist of population growth, technological development, economic development, and policy. These driving forces result in the generation of pressures (P) on the environment that are expressed as human occupation and exploitation of the environment. Examples of pressures are energy production, manufacturing, service industries, transportation, tourism, agriculture, forestry and waste release (Corvalan et al., 1996; WHO, 1999).

The environment responds to these pressures. This response is known as the state (S) of the environment. The state of the environment is expressed in terms of the availability and quality of natural resources, the amount of environmental pollution that exists, and the occurrence and magnitude of natural hazardous events. When a negative environmental state exists, individuals and the community are exposed to environmental hazards. This is the exposure (E_1) component of the DPSEEA framework. According to the National Academy of Sciences (1991), an exposure is an event that occurs when there is contact at a boundary between humans and environmental contaminants of a specific concentration for a specific time period. This environmental exposure leads to various health effects (E_2) that differ depending on the environmental hazard present. These health effects are measured through epidemiological studies of morbidity and mortality. The actions (A) that are taken to eliminate or reduce exposure to environmental hazards are hazard management, environmental improvements through pollution control, education and awareness training, treatment rehabilitation, and economic and social policy changes.

Environmental Risk Assessment

The National Academy of Sciences (1983) defines risk assessment as the collection of factual information to define the health effects of exposure

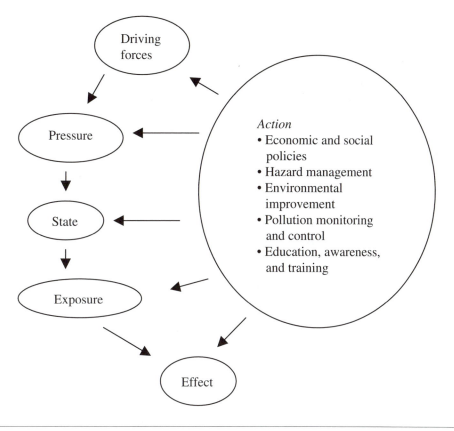

Figure 7.2   The DPSEEA Framework

of animals or populations to hazardous materials and situations. An environmental risk assessment uses a systematic approach to organize, collect, and analyze scientific data on environmental hazards in relation to their potential effects on humans. The Environmental Protection Agency (EPA) provides a four-step process to an environmental risk assessment: hazard identification, exposure assessment, dose-response assessment, and risk characterization (Hertz-Picciotto, 1995; Environmental Protection Agency [EPA], 1986). Figure 7.3 presents the risk assessment model.

The determination as to whether a population has been exposed to a hazardous environmental agent and the determination of whether that agent is harmful to humans is considered the first step, hazard identification, in an environmental risk assessment. Hazard identification first establishes whether or not an exposure actually occurred and the nature of events surrounding such an exposure. Second, a determination is made regarding the likelihood that individuals within the community actually had contact with the hazardous agent. Lastly, the question of whether such an exposure has the ability to cause harm to humans is determined from evidence-based research and practice.

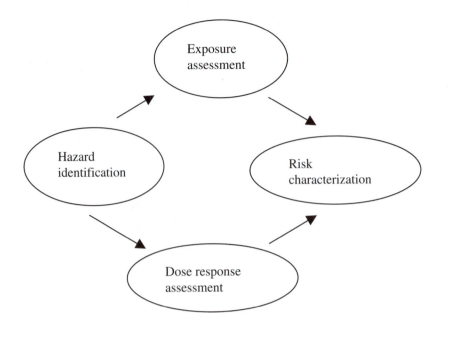

Figure 7.3   The Environmental Protection Agency Risk Assessment Model

The second step, exposure assessment, consists of identifying the hazardous agent, the route of exposure, and the amount and duration of exposure that may have occurred or may still be occurring. Questions that the exposure assessment attempts to answer are (a) who was exposed and/or what was contaminated? (b) does the exposure occur through breathing air, drinking water, skin contact, or how? (c) how much exposure occurred? and (d) how often and for how long did the exposure occur? An essential function of the public health nurse in the exposure assessment process is the conducting of an exposure history. An exposure history creates a sense of awareness in community members, assists in an accurate medical diagnosis, and identifies potential hazards. Table 7.3 provides the components of an exposure history.

Dose-response assessment is the third step in the environmental risk assessment process. Dose-response assessment is dependent on evidence-based or research-based scientific data regarding the known relationships that exist between the environmental hazard and its adverse effects on humans. Frequently, the public health nurse will consult with a toxicologist to critically analyze the relationship between the hazardous agent identified, the information in the exposure assessment, and the morbidity or mortality findings present in the individuals or community. This dose-response assessment validates the magnitude of the actual risk that the environmental agent may present, based on the information collected during the exposure assessment process.

Table 7.3   Exposure History

Home Assessment
- Location of home
- Physical materials used to construct home
- Heating and cooling systems

Hazardous Agents in the Home
- Indoor air quality
- Common household products
- Pesticides and lawn care products
- Lead products and waste
- Recreational hazards
- Water supply
- Soil contamination

Work History
- Health and safety practices at work
- Description of prior and current jobs

Biological Marker Assessment
- Blood specimens
- Urine specimens
- Hair or nail specimens

Finally, all the data from the hazard identification, exposure, and dose-response assessment are synthesized to predict the quantitative risk expected from the environmental exposure in the defined population. Risk characterization is the final determination of the potential or actual adverse health effects that can or will be experienced by the at-risk population based on the known agent, amount of exposure, and the known adverse effects of exposure to that particular agent at the exposure doses reported. In addition to this environmental risk assessment model, the Agency for Toxic Substances and Disease Registry (ATSDR) obtains information from the EPA and other public health agencies during an environmental investigation using a public health assessment (PHA) framework.

PHA: Environmental Investigation Framework

ATSDR (1994) defines a PHA during an environmental investigation as the evaluation of data on the release of hazardous agents into the environment as a means to assess any past, current, or future impact on the public's health; to develop health advisories or recommendations; and to identify studies or public health actions that are needed to mitigate or prevent adverse human effects. This evaluation data is used to assess how an environmental risk may have occurred through an analysis of the human exposure pathways: (a) the source (landfill, spill), (b) transport media (ground, air), (c) exposure point (drinking water, food source), (d) route of exposure (ingestion, inhalation, skin contact), and (e) receptor population (individuals, children, families). Table 7.4 outlines some categories of environmental data collected in the public health assessment environmental investigation.

Risk Communication

Risk communication is a community-level, population-based, public health, educational intervention designed to disseminate information among interested community members about the nature, magnitude, significance, or control of environmental hazards (U.S. Army Center for Health Promotion and Preventive Medicine, 2001, 2003) once the environmental risk assessment is initiated and again at its completion. Risk communication is necessary to provide community members with a foundation for understanding their individual level of environmental risk. This involves the communication of highly scientific and technical information to community members, who are generally concerned and anxious (U.S. Army Center for Health Promotion and Preventive Medicine, 2001, 2003). The environment in which risk communication occurs is usually low in trust and high in concern.

Elements of risk communication consist of the message, the messenger, the community members (audience) and the environmental context. These elements are mixed together through several communication channels to deliver the risk communication message to community members. Public health professionals have several channels through which risk communication can be directed: community members (community meetings, fliers, direct mailings), coworkers (meetings, hotlines, news releases), elected officials (phone calls, personal visits, invitation to community meetings), environmental activists (fact sheets, involvement in community meetings, advance notices), and the media (radio, television, personal interviews, news conferences). Risk communication guidelines have been proposed by the ATSDR. Table 7.5 presents a summary of risk communication principles (ATSDR, 1997; Covello & Allen, 1988).

Summary

Key issues in environmental health assessment are as follows.

- The symbiotic, reciprocal, and dependent relationship between the environment and individuals is considered the associative factor that links environmental hazards to all aspects of human life.
- Environmental assessment must be a component of a community assessment.
- A personal health perspective definition of environmental health is the freedom from illness or injury related to exposures to toxic agents and other environmental conditions that may cause a detrimental health effect in the individual.

Table 7.4   Public Health Assessment Environmental Investigation Framework: Selected Elements

Site Data
- Name, address, location
- Type of site—home, mine, landfill, spill
- Description of problems

Site History
- Description of previous EPA actions or hazardous releases
- Physical barriers to prevent pollution

Geographic and Demographic Data
- Political geography
- Distance from site to closest residence
- Population characteristics within 1 mile
- Sensitive demographic characteristics—schools, day care facilities, hospitals, homes, rivers, streams, lakes

Relationship to Community
- On-site activities
- Community relations plans
- Presence of physical barriers

Substances Identified
- List of chemicals and amounts present

Analytical Information
- Results of samples collected
- Sample storage protocols

Soil Exposure Pathway
- Type of soil sample
- Exact location with maps and dates

Surface Water Pathway
- Site of location
- Type and location of sample
- Relationship to groundwater
- Location of all downstream surface water intakes
- Contaminant concentrations and pH

Sediment Exposure Pathway
- Description of location of samples with maps
- Type of sample collected and depth of sampling points

Groundwater Pathway
- Well water survey
- Assessment of water sources
- Hydrogeology assessment
- Groundwater analysis

Air Exposure Pathway
- Ambient air
- Air emissions
- Soil gases
- Indoor air quality
- Indoor dust

Food-Chain Exposure Pathway
- Food sources
- Point of origin of food source
- Relationship of food chain to other exposure pathways

Table 7.5   Principles of Risk Communication

Cardinal Rules of Risk Communication
- Accept and involve the public as a partner
- Plan carefully and evaluate your communication
- Listen to the public's concerns
- Communicate openly and honestly
- Use credible sources
- Identify and meet the media's needs
- Speak clearly and compassionately

Pitfalls to Avoid
- Expression of nonverbal messages inconsistent with verbal message
- Attacking a person rather than the issue
- Speculating on an issue
- Promising things that are undeliverable
- Blaming others rather than taking responsibility
- Assuming something you say is "off the record"
- Lengthy and technical presentation

- The interrelationships that exist between an individual, the community, the presence or absence of environmental hazards, and the detrimental effects of such hazards are the ultimate determinants of a healthy environment.
- Environmental health indicators can be used to monitor trends in the environment, identify potential health risks, monitor trends in health status, compare communities in terms of environmental health status, monitor and assess the effectiveness of environmental health policies, and provide data on associative linkages between the environment and health.
- Environmental hazards are classified as either physical, biological, chemical and gaseous, mechanical, psychosocial, or organizational.
- Physical environmental hazards consist of radiation, noise, waste disposal, and accidents.
- Infectious agents, plants, insects, rodents, and animals are biological hazards.
- Chemical and gaseous agents can leach into the soil and water or concentrate in the air.
- Mechanical hazards include exposure to continuous vibrations, repetitive motions, lifting, and poor ergonomic workplace designs.
- Psychological and social hazards in the environment consist of socioeconomic and cultural differences, societal and intimate partner violence, overcrowded conditions, and traffic.
- Organizational hazards are those potential threats created in an environment through the existence of institutions, organizations, and other systematic social structures.
- An ecological approach views environmental health as the product of the interrelationships of the individual ecosystem and subsystems of the larger ecosystem, such as family, community, culture, and physical and social environments.

- The four subsystems of the ecological approach are ontogenetic, microsystem, exosystem, and macrocultural.
- The framework known as DPSEEA stands for *d*riving forces that motivate environmental forces; generation of *p*ressures on the environment; *s*tate of the environment; *e*xposure, or the intersection between individuals and hazards in the environment; the health *e*ffects that result from exposure; and *a*ctions taken to alter environmental hazards and health consequences.
- Risk assessment involves the collection of factual information to define the health effects of exposure of animals or populations to hazardous materials and situations.
- An environmental risk assessment uses a systematic approach to organize, collect, and analyze scientific data on environmental hazards in relation to their potential effects on humans.
- The EPA's four-step process for an environmental risk assessment is hazard identification, exposure assessment, dose-response assessment, and risk characterization.
- Risk communication is a community-level, population-based, public health, educational intervention designed to disseminate information among interested community members about the nature, magnitude, significance, or control of environmental hazards.
- Elements of risk communication consist of the message, the messenger, the community members (audience), and the environmental context.

References

Agency for Toxic Substances and Disease Registry. (1994). *Environmental data needed for public health assessments: A guidance manual.* Retrieved June 12, 2003, from http://www.atsdr.cdc.gov/ednpha.html

Agency for Toxic Substances and Disease Registry. (1997). *A primer on health risk communication principles and practices.* Retrieved June 12, 2003, from http://www.atsdr.cdc.gov/HEC/primer.html.

Corvalan, C., Briggs, D., & Kjellstrom, T. (1996). Development of environmental health indicators. In D. Briggs, C. Corvalan, & M. Nurmine (Eds), *Linkage methods for environmental and health analysis: General guidelines* (pp. 19-53). Geneva, Switzerland: UNEP, USEPA, and WHO.

Covello, V., & Allen, F. (1988). *Seven cardinal rules of risk communication.* Washington, DC: United States Environmental Protection Agency, Office of Policy Analysis.

Department of Health and Human Services. (1998). *Evaluating the environmental health workforce.* Rockville, MD: Author.

Environmental Protection Agency. (1986). Guidelines for cancer risk assessment. *Federal Register, 51,* 33992.

Green, L., & Kreuter, M. (1999). *Health promotion planning: An educational and ecological approach* (3rd ed.). London: Mayfield.

Hertz-Picciotto, I. (1995) Environmental risk assessment. In E. Talbott & G. Craun (Eds.), *Introduction to environmental epidemiology* (pp. 23-38). New York: CRC Lewis.

Institute of Medicine. (1995). *Nursing, health, and the community.* Washington, DC: National Academy Press.

National Academy of Sciences. (1983). *Risk assessment in the federal government: Managing the process.* Washington, DC: National Academy Press.

National Academy of Sciences. (1991). *Human exposure assessment for airborne pollutants: Advances and opportunities.* Washington, DC: National Academy Press.

National Center for Environmental Health, Centers for Disease Control and Prevention, & American Public Health Association. (2001). *Environmental health competency project: Recommendations for core competencies for local environmental health practitioners.* Washington, DC: APHA.

Sormanti, M., Pereira, L., El-Bassel, N., Witte, S., & Gilbert, L. (2001). The role of community consultants in designing an HIV prevention intervention. *AIDS Education and Prevention, 13*(4), 311-328.

U.S. Army Center for Health Promotion and Preventive Medicine. (2001). *Just the facts: Health risk communication* (USACHPPM Publication No. 39-001-0701). Retrieved June 14, 2003, from http://chppm-www.apgea.army.mil/documents/FACT/39-001-0701.pdf

U.S. Army Center for Health Promotion and Preventive Medicine. (2003). *Risk communication capability.* Retrieved June 14, 2003, from http://chppm-www.apgea.army.mil/usachppmtoday/032001/032001hrc1.asp

World Health Organization. (1999). *Environmental health indicators: Framework and methodologies.* Retrieved June 14, 2003, from http://www.northampton.ac.uk/ncr/who/

8

Community Assessment and Analysis

A community assessment provides valuable population-level data on the health conditions and risk factors present in a community. These data guide public health program planning. In addition, the assessment provides a profile of the community's assets and needs to achieve a level of community competence. (Community competence is the ability of the community to engage in effective problem solving to meet the community's needs. For more details, refer to chapter 10). A comprehensive community assessment should integrate behavioral and environmental assessments as well as assessments of public health organizations and community-based organizations. This chapter focuses on the community assessment process by defining community assessment; proposing community assessment models; identifying data collection sources and methods; and proposing various community assessment processes, such as geographic information systems, community profiling, and needs assessments.

Introduction

The first step in identifying community-level, population-based health problems is the conducting of a community assessment. A community assessment involves the collection of data and information about various characteristics of a population within a defined community. A multidimensional approach to community assessment uses multiple assessment strategies (behavioral, public health agency, and environmental), multiple data sources, and multiple data collection (primary and secondary) methods (Plescia, Koontz, & Laurent, 2001). Community health assessments are dependent on valid, reliable, and accessible public health data.

Community Assessment Defined

A community assessment is defined as the process of collecting data (from primary and secondary data sources) and information regarding demographics, health status, and the infrastructure of a defined community. Health trends and community priorities are established based on community assessment data. A community assessment is conducted as a foundation for identifying community-level strengths (assets) and weaknesses, planning interventions and programs, and evaluation of community interventions and programs. A community assessment is a comprehensive analysis of the community, with behavioral, public health agency, and environmental health assessment data frequently incorporated into the analysis.

The focus of a community assessment is on those populations that are integral to the community. The parameters of the community assessment are established by identifying the community of interest. The community is typically identified through either geopolitical affiliations or common interests.

Community Assessment Models

Community assessment models provide the framework for the collection of community assessment data and information. These frameworks provide the structure to ensure that community assessment data are collected in a systematic manner consistent with the theoretical premises of the respective models. Public health nurses must select the appropriate model based on their definition of community, types of data needed, and the potential use of the data for program planning.

Community as Partner

The community-as-partner model focuses on the philosophical orientation of primary health care as defined by WHO. Anderson and McFarlane (1996) use a total person approach to assess problems. Major components of the community-as-partner model are the community assessment wheel and the nursing process. Only the community assessment wheel, which is the community assessment component, is pertinent to the discussions in this chapter.

The community assessment wheel has a core and eight subsystems. At the core of the model are the community residents, who are described by demographics, values, beliefs, and common history. There is an influential interrelationship that exists between the core community residents and the eight subsystems that surround the core community. The eight subsystems are physical environment, education, safety and transportation, politics and government, health and social services, communication, economics, and recreation (Anderson & McFarlane, 1996).

This model is based on Betty Neuman's (1989) nursing theory. The total community is surrounded by a normal line of defense that represents the level of health obtained by the community, such as immunization rates (represented as a solid line in the model). Outside of the normal line of defense is a flexible line of defense or buffer zone that protects the community. The eight subsystems are divided by broken lines indicating that each subsystem influences and is influenced by the other subsystems. The core population (in the center of the assessment wheel) is surrounded by broken lines and flexible lines of resistance that extend into the subsystems. These represent the lines of resistance throughout the subsystems. Stressors produced from within the community or external to the community can penetrate the normal lines of defense of the community. Disequilibrium occurs once a stressor penetrates or exists within the normal lines of defense. At this point, the health of the core community is dependent on the flexible lines of resistance. A community assessment using this model focuses on assessing the core community, the eight subsystems, the normal lines of defense, flexible lines of defense, and lines of resistance.

Community Health Assessment Tool

The community health assessment tool (CHAT) was developed based on Gordon and Kucharski's (1987) 11 functional health patterns. These functional health patterns provide the framework for the CHAT. They are (a) community health and safety efforts; (b) the adequacy of the community's nutritional efforts; (c) waste management in the community; (d) community transportation and recreation systems; (e) community cycles and rhythms; (f) community decision-making processes; (g) community self-perception and opinion; (h) informal and formal roles defined by the community; (i) community reproductive functions, resources, and family structure; (j) community support services; and (k) cultural, ethical, and spiritual community needs (Gordon & Kucharski, 1987; Krieger & Harton, 1992).

Epidemiological Model

Agent, host, and environment are the essential components of the epidemiological triangle. The agent is the offending organism or event that predisposes an individual to disease. The host is the person who is susceptible to the disease. The environment consists of the biological, physical, and social conditions necessary for a disease process to occur (Mausner & Kramer, 1985).

The epidemiological model components, agent, host, and environment, provide the essential components from which data are collected in a community assessment. Data is collected about each component, and the relationships that exist between each component provide the summative analysis of the community assessment process. Community-level interventions are directed at each component and at the relationships between the components that are identified as community problems.

General Ethnographic and Nursing Evalution Studies in the State

Epidemiological and ethnographic data are integrated into a comprehensive community analysis in the general ethnographic and nursing evaluation studies in the state (GENESIS) model. The purpose of the GENESIS model is to identify community residents' perceptions of their health needs and to describe health problems and related factors that influence this health status. Essential components of the GENESIS model are history, culture, politics, health services, social services, education, environment, economics, and employment.

The GENESIS model uses epidemiological and qualitative data. Epidemiological data consist of health indexes such as morbidity and mortality data. Qualitative data is collected to gain an understanding of the community's perception of members' beliefs, values, strengths, and needs (Counts & Boyle, 1987; Russell, Gregory, Wotton, Mordoch, & Counts, 1996).

Community Identification Process

Another qualitative community assessment model is the community identification process (CID). This model involves collecting information on how community members view themselves and their world, as a means to best affect beliefs and behaviors. It can be used with other quantitative data collection measures. The CID is a rapid assessment model that focuses on (a) defining the population, (b) creating taxonomies and acquiring materials, (c) surveying internal knowledge, (d) summarizing internal knowledge, (e) developing an external knowledge base, (f) integrating information and refining segments, (g) interviewing key gatekeepers and opinion makers and observing the community, (h) interviewing key participants, and (i) analyzing and interpreting the data (Tashima, Crain, O'Reilly, & Elifson, 1996).

Helvie's Energy Theory for Community Assessment

Helvie's (1998) energy theory is a system theory that focuses on energy as the capacity to do work. Three types of energy in the community are identified: bound, kinetic, and potential. The community and individuals are considered as changing energy fields that affect and are affected by energy exchanges with the environment. The internal environment is the community's subsystems; the external environment relates to other communities, the state, and the nation as they exchange energy with the community. These energy exchanges are considered to influence the health of the population and determine the placement of the population on an energy or health continuum. The community assessment process, according to this theory, consists of a comparison of past and present energy balances with other energy system states at other levels, such as comparing the community energy system to state or national energy systems (Helvie, 1998).

Assets Mapping Approach

The assets mapping approach focuses on the positive aspects of a community rather than on its deficits. Data collected using the assets approach are used to construct a map of assets and capacities. The community assets are mapped according to building blocks—primary, secondary, and potential. Primary building blocks are the assets located in the community and controlled by individuals who live in the community. Secondary building blocks are assets located in the community but controlled by forces outside the community. Potential building blocks are assets located outside the community and controlled outside the community. These building blocks form the basis for data collection (Kretzmann & McKnight, 1997; McKnight & Kretzmann, 1997).

The primary building blocks of the community are assessed along two categories: individual and organizational. Individual assets consist of skills, talents, individuals' personal experiences, individual businesses, personal income and property, and special talents of labeled individuals (elderly, disabled, mentally challenged). Individual assets are assessed using the Individual Capacity Inventory developed by McKnight and Kretzmann (1997). Community associations and organizations are assessed to determine the community's organizational assets.

Secondary building blocks are assessed along three aspects of the community: private and nonprofit organizations, physical resources, and public institutions and services. In the category of private and nonprofit organizations, the assets of higher education institutions, hospitals, and social service agencies are assessed. Physical resources consist of vacant land and buildings, commercial or industrial structures, housing, and utility services (energy and waste). Public institutions and services consist of public schools, police and fire departments, recreational parks, and libraries (Kretzmann & McKnight, 1997; McKnight & Kretzmann, 1997).

Potential building blocks are also assessed along three aspects of the community: welfare and public capital improvement expenditures, and public information (Kretzmann & McKnight, 1997; McKnight & Kretzmann, 1997). The assets mapping approach builds a community's capacity to meet its identified needs. This approach identifies community strengths that can be used to develop or build more community capacity to create a competent community. (Community capacity refers to the community having the necessary resources and ability to meet its needs.)

Data Collection Sources

Community assessment involves the systematic acquisition of data from multiple data sources in the community. Data can be collected from three levels or sources of data: federal, state, and local. Data collection involves the gathering of both primary and secondary data. Primary data collection consists of data collection methods that the community health professional generates from original data sources through methods such as observation, surveys developed or administered during the assessment process, interviews, and focus groups. Secondary data are extracted from published reports and documents, health survey results, statistical and census data, meeting minutes, association and organization annual reports, health-care report cards, and other health records (Helvie, 1998). Table 8.1 provides a list of data sources at the national, state, and local levels.

Data Collection Methods

Community assessment data are generated through multiple methods. Data collection methods vary in technique and in the types of data generated. This section summarizes the major data collection methods used in community assessment: collection from archival material, windshield and walking surveys, observation, interviews, focus groups, surveys, Delphi technique, and public forums.

Archival Data

Archival data are used as a secondary data source. Archival data consist of information in previously published reports or databases, which must be extracted and analyzed. Archival data provide a source from which to compare trends in community assessment data.

Windshield and Walking Surveys

A "windshield survey" is performed by riding through a community and astutely assessing various dimensions of that community (see Appendix F). A "walking survey" is performed by walking through the community and astutely assessing the same dimensions. Observations are made using the

Table 8.1   National, State, and Local Data Sources

National Data Sources

Agencies
- National Census for Health Statistics
- Centers for Disease Control and Prevention
- National Institutes of Health
- Environmental Protection Agency
- Health Care Financing Administration
- Health Resources and Services Administration
- Substance Abuse and Mental Health Services Administration
- Bureau of Labor Statistics
- Agency for Toxic Substances and Disease Registry

National Surveys, Data Sets and Reports
- National Mortality Followback Survey
- National Health Interview Survey
- National Health and Nutrition Examination Survey
- National Maternal and Infant Health Survey
- National Health Care Survey
- National Hospital Discharge Survey
- National Nursing Home Survey
- National Home and Hospice Care Survey
- National Hospital Ambulatory Medical Care Survey
- National Notifiable Diseases Surveillance System
- Youth Risk Behavior Surveillance Survey
- Behavioral Risk Factor Surveillance System
- HIV/AIDS Surveillance Reports
- U.S. Census Bureau
- National Immunization Survey
- National Household Surveys on Drug Abuse
- Drug Abuse Warning Network
- Survey of Mental Health Organizations
- Hazardous Substance Release/Health Effects Database

State Data Sources

State Vital Statistics
- Birth certificate data
- Death certificate data
- Fetal death certificate data

Disease Registries
- National Cancer Institute Surveillance, Epidemiology and End Results

State Health Report Cards

Local Data Sources
- Chamber of commerce
- County government
- Police and fire department
- Regional transportation authority

human senses of sight, hearing, taste, smell, and touch. Windshield and walking surveys should be conducted during a variety of time periods so that a general feel for the community may be obtained. Windshield and walking surveys provide a good first assessment of the community. These kinds of surveys provide a broad assessment of the community and also provide the assessor with a general feel for the community, as well as identifying areas for further investigation.

Participant Observation

Observations are made during the windshield and walking surveys by the assessor as an outsider looking into the community. In contrast, as a participant observer, the assessor engages in the life of the community and observes the community dynamics and individual interactions of community members from within. Observers gather information using their human senses. Observers are challenged with collecting data about the community and learning from community members without influencing community behaviors.

Interviews

Interviews are a one-to-one interaction between the assessor and a community informant. An interview is a conversation with the defined purpose of soliciting information. Key informants in the community are individuals with positions in the community that provide them with unique insights regarding the community. Key community informants may be public officials, health-care professionals, religious leaders, prominent business leaders, and informal community leaders.

Interviews can be performed face to face or by telephone. Face-to-face interviews provide the interviewer with an opportunity to monitor nonverbal behavior, control the physical environment, record spontaneous answers, know who exactly is answering, and ensure that the interview is complete. Face-to-face interviews are expensive and time consuming. Telephone interviews are conducted via a telephone conversation, which should be brief.

The interviewer uses structured or unstructured questions to elicit community assessment data. Key informant interviews may be recorded via an audiotape, with the informant's permission. The interviewer may also record field notes during the interview regarding verbal and nonverbal communication. The audiotape is transcribed verbatim. The written narrative text of the interview is analyzed using various qualitative analytic procedures such as thematic and discourse analysis.

Focus Groups

A focus group is a small group discussion, conducted by a trained facilitator, which focuses on a specific discussion topic. This technique is used to collect qualitative data. Focus groups are considered to provide a broader depth and breadth of understanding on the discussion topic. Participants are selected for their homogeneity in relation to certain characteristics. Focus groups usually consist of 8 to 10 members, rarely more than 12 (Kreuger, 1994).

A focus group guide is developed as a tool for the group facilitator to follow. The focus group guide assists the group facilitator in keeping group discussions focused in a certain area. Probing questions or areas to be examined are outlined in the guide. The group facilitator uses open-ended questions. Further clarification and exploration of an area of discussion is conducted through spontaneous probing by the group facilitator.

A comoderator sometimes attends the focus group sessions. This comoderator notes nonverbal communication in relation to the topics being discussed when the behavior occurs. Additionally, the comoderator draws a seating chart to note the position of focus group participants in relation to each other. Focus groups are audiorecorded, with the participants' permission. The audiotape is transcribed verbatim into a narrative text. The narrative text is analyzed using qualitative analysis methods such as thematic analysis and discourse analysis.

Surveys

A survey is a method of collecting data through questionnaires. A survey is an excellent tool with which to collect data regarding demographic information, knowledge, attitudes, and behaviors. Questionnaires can be self-administered by community constituents or administered by a trained data collector. Surveys can be handed to community members; read to residents, with a data collector recording the responses; or mailed to community members with a self-addressed, stamped envelope provided.

Surveys can consist of open-ended or closed-ended questions. Open-ended questions provide community members with a question to which they respond using a declarative statement or explanation. Closed-ended questions provide fixed responses from which the community member selects an answer to the question on the survey. Closed-ended questions consist of true-false, multiple-choice, or Likert-scale questions.

"Concern surveys" are a special type of survey conducted during a community assessment. Concern surveys are administered to community members to identify what they consider the most important issues facing their community. A community concern survey involves community members early, asks community members to identify problems, increases community member participation, assists in developing community coalitions around specific community concerns, focuses the community agenda in relation to the community's concerns, and builds community consensus (Shriner & Fawcett, 1988).

Delphi Technique

The Delphi technique is a method of data collection used to obtain a consensus opinion from a group of experts on a specific problem or concern. The Delphi technique has been used to establish national priorities, such as research priorities, and in community assessments, to elicit data from community members who are considered not necessarily experts but knowledgeable about the community.

Three characteristics of the Delphi technique are anonymity, iteration with controlled feedback, and statistical group response (Couper, 1984). Anonymity is the maintenance of no linkages between the individual responses and the respondent's identity. Iteration with controlled feedback consists of data collection occurring in rounds. Questions are sent to the experts in the first round of data collection, and their responses are analyzed and given to back to them with their own response and the group's responses in a prioritized manner. The respondents then again respond to the questions provided, taking into account the new categorical prioritization. This iterative process continues until a reasonable group consensus emerges, which typically takes two to four rounds. The reporting of a group score and a ranking for each item prioritized is the statistical group response. The Delphi technique is a method with which to generate community consensus on issues and create a prioritized agenda for community action.

Community Forums

A community forum is a meeting that is publicized throughout the community in which constituents may discuss important issues or concerns, identify problems, and engage in problem-solving discussions. The community forum is similar to town hall meetings. A community forum provides community members from various backgrounds with an opportunity to express their opinions and serves as an initial step to understanding the community's needs and resources.

Questions addressed at community forums are general and nonspecific in nature. Table 8.2 outlines some questions that can be included in community forums.

Meetings should be held at different sites throughout the community at various times. Community members should also be personally recruited.

Table 8.2   Sample Community Forum Questions

- What are some of the problems in the community?
- Who is affected?
- Are there related issues of concern? How widespread are these concerns?
- Who will oppose efforts to prevent or resolve the problems?
- How can these barriers be overcome?
- What resources are available in the community?
- What resources are needed in the community?
- What local community members, groups, institutions, or organizations can help with the problems and concerns?

Group sizes should be no larger than 30 to 40 members. If permitted, the meeting should be audiorecorded. The audiotape can be transcribed for further analysis. One group facilitator should be responsible for recording verbal and nonverbal communications of attendees.

The Geographic Information System

The geographic information system (GIS) permits the integration, storage, retrieval, analysis, and communication of data, with spatial or geographic components displayed on community maps (Melnick & Fleming, 1999). GIS assists in the epidemiological correlation of variables of person, place, and time typically used to analyze and identify problems. GIS is a tool used to plot data on maps as a means of understanding and displaying diseases or risk factors in relation to geographic and demographic data.

This technology is frequently used as a tool for understanding and displaying in map form a disease or disease risks that are related to environmental exposures. GIS technology is being used to explore other nonenvironmental diseases that cluster geographically. Childhood immunization rates, homicides, high-risk pregnancies, and motor vehicle accidents have been geographically displayed.

In addition to serving as a community assessment tool, GIS is a program planning tool that can be used to assist with the development and administration of specific programs targeting geographically identified needs (Melnick & Fleming, 1999). GIS has the ability to assess variations in the demographic, socioeconomic, and health characteristics of a population by overlaying a wide variety of other characteristics. The overlaying of population-based data on various characteristics provides a graphic picture of potential associations that exist with the characteristics under assessment in targeted populations in a community. Geographical displays of population-based data can be charted over time by comparing geographical maps, thus displaying trends and providing outcome-related data for program evaluation purposes.

Community Profiling

Community profiling is the term used to describe the broadest type of community assessment, which varies in scope to include needs, resources, and a range of issues that affect a community. It refers to a diverse range of projects that are initiated by a variety of different organizations. Hawtin, Hughes, and Percy-Smith (1999) define community profiling as

> A *comprehensive* description of the needs of a population that is defined, or defines itself, as a *community*, and the *resources* that exist within that community, carried out with the *active involvement of the community* itself, for the purpose of developing an action plan or other means of improving the quality of life in the community. (p. 5)

A community profile is considered comprehensive in nature because of its focus on both needs and resources in a defined community. A good community profile is considered to include the active involvement of community members. Community empowerment is expected to result from community members working together toward a common goal. Hawtin et al. (1999) describe three tiers of community involvement: core, volunteers, and wider community. The core group ensures that the community profiling is planned and managed. Volunteers are a pool of community members who want to do something different or to offer their special skills to benefit the community. Wider community means the involvement of the entire community, even if it is only when they are informed that a community profile will be conducted and given periodic updates on its progress. The wider community is an excellent communication channel through which to disseminate the results of the community profile.

Community profiling consist of six stages: (a) preparing the ground, (b) setting aims and objectives, (c) deciding on methods, (d) fieldwork, (e) reporting, and (f) action. Table 8.3 provides a detailed outline of the community profiling steps (Hawtin et al., 1999).

Community Analysis

After the community assessment data is collected, the assessor conducts a community analysis of the data. Community analysis is the second phase of the integrated community assessment process. Community assessment data can be analyzed using criteria to discern the significance of a problem. Some community analysis criteria are frequency of occurrence, duration of problem, severity of problem, magnitude or scope of problem, seriousness, legality, and community perception. Helvie (1998) defines community analysis as the classification, summation, interpretation, and validation of data as a means to construct community diagnoses and establish community health priorities.

Table 8.3   Community Profiling Steps

Preparing the Ground
- Create a steering group
- Initial planning
- Develop contacts
- Share learning experiences with others
- Identify resources
- Engage consultants or professional researchers
- Develop a management structure

Setting Aims and Objectives

Deciding on Methods

Fieldwork
- Develop or produce data collection instruments
- Train staff in data collection methods
- Collect new data
- Record data
- Analyze data

Reporting
- Write fieldwork analysis
- Produce draft profile
- Receive consultation regarding draft
- Amend profile
- Produce final profile
- Disseminate profile findings

Action
- Receive consultation on key issues, priorities, and potential actions
- Draft a community action plan
- Produce community action plan
- Disseminate community action plan
- Implement community action plan
- Monitor and evaluate community action plan

This community analysis process of classification, summation, interpretation, and validation provides a comprehensive examination of the data collected. Classification consists of sorting and classifying data into some meaningful system. Summation consists of placing data into categories on a data analysis sheet. Summation can consist of a list or narrative statements about the data collected. Interpretation involves a comparative analysis of the community assessment data collected, with established standards, state and national statistics, and the community's own historical data from previous years or community assessments. From these comparisons, inferences are hypothesized regarding the meanings of the community assessment data. Validation is the final step of the community analysis process. Validation consists of further data collection as a measure to close gaps, clarify, or resolve any incongruities that exist in the data collected (Helvie, 1998).

Integrated Community Assessment Process

Based on the community assessment models, data sources, and data collection methods presented earlier, I propose an integrated community assessment process. The integrated community assessment process consists of the systematic collection of population-based data in a defined community using primary and secondary data collection methods to identify community assets and deficits. The culmination of the integrated community assessment process is a community diagnosis, the planning of community interventions, and evaluation of these interventions.

The integrated community assessment process consists of six phases (see Appendix F). Phase 1 consists of community assessment data collection. Primary and secondary data collection is used to identify assets and deficits that exist within the community. Appendix F presents a tool that can be used to conduct the integrated community assessment with components and areas of inquiry identified to complete the assessment. Phase 1 has three parts: a narrative description of the community, a windshield or walking survey, and archival community data collection.

Community assessment data analysis occurs during phase 2. Comprehensive review, critique, and analysis of all data are completed to develop a list of assets, deficits, and needs. Helvie's (1998) steps of data analysis—classification, summation, interpretation, and validation—are recommended to formulate a list of assets, deficits, and potential interventions based on the data collected.

Writing a community diagnosis is phase 3. Community diagnosis consists of listing community asset and diagnosis statements that provide direction for developing community interventions and evaluating such interventions. Community interventions are proposed to strengthen the assets or eliminate the deficits identified in the community assessment. For each community diagnosis statement, corresponding objectives, interventions, timelines, and evaluation methods are presented in phase 4, which is known as the proposed multilevel intervention phase. Phase 5 is the report writing phase. The report generated in phase 5 can also have an oral component. A written report that comprehensively summarizes the community assessment data is the final product of phase 5. The integrated community assessment approach culminates with an evaluation of the community assessment process: what worked, what did not work, what other data sources should be included in the future, and what other methods should be used. The evaluation of the integrated community assessment process is phase 6.

Needs Assessment Approach

A needs assessment is considered a specialized and focused assessment of a particular need. A need is considered to exist if there is a discrepancy between "what is" (actual state) and "what should be" (target state). Witkin and Altschuld (1995) define a needs assessment as

> A systematic set of procedures undertaken for the purpose of setting priorities and making decisions about program or organizational improvement and allocation of resources. The priorities are based on identified needs. (p. 4)

Some reasons to conduct a needs assessment are to (a) provide supporting data to justify a new or improved program or service; (b) provide data to justify discontinuation of a program or service; (c) recommend organizational change in purpose, direction, management, operations, or personnel; (d) determine solutions or actions to rectify a problem; (e) periodically reappraise services and activities within a program; and (f) validate the current target populations (Petersen & Alexander, 2001; Witkin & Altschuld, 1995).

Community-based public health programs should continually ensure public accountability. A method of ensuring this public accountability is to validate that existing programs or services are directed at and meeting the needs of the targeted community population. This can be accomplished through an ongoing needs assessment process focusing on the following questions:

- What is the target population?
- What are the target population's needs?
- Which groups within the target population have what types of needs?
- Where are the needs geographically in the community?
- What are the current programs or services directed to meet those needs, by whom, and where?
- What new or unmet needs continue to exist in the target population?
- What has changed since the establishment of existing programs? (Petersen & Alexander, 2001)

Levels and Types of Need

A needs assessment identifies a population's present needs and desires within a specific community context. From the needs assessment process, statements of need are derived and prioritized later for community action. Witkin and Altschuld (1995) identified three levels of need that exist within a community – primary (level 1), secondary (level 2), and tertiary (level 3).

The primary needs level consists of the service receivers (students, clients, information users, commuters, potential customers) among whom the need exists. The people in level 1 are the individuals who will ultimately benefit from the fulfillment of community needs. Level 1 is generally the initial focus of a needs assessment. The secondary needs level consists of service providers and policy makers (teachers, parents, social workers, health-care

Table 8.4   Three-Phase Needs Assessment (NA) Process

Preassessment
- Develop a management plan for the NA
- Define NA purpose
- Define boundaries of NA
- Identify major areas or issues of NA
- Identify existing data sources
- Determine data to collect, data sources, data collection methods, and potential uses of data

Assessment
- Collect data
- Establish preliminary priorities of needs from levels 1, 2, and 3
- Compile all data and begin analyzing and synthesizing data

Postassessment
- Complete data analysis and synthesis to bridge gap between what is known and what is needed
- Set priorities for needs
- Identify potential solutions
- Develop an action plan to implement interventions
- Evaluate the NA process
- Disseminate results

SOURCE: Witkin and Altschuld (1995).

professionals, administrators). A needs assessment directed at level 2 may focus on the educational or training needs of service providers and policy makers to ensure that the solutions to the need can be delivered. The tertiary needs level consists of resources or solutions (buildings, facilities, equipment, technology, transportation, salaries and benefits, program delivery systems) to the need. Needs assessments at levels 2 and 3 are the result of level 1 needs assessments. For example, once needs are identified at the consumer level (level 1), an assessment of service providers' abilities to deliver the needed program or services and an assessment of the resources that are available generally occur.

In addition to needs existing on various levels, there are various types of needs that exist. Petersen and Alexander (2001) describe four types of needs: comparative; expected, wanted, desired or felt; expressed; and extrapolated. Community health experts define comparative needs based on comparison data. Comparative needs are defined based on data gathered to assist in meeting a targeted state or expected minimal standards defined by experts. Expected, wanted, desired, or felt needs are defined by the target population, the public, policy makers, or community stakeholders. These are the needs that these individuals expect or want to be delivered. Expressed needs are demands for specific services. Demands for these needs are expressed through the support of legislation or policies or electing representatives who plan to address an expressed need. Extrapolated needs can be determined when data from one target population are applied to another to ascertain the community's needs.

Table 8.5   Petersen and Alexander's Stages of Needs Assessment

Start-up Planning Stage
- Establish organizational structure
- Identify potential users
- Identify stakeholders
- Identify overall target population
- Identify the types of needs to be assessed

Operational Planning Stage
- Establish who will determine needs indicators and data sources
- Establish who will produce data reports
- Determine methods of collecting data and ranking priorities
- Determine the organization and management of meetings
- Determine methods to resolve conflicts and reach consensus
- Determine coalition-building strategies

Data Stage
- Identify indicators of needs
- Identify available data needed and sources
- Create a resource inventory
- Assemble data

Needs Analysis Stage
- Prioritize needs
- Determine populations with specific needs
- Identify potential solutions
- Reassess needs in consideration of potential solutions
- Identify resources available to meet needs
- Reach consensus on solutions

Program and Policy Development Stage
- Develop plans to translate need statements into policy statements
- Secure approval of policy plans
- Communicate results of needs assessment
- Collaborate with advocacy groups to promote policies
- Develop plans to monitor and evaluate proposed solutions

Resource Allocation Stage
- Develop tenets to determine funding formulas
- Reach consensus on need indicators and funding formulas
- Construct initial funding proposals
- Present funding proposals to stakeholders

SOURCE: Petersen and Alexander (2001).

Needs Assessment Phases

A needs assessment is a systematic approach that can be described to occur in a series of phases using various data collection methods. Witkin and Altschuld (1995) propose a three-phase needs assessment process consisting of preassessment, assessment, and postassessment. The preassessment phase is an exploratory phase to determine what is known, decide on assessment boundaries, identify major issues of concern, define the purpose of the needs assessment, identify potential data sources, define the method of data collection, and determine what types of decisions will be made from the needs assessment. The assessment phase consists of the actual data collection process, and preliminary priorities are set. The postassessment phase consists of analyzing and synthesizing the data into an action plan to address the identified community needs. Table 8.4 summarizes this process.

Petersen and Alexander (2001) propose a process with an emphasis on the careful planning of a needs assessment. Planning the approach and organizing the way in which the needs assessment will be conducted is seen as a vital prerequisite to the process. Table 8.5 summarizes Petersen and Alexander's stages in the needs assessment process.

Both needs assessment approaches use multiple data collection methods identified earlier in this chapter. Community member surveys are frequently used to collect needs assessment data, alone or in combination with interviews or focus groups.

Summary

Key issues in community assessment and analysis are as follows.

- A community assessment involves the collection of data and information about various characteristics of a population within a defined community.
- A multidimensional approach to community assessment uses multiple assessment strategies (behavioral, public health agency, and environmental), multiple data sources, and multiple data collection (primary and secondary) methods.
- A community assessment is defined as the process of collecting data (from primary and secondary data sources) and information regarding the demographics, health status, and infrastructure of a defined community.
- Community assessment models provide a framework for the collection of community assessment data and information.
- The community-as-partner model focuses on the philosophical orientation of primary health care.
- The community assessment wheel has a core and eight subsystems. The community residents are at the core of the model. The eight subsystems are physical environment, education, safety and transportation, politics and government, health and social services, communication, economics, and recreation.
- CHAT was developed from Gordon and Kucharski's (1987) 11 functional health patterns.

- The 11 CHAT functional health patterns are (a) community health and safety efforts; (b) the adequacy of the community's nutritional efforts; (c) waste management in the community; (d) community transportation and recreation systems; (e) community cycles and rhythms; (f) community decision-making processes; (g) community self-perception and opinion; (h) informal and formal roles defined by the community; (i) community reproductive functions, resources, and family structure; (j) community support services; and (k) cultural, ethical, and spiritual community needs.
- Agent, host, and environment compose the essential components of the epidemiological triangle model for community assessment.
- Epidemiological and ethnographic data are integrated into a comprehensive community analysis in the GENESIS model.
- Essential components of the GENESIS model are history, culture, politics, health services, social services, education, environment, economics, and employment.
- The intention of CID is to provide information on how community members view themselves and their world, as a means to affect beliefs and behaviors.
- CID is a rapid assessment that focuses on (a) defining the population, (b) creating taxonomies and acquiring materials, (c) surveying internal knowledge, (d) summarizing internal knowledge, (e) developing an external knowledge base, (f) integrating information and refining segments, (g) interviewing key gatekeepers and opinion makers and observing the community, (h) interviewing key participants, and (i) analyzing and interpreting the data.
- Helvie's (1998) energy theory is a system theory that focuses on energy as the capacity to do work. Three types of energy in the community are identified: bound, kinetic, and potential.
- The assets mapping approach focuses on the positive aspects of a community rather than the deficits.
- Community assets are mapped according to primary, secondary, and potential building blocks.
- The primary building blocks of the community are assessed along two categories, individual and organizational.
- Secondary building blocks are assessed along three aspects of the community: private and nonprofit organizations, physical resources, and public institutions and services.
- Potential building blocks are also assessed along three aspects of the community: welfare and public capital improvement expenditures, and public information.
- Community assessment data can be collected from three levels or sources of data: federal, state, and local.
- Primary data collection consists of data collection methods such as observation, surveys developed or administered during the assessment process, interviews, and focus groups.

- Secondary data collection consists of extracting data from published reports and documents, health survey results, statistical and census data, meeting minutes, association and organization annual reports, health-care report cards, and other health records.
- Archival data consists of data from previously published reports or databases, which is extracted and then analyzed.
- A windshield survey is performed by riding through a community and astutely assessing various dimensions of that community.
- A participant observer engages in the life of the community and observes community dynamics and the individual interactions of community members.
- Interviews are a one-to-one interaction between the assessor and a community informant.
- A focus group is a small group led by a trained facilitator that focuses on a specific discussion topic.
- A survey collects data through questionnaires.
- Concern surveys are administered to community members to identify what they consider are the most important issues facing their community.
- The Delphi technique is a method of data collection in which a consensus opinion is obtained from a group of experts on a specific problem or concern.
- A community forum is a meeting that is publicized throughout the community in which constituents may discuss important issues or concerns, identify problems, and engage in problem-solving discussions.
- GIS permits the integration, storage, retrieval, analysis, and communication of data with spatial or geographic components displayed on community maps.
- GIS is a tool used to plot data on maps as a means to understanding and displaying diseases or risk factors in relation to geographic and demographic data.
- Community profile is the term used to describe the broadest type of community assessment, which varies in scope to include needs, resources, and a range of issues that affect a community.
- The community profiling stages are (a) preparing the ground, (b) setting aims and objectives, (c) deciding on methods, (d) fieldwork, (e) reporting, and (f) action.
- After the community assessment data is collected, the assessor conducts a community analysis of the data.
- Community analysis criteria are frequency of occurrence, duration of problem, severity of problem, magnitude or scope of problem, seriousness, legality, and community perception.
- The integrated community assessment process consists of six phases: data collection, data analysis, community diagnosis, proposal of multilevel interventions, a written or oral report with recommendations, and evaluation of the assessment process.

- A needs assessment is considered a specialized and focused assessment of a specific need.
- The purposes of a needs assessment are to (a) provide supporting data to justify a new or improved program or service; (b) provide data to justify discontinuation of a program or service; (c) recommend organizational change in purpose, direction, management, operations, or personnel; (d) determine solutions or actions to rectify a problem; (e) periodically reappraise services and activities within a program; and (f) validate the current target populations.
- Three levels of needs assessment that exist within a community are primary (level 1), secondary (level 2), and tertiary (level 3).
- There are four types of needs that can be identified in a needs assessment: comparative; expected, wanted, desired or felt; expressed; and extrapolated.
- Three phases of a needs assessment process are preassessment, assessment, and postassessment.

References

Anderson, E., & McFarlane, J. (1996). *Community as partner: Theory and practice in nursing*. Philadelphia: J. B. Lippincott.

Counts, M., & Boyle, J. (1987). Nursing, health, and policy within a community context. *Advances in Nursing Science*, 9(3), 12-23.

Couper, M. (1984). The Delphi technique: Characteristics and sequence model. *Advances in Nursing Science*, 7(1), 72-77.

Gordon, M., & Kucharski, P. (1987). A new look at the community: Functional health pattern assessment. *Journal of Community Health Nursing*, 4, 21-27.

Hawtin, M., Hughes, G., & Percy-Smith, J. (1999). *Community profiling: Auditing social needs*. Philadelphia, PA: Open University Press.

Helvie, C. (1998). *Advanced practice nursing in the community*. Thousand Oaks, CA: Sage.

Kretzmann, J., & McKnight, J. (1997). *Building communities from the inside out: A path toward finding and mobilizing a community's assets*. Chicago, IL: ACTA.

Kreuger, R. (1994). *Focus groups: A practical guide for applied research* (2nd ed.). Thousand Oaks, CA: Sage.

Krieger, N., & Harton, M. (1992). Community health assessment tool: A pattern approach to data collection and diagnosis. *Journal of Community Health Nursing*, 9, 229-234.

Mausner, J., & Kramer, S. (1985). *Epidemiology: An introductory text* (2nd ed.) Philadelphia, PA: Saunders.

McKnight, J., & Kretzmann, J. (1997). Mapping community capacity. In M. Minkler (Ed.), *Community organizing and community building for health* (pp. 157-172). New Brunswick, NJ: Rutgers University Press.

Melnick, A., & Fleming, D. (1999). Modern geographic information systems: Promises and pitfalls. *Journal of Public Health Management and Practice*, 5(2), i-iii.

Neuman, B. (1989). *The Neuman systems model* (2nd ed.). Norwalk, CT: Appleton & Lange.

Petersen, D., & Alexander, G. (2001). *Needs assessment in public health: A practical guide for students and professionals*. New York: Kluwer Academic/Plenum.

Plescia, M., Koontz, S., & Laurent, S. (2001). Community assessment in a vertically integrated health care system. *American Journal of Public Health*, *91*(5), 811-813.

Russell, C., Gregory, D., Wotton, D., Mordoch, E., & Counts, M. (1996). ACTION: Application and extension of the GENESIS community analysis model. *Public Health Nursing*, *13*(3), 187-194.

Shriner, K., & Fawcett, S. (1988). Development and validation of a community concern report method. *Journal of Community Psychology*, *16*, 306-316.

Tashima, N., Crain, C., O'Reilly, K., & Elifson, C. (1996). The community identification (CID) process: A discovery model. *Qualitative Health Research*, *6*(1), 23-48.

Witkin, B., & Altschuld, J. (1995). *Planning and conducting needs assessments: A practical guide*. Thousand Oaks, CA: Sage.

Part III

Public Health: Community Health Interventions and Program Planning

9

Cultural Competence

Public health nursing is experiencing challenges in providing quality public health services to diverse populations with various spiritual and cultural perspectives. Culturally competent care provides the public health nurse with a framework to use in meeting the holistic and public health needs of diverse populations. This chapter focuses on defining culture and cultural assessments, presenting a community-based transcultural nursing perspective, providing cultural competencies, and describing the development of cultural competence.

Introduction

The public health system is continually challenged with providing health care services to diverse populations that may be culturally homogenous or heterogeneous within the same community. This increasing diversity is the result of the increasing migration of immigrants and refugees, demographic shifts in racial and ethnic groups, and the emergence of minority populations that were, historically, the majority population in their country of origin or in communities that have encountered a dramatic racial demographic shift (e.g., a community that was primarily white and now is populated by a majority of African Americans or Latinos). The public health infrastructure is challenged with providing health-care services to meet the multiple needs and exploit the assets of these culturally specific populations. To effectively deliver health-care services to diverse groups, public health professionals must be culturally competent in assessing, planning, implementing, and evaluating public health interventions. This chapter will explore the multiple dimensions of culture, community-based transcultural nursing, cultural diversity, and cultural competence.

Culture

Culture is defined as an integral pattern of shared traditions and human behavior that includes the history, folklore, thought, communication (language), actions, customs, beliefs, and values of a group of people in a population (Brownlee, 2003; National Center for Mental Health Services and Substance Abuse & Mental Health Services Administration, 2000). Public health nurses view culture from either an emic or an etic perspective. The emic view is the insider's perspective as to what is culturally important to know and believe; the etic view is an outsider's perspective and views of a specific culture. The difference in emic and etic perspectives can create cultural dilemmas for public health nurses.

The multiple cultural perspectives generated from either the emic or the etic perspective create a set of culturally relevant experiences and feelings for public health nurses—ethnocentrism, cultural imposition, cultural ignorance, cultural bias, culture shock, cultural pain, cultural variation, cultural barriers, stereotyping, culture boundness, cultural backlash, enculturation, and acculturation. Table 9.1 provides summary definitions of these cultural concepts.

Community-Based Transcultural Nursing

Population-based public health nursing is dependent on culturally relevant care provided to diverse populations within the community. Leininger (2001) proposes that community-based transcultural nursing is essential to the future of public health nursing. Community-based transcultural nursing provides a framework from which to deliver culturally competent care to diverse populations. Leininger describes community-based transcultural nursing as "the creative use of transcultural nursing concepts, principles, research, knowledge, and practices that focus on large overall designated communities or geographic contexts in order to provide culturally competent nursing care" (p. 220). Attention to culturally competent nursing care is essential because all humans are culturally grounded every day by their words, decisions, and behaviors. Human behavior is grounded in cultural values, beliefs, and cultural community lifeways (Leininger, 2001).

Transcultural nursing exists on both the macro- and microlevels. Leininger (2001) described the macrocultures as the larger cultural designations. Macrocultures can be defined by a geographic orientation or racial or ethnic perspective, such as North American (geographic) or African American (racial and ethnic). Microcultures are the smaller cultural designations. Microcultures can be defined also by a geographic orientation or common interest or aggregate perspective, such as that of the American South (geographic) or gay or lesbian (common interest or aggregate perspective). Knowing the cultural perspective that a population uses to

Table 9.1 Culturally Relevant Concepts

Ethnocentrism	Belief that one's own culture is the best and most superior
Cultural imposition	Results from ethnocentrism: One cultural group forces or imposes its cultural values, beliefs, and behaviors onto another group
Cultural ignorance	Insufficient cultural knowledge to provide culturally competent care
Cultural blindness	Ignoring all cultural differences and acting as though cultural differences do not exist
Culture shock	A state of disorientation, helplessness, discomfort, or inability to function resulting from the strangeness or unfamiliarity experienced in another culture
Cultural pain	Discomfort or pain experienced by an individual or group resulting from offensive comments or actions by another individual or cultural group
Cultural variation	Diversity that exists within and between cultural groups
Cultural barriers	Obstacles that interfere with or alter care due to cultural rules and obligations
Stereotyping	Labeling individuals or groups with perceived characteristics
Culture bound	Individuals are considered culture bound when they have become limited to their own cultural values, beliefs, and actions and have little or no ability to appreciate other cultural viewpoints
Cultural backlash	The repercussions that develop when an individual or group from another culture adopts another culture's values, beliefs, or actions
Enculturation	Developmental process in which children acquire cultural knowledge and internalize a culture's values, beliefs, and actions
Acculturation	Change of cultural values, beliefs, and actions over time resulting from the experience of living in a multicultural society
Multiculturalism	Integration of multiple cultures into one society in such a way that each cultural group maintains its cultural identity but has a sense of belonging to the larger society; acceptance of diverse cultures to ensure harmony and cross-cultural understanding

identify itself assists the public health nurse in understanding cultural values, beliefs, and behaviors.

Leininger (2001) also describes some fundamental issues that must be understood to deliver transcultural nursing care:

- Culture is stable, but changes over time.
- Human behavior is strongly influenced by cultural patterns, norms, and practices.
- Cultural values and beliefs have intercultural and intracultural variations.
- Cultural rituals, symbols, and practices are important in understanding a culture.
- Total lifeways must be studied to understand people's cultural belief systems and practices, including religious practices, politics, economics, technologies, and kinship relationships.
- Communication, space, and time patterns are culturally derived.

- Cultural gatekeepers are essential to understanding and conducting cultural assessments (gatekeepers are individuals who control access, formally or informally, to a community or population).
- Transcultural care needs vary among communities with similar cultures.
- Subcultures are present within the dominant culture of a community.

In community-based transcultural nursing, the goal is to enter the client's world and deliver culturally competent public health nursing care that meets the population's public health needs. To meet these needs in a culturally competent and sensitive manner, public health nurses must respect the cultural environment in which they are practicing. Leininger (2001) provides some principles of transcultural nursing to assist nurses in the delivery of culturally competent nursing care:

- All human cultures have diverse living, caring, and healing modes that must be learned if they are to work effectively.
- Care is a basic human need and the essence of nursing.
- It is a prerequisite in transcultural nursing that nurses be culturally aware of their own culture.
- People have a right to their own cultural values, beliefs, and practices.
- Transcultural nursing focuses on comparative values, beliefs, and practices as a means to provide adequate health-care service.
- Nurses must combine the use of humanistic and scientific cultural knowledge in the provision of care.
- Knowledge of cultural variation enables nurses to respect clients and assist them to maintain their well-being.
- A willingness to enter the client's cultural world as an engaged partner is essential to an effective nurse-client or nurse-family relationship.
- Nurses must listen, respect, and be attentive to clients' different cultural values and beliefs.
- Speaking in the client's cultural language facilitates an understanding of the client's needs.
- Nurses must continually strive to understand clients' cultural lifeways and values.
- Worldviews, environmental contexts, and social structures shape each culture's healing and health practices.
- Every culture has two health-care systems: the generic (indigenous, traditional, or folk) and professional. Nurses must understand the value systems and cultural beliefs regarding both systems.
- Each culture has its own manner of promoting and maintaining health, death, and unfavorable sociocultural conditions.
- Nurses must understand the major differences between Western and non-Western health-care practices to plan public health programs.

Attention to these transcultural nursing principles prepares the public health nurse with an element of cultural sensitivity from which to conduct a cultural assessment. To understand intercultural and intracultural values, beliefs, and practices and to deliver culturally specific and sensitive care, public health nurses must conduct a cultural assessment.

Cultural Assessment

Culture defines who individuals are and what they value, believe, and think. Culture dictates an individual's way of life in a community. A clear understanding of individuals and groups within a population is necessary to adequately develop and plan public health programs for culturally diverse populations. This is accomplished through the integration of cultural assessment into behavioral, environmental, and public health assessments. Additionally, cultural assessment should be integrated into the development of community-level interventions and public health programs.

Cultural assessment provides a contextual understanding of an individual or population's values, beliefs, and behaviors. Giger and Davidhizar (1999) identified six cultural phenomena that provide information on the organization of a population's cultural values, beliefs, and behaviors: environmental control, biological variation, social organization, communication, space, and time orientation. Environmental control refers to the culture's beliefs regarding ability to plan activities that control nature or direct environmental factors. Biological variations are the physical and genetic differences that occur from one cultural group to the next, such as body build and structure, skin color, disease susceptibility, and nutritional variations. Social organization consists of the support networks recognized to be of significance to the cultural group. Common social organization variations are the family unit and religious or ethnic social groups. Communication consists of patterns of oral, nonverbal, and written communication, which vary among cultures. These patterns may include pronunciation, word meaning, voice tone and quality, eye contact, gestures, facial expression, body posture, silence, and interjection during conversations. Space consists of an individual's perception of his or her personal space (that area an individual needs between him- or herself and another individual to feel comfortable). Space zones have been identified as intimate (up to 1½ feet), personal distance (1½ to 4 feet), social distance (4 to 12 feet), and public distance (12 feet or more). The last cultural phenomenon to explore during an assessment is time orientation. Cultures vary in their perception of time; a culture may be future oriented or present oriented. These six cultural phenomena provide a framework from which to assess cultural variations among cultural groups.

In addition to these phenomena, Boyle (1995) identifies seven components of a cultural assessment. The seven cultural components of a cultural assessment are (a) family and kinship systems; (b) social life; (c) political systems; (d) language and traditions; (e) worldview, value orientations, and cultural norms; (f) religion; and (g) health beliefs and practices.

Cultural Competence Defined

Cultural competence is described as acceptance of and respect for difference, a continuing self-assessment regarding culture, regard for and attention to the dynamics of difference, engagement in ongoing development of cultural knowledge, and the resources and flexibility within service models that make it possible to work toward better meeting the needs of minority populations (National Center for Mental Health Services and Substance Abuse & Mental Health Services Administration, 2000). Cultural competence promotes trust, respect, mutual understanding, novel and innovative ideas and strategies, creativity, multiple worldviews, participation, empowerment, and cooperation.

Cultural competence consists of both knowledge-based theory and interpersonal skills (Campinha-Bacote, Yahle, & Langekamp, 1996). Cultural competence extends beyond cultural sensitivity and awareness. The American Association of Nurses (AAN) Expert Panel (1992) proposed four recommendations to guide cultural competence. Nursing care based in cultural competence must be

- Designed specifically for the individual
- Based on an individual's cultural uniqueness
- Self-empowering, promoting individual decision making
- Sensitive to the individual's cultural uniqueness

Cultural competence can exist on an individual or organizational level. Brownlee (2003) describes a culturally competent organization as an entity that transforms differences among various groups of people into standards, policies, and practices that are effectively integrated to accomplish the organization's mission and goals. Organizational cultural competence is dependent on a shared vision and a desired outcome among culturally diverse groups. Public health infrastructure necessitates the existence of culturally competent public health professionals and public health agencies or organizations.

Principles of Cultural Competence

Five essential principles are considered to define the model of cultural competence: valuing diversity, conducting a cultural self-assessment, understanding the dynamics of differences, institutionalizing cultural knowledge, and adapting to diversity. Valuing diversity means acceptance and respect for differences within and between cultural groups. Cultural self-assessment consists of being knowledgeable and aware of your own culture and conscious of others' cultures. Understanding the dynamics of differences consists of an awareness of how different values, beliefs, traditions, and behaviors affect the interaction of individuals within a group. Integration of cultural knowledge into multiple facets of an organization promotes institutionalization of cultural knowledge. The recognition, respect, and integration of differing values into an organizational system to meet the needs of diverse groups and the organization is the essence of adapting to cultural diversity (Brownlee, 2003).

Cultural and Linguistic Competence

Cultural and linguistic competence is described as the congruence between attitudes, behaviors, and policies that exist within individual health-care professionals, a system, or an organization and that promote effectiveness in cross-cultural situations (Office of Minority Health, 2001). This competence implies that public health nurses should have the capability to function effectively within an organizational context providing care that is consistent with the served population's language, cultural beliefs, behaviors, and needs.

The Office of Minority Health developed standards for culturally and linguistically appropriate services (CLAS) as a measure to ensure that all individuals who enter the health-care system receive equal, fair, quality health care (Ross, 2001). Additionally, these standards create accountability within organizations for providing equitable and quality health-care services. Health-care consumers and policy makers can use these standards to hold public health agencies accountable for providing culturally and linguistically competent care. These standards focus primarily on culture and language, since these are considered two integral components that define individuals within the larger population.

The 14 CLAS standards are organized into three themes: culturally competent care, language access services, and organizational supports for cultural competence. Table 9.2 presents the Office of Minority Health Cultural and Linguistic competencies (Ross, 2001).

The Development of Cultural Competence

The development of cultural competence is an ongoing process that consists of life-long cultural learning. The development of cultural competency skills is knowledge based; personal experiences are combined with interpersonal skills. Skills necessary for cultural competence are self-awareness, open

Table 9.2   Office of Minority Health Culturally and Linguistically Appropriate Services
(CLAS) Standards

Cultural Competence Themes

Health-care organizations should ensure that patients and consumers receive effective, understandable,
and respectful care that is consistent with their cultural health beliefs and practices and preferred
language.

Health-care organizations should implement strategies to recruit, retain, and promote a diverse staff and
leadership that are representative of the demographic characteristics of the service area at all
organizational levels.

Health-care organizations should ensure that there is ongoing education and training in CLAS delivery
for all disciplines and staff.

Language Access Services Themes

Health-care organizations must offer and provide language assistance services at no cost to each patient
and consumer in a timely manner during all hours of operation.

Health-care organizations must provide written notices of their patient rights in their patients' preferred
language, both verbal and written.

Health-care organizations must ensure that interpreters and bilingual staff are competent to provide
language assistance services. Family and friends of patients should not be used to provide
interpretation services (except at the request of the patient or consumer).

Health-care organizations must make available patient-related materials and signage in the common
languages of groups represented in the service area.

Organizational Supports for Cultural Competence Themes

Health-care organizations' strategic plans should have clear goals, policies, operational plans, and
management accountability or oversight mechanisms to provide culturally and linguistically
appropriate services.

Health-care organizations should conduct initial and ongoing organizational self-assessments of CLAS
and related services.

Health-care organizations should ensure that data on the individual patient's or consumer's race,
ethnicity, and spoken and written languages are collected in health records, integrated into the
organization's management information systems, and periodically updated.

Health-care organizations should maintain a current demographic, cultural, and epidemiological profile of
the community to accurately conduct program planning.

Health-care organizations should develop participatory, collaborative partnerships with communities
using both formal and informal mechanisms that facilitate community and patient involvement.

Health-care organizations should ensure that conflict and grievance resolution processes are culturally
and linguistically sensitive, with a proactive stance to identify, prevent, and resolve cross-cultural
conflicts or complaints by patients and consumers.

Health-care organizations should inform the public of their progress and successful innovations in
implementing CLAS standards and should provide public notice in their communities about the
availability of this information.

SOURCE: Ross (2001).

mindedness, respect for individual differences, willingness and readiness to
learn, effective communication skills, nonjudgmental practices, and creativity (Grossman, 1994). In addition to these personal skills, Orlandi (1992)

proposed a three-stage process for cultural competence development. The three stages consist of cultural incompetence, cultural sensitivity, and cultural competence. Each stage consists of four dimensions: cognitive, affective, psychomotor, and overall effect.

Campinha-Bacote et al. (1996) proposed another model that provides some explanation for the development of cultural competence. The components of this model are cultural awareness, cultural knowledge, cultural skill, and cultural encounter. Cultural awareness is being conscious of, having an appreciation for, and being sensitive to another individual's values, beliefs, practices, lifestyles, and problem-solving strategies. Cultural knowledge is a critical element for multiculturalism. It involves learning about another individual's culture from both the etic and emic perspectives. The emic perspective can be accomplished by an outsider through an acculturation process of living within the culture and adopting specific cultural values and norms. The third component of this model is cultural skill. Cultural skill is the cumulative synthesis and integration of cultural awareness and cultural knowledge in public health practice with the purpose of meeting the individual's needs. The final component of this model is cultural encounter. The cultural encounter extends cultural skill to all levels of public health care provided. Cultural encounter is the ability to provide culturally competent care in all public health interactions.

The model proposed by Campinha-Bacote et al. outlines the various stages through which the public health provider progresses in the development of cultural competency skills. In today's multicultural society, public health practitioners are expected to be culturally competent early in their professional career. To provide a culturally competent public health workforce, public health curriculums should include cultural competence as a theme.

The Cultural Competence Training Model

The curricular themes of cultural information and cultural competency skills should span the entire educational curriculum as a common concept for public health-care providers. Berlin and Fowkes (1983) proposed LEARN (*l*isten to the patient, *e*xplain your perceptions, *a*cknowledge differences, *r*ecommend treatment, *n*egotiate an agreement) as a model with which to train physicians in cultural competency skills. This model is simple but can assist in creating that cultural consciousness that is recommended for all public health providers. Table 9.3 presents the LEARN model.

Organizational Linguistic Competence

Language tranfers information and transmits the essence of an individual's culture throughout generations. The spoken and written word provides

Table 9.3   The LEARN Model

Listen to the patient's perception of the problem with sympathy and understanding.

Explain your perceptions of the problem and your treatment plan.

Acknowledge and discuss differences and similarities between your perceptions and the client's.

Recommend treatment that is within the client's cultural parameters.

Negotiate an agreement for treatment that is consistent with the client's cultural framework.

SOURCE: Berlin and Fowkes (1983).

Table 9.4   Public Health Organization Linguistic Competence Checklist

Does your organization have....
- A mission statement that articulates principles, rationale, and values regarding linguistic and culturally competent services
- Policies and procedures that support recruitment, hiring, and retention to achieve a diverse and linguistically competent staff
- Position descriptions and personal performance measures that include skills related to linguistic competence
- Policies and resources that support in-service training or professional development related to linguistic competence
- Polices, procedures, and fiscal planning that ensure the availability of translation and interpretation services
- Policies and procedures that evaluate the quality and appropriateness of interpretation and translation services
- Polices and procedures that evaluate populations' satisfaction with interpretation and translation services
- Policies and procedures regarding the translation of patient information materials and forms (such as consent forms, educational materials) that meet populations' literacy needs
- Policies and resources that support community outreach initiatives for individuals with limited English proficiency
- Policies and procedures that support the review of demographic surveillance data to assess trends and needs for interpretation and translation services

SOURCE: National Center for Cultural Competence (2001).

public health practitioners with a means of understanding cultural expressions and behaviors. Individual language expression is a part of cultural competency skills. Linguistic competence is one antecedent for cultural competence. As a means of providing culturally competent care, public health organizations must focus on linguistic competence as one component of cultural competence. This kind of communication can occur through individuals having bilingual ability, through translation, or through interpretation.

Translation refers to the conversion of written materials from one language into another language. Interpretation consists of the oral restating in one language by an individual with bilingual ability of what was said in another language (National Center for Cultural Competence, 2001). The

National Center for Cultural Competence provides a checklist of 10 areas that an organization can use to assess its linguistic competence. Table 9.4 presents a linguistic competence checklist that can be used by public health organizations.

Summary

Key issues in cultural competence are as follows.

- Culture is defined as an integral pattern of shared traditions and human behavior that includes the history, folklore, thought, communication (language), actions, customs, beliefs, and values of a group of people in a population.
- The emic view is the insider's perspective of what is culturally important to know and believe.
- The etic view is an outsider's perspective on and views of a specific culture.
- Community-based transcultural nursing is the creative use of transcultural nursing concepts, principles, research, knowledge, and practices that focus on large overall designated communities or geographic contexts so that culturally competent nursing care may be provided.
- Macrocultures are the larger cultural designations.
- Microcultures are the smaller cultural designations.
- A clear understanding of individuals and groups within a population is necessary to adequately develop and plan public health programs for culturally diverse populations.
- Cultural assessment should be integrated into the development of community-level interventions and public health programs.
- Cultural assessment provides a contextual understanding of an individual or group's values, beliefs, and behaviors.
- Six cultural phenomena that provide information on the organization of a population's cultural values, beliefs, and behaviors are environmental control; biological variation; social organization; and communication, space, and time orientations.
- Seven cultural components of a cultural assessment are family and kinship systems; social life; political systems; language and traditions; worldview, value orientation, and cultural norms; religion; and health beliefs and practices.
- Cultural competence is described as an acceptance of and respect for difference, a continuing self-assessment regarding culture, a regard for and attention to the dynamics of difference, engagement in ongoing development of cultural knowledge, and resources and flexibility within service models to work toward better meeting the needs of minority populations.

- A culturally competent organization is an entity that transforms differences among various groups of people into standards, policies, and practices that are effectively integrated to accomplish the organization's mission and goals.
- The five essential principles that are considered to define the model of cultural competence are valuing diversity, conducting a cultural self-assessment, understanding the dynamics of differences, institutionalizing cultural knowledge, and adapting to diversity.
- Cultural and linguistic competence is described as the congruence between attitudes, behaviors, and policies that exists within individual health-care professionals, systems, or organizations that promotes effectiveness in cross-cultural situations.
- The three themes of CLAS standards are culturally competent care, language access services, and organizational supports for cultural competence.
- The maintenance of cultural competence is an ongoing process that consists of life-long cultural learning.
- Skills necessary for cultural competence are self-awareness, open mindedness, respect for individual differences, willingness and readiness to learn, effective communication skills, nonjudgmental practices, and creativity.
- The three-stage process for cultural competence development consists of cultural incompetence, cultural sensitivity, and cultural competence.

References

American Association of Nurses Expert Panel on Culturally Competent Health Care. (1992). Culturally competent health care. *Nursing Outlook, 40,* 277-283.

Berlin, E., & Fowkes, W. (1983). A teaching framework for cross-cultural health care. *Western Journal of Medicine, 139,* 934-938.

Boyle, J. (1995). Alterations in lifestyle: Transcultural concepts in chronic illness. In M. Andrews & J. Boyle (Eds.), *Transcultural concepts in nursing care* (2nd ed., pp. 237-252). Philadelphia, PA: Lippincott.

Brownlee, T. (2003). Building culturally competent organizations. *The Community Tool Box.* Retrieved June 13, 2003, from http://ctb.lsi.ukans.edu/tools/EN/sub_section_main_1176.htm.

Campinha-Bacote, J., Yahle, T., & Langenkamp, M. (1996). The challenge of cultural diversity for nurse educators. *Journal of Continuing Education in Nursing, 27,* 59-64.

Giger, J., & Davidhizar, R. (1999). *Transcultural nursing: Assessment and intervention* (3rd ed.). St. Louis, MO: Mosby.

Grossman, D. (1994). Enhancing your cultural competence. *American Journal of Nursing, 94*(7), 58-62.

Leininger, M. (2001). Transcultural nursing care in the community. In K. Lundy & S. Janes (Eds.), *Community health nursing: Caring for the public's health* (pp. 218-233). Boston, MA: Jones and Bartlett.

National Center for Cultural Competence. (2001, January). Linguistic competence in primary health care delivery systems: Implications for policy. *Policy Brief,* p. 2.

National Center for Mental Health Services and Substance Abuse & Mental Health Services Administration. (2000). *Cultural competence standards.* Washington, DC: Department of Health and Human Services.

Office of Minority Health. (2001). *Assuring cultural competence in health care: Recommendations for national standards and an outcomes-focused research agenda.* Retrieved June 13, 2003, from http://www.omhrc.gov/CLAS/cultural1a.htm

Orlandi, M. (1992). *Cultural competence for evaluators.* Washington, DC: Department of Health and Human Services.

Ross, H. (2001, February/March). Office of Minority Health publishes final standards for cultural and linguistic competence. *Closing the Gap: A Newsletter of the Office of Minority Health,* pp. 1-3.

10

Community Development

Community development is the catalyst needed to create community-level change. Effective community development creates a competent community that assists public health nurses in promoting the public's health by meeting the community's needs. This chapter focuses on providing a community development paradigm, describing the concept of community organization and models and strategies to effect community development, discusses community change models, and concludes with a community competence framework.

Introduction

Promoting the health of a community is a mechanism to affect the public's health. Public health nurses focus on the provision of health-care services to a population of individuals that exists within a defined community, whether the community is a geopolitical or common-interest community. New paradigmatic approaches to community-based and population-based public health practice focus on increasing a community's competence as a means of ensuring that public health needs and the nation's Healthy People 2010 objectives are achieved.

A Community Development Paradigm

The greatest assets of a community are the community members and groups that exist within the community. The current paradigm in public health is the promotion of assets building, with a concentration on mobilizing community members. This paradigm focuses on empowering community members and building organizational capacities as a measure to provide public health services and effect community level change. This change in the public health paradigm is frequently referred to as a shift from agency-based delivery of services to a holistic and community-based paradigm (Veazie et al., 2001).

The community-based paradigm promotes decentralization of public health decision making by engaging community members in all phases of public health assessment, program planning, implementation of interventions, and evaluation. Community members are identified as the key stakeholders in the public health system, with the ultimate goal of community development processes that will develop a competent community. Through community organizational processes, public health professionals maximize the individual, group, institutional, and organizational assets as a means to achieve the community's identified goals. At the center of these public health efforts are community members and community-based organizations that are indigenous to the community and focus on implementing community-level interventions and public health programs that promote the health of the community. In a sense, the community is the object of the intervention and the community's populations and organizations are those intervening.

Community Organization

Community organization efforts are consistent with the community-based paradigm for public health. Additionally, community organization is a means of effecting community-level change. By definition, community organization involves a process that empowers and mobilizes individual community members and groups to achieve the community's identified goals (Swanson & Albrecht, 1993). Bracht (1990) defines community organization as

> A planned process to activate a community to use its own social structure and any available resources (internal-external) to accomplish goals, decided primarily by community representatives. . . . interventions are organized . . . from within the community to attain and then sustain community improvement. (p. 67)

These definitions are consistent with the community-based paradigm of public health. Both focus on community organization as a process that actively engages community members to use their own assets to achieve the goals defined by the community. Public health nurses are challenged with effectively assisting community members to define their goals in a manner that focuses on an identified need and also achieves Healthy People 2010 objectives.

Effective community organization promotes a greater understanding of the community, generates and uses the power dynamics that exist within the community, articulates issues of concern to the community, engages community members, maximizes community resources, and promotes communication within various populations that exist within the community. A critical element of community organization efforts is to accurately identify community issues that are important and relevant to the community members. The community-based paradigm that provides the present context for community organization is considered to be a bottom-up or grassroots approach to community development.

Community organization is achieved through several strategies and interventions. Organization of the community occurs through community engagement, community empowerment, capacity building, and coalition building. These community organization strategies will be discussed later in this chapter. Four models are used to effect community organization: social planning, local community development, social action, and community partnerships. Community partnerships are a model, but also a process, and each of these will be presented separately later in this chapter.

Community Organization Models _____

Three of the four community organizational models to be presented are social planning, local community development, and social action.

Social Planning

Social planning is a top-down approach to community organization. This model proposes that an expert public health practitioner with technical skills implement community-level change. Recommendations for community-level change using this model are imposed on the community rather than defined by or with community members. Using this model, the public health nurse assesses, develops, plans, implements, and evaluates interventions with minimal input from the community. The social planning model is not consistent with the current community development paradigm of community engagement and participation.

Local Community Development

Local community development is also known as the community development model. The United Nations International Children's Emergency Fund (UNICEF) and the World Health Organization Joint Committee on Health Policy (1981) defined community development as "a process designed to improve conditions of economic and social progress for the whole community with its active participation and the fullest possible reliance on the community's initiative" (p. 8). Community development is a bottom-up or grassroots approach to community organization. This model proposes that community members identify their issues, participate in decision-making processes, and determine the community-level interventions needed and strategies to be used to effect community-level change. One intention of this model is to bring community members from various spectrums within the community together to build community competence and consensus through community partnering. This model uses democratic and cooperative measures to engage community members. Engaging community members actively develops the indigenous leadership within the community that will later foster community competence.

Social Action

Social action is another grassroots model. Social action is the most politically focused model. This model assumes that there is inequity or disparity in the power distribution within the community that affects the community's health. An assumption of this model is that disadvantaged or vulnerable populations exist within the community and need assistance with organization. This model focuses its interventions on mobilizing or redistributing community resources from the larger community or society to the disadvantaged or vulnerable community population. Interventions using this model include political processes, advocacy, policy development or change, and redistribution of power within the community.

The Community Partnership Model and Process

Community partnership is considered both a model and process. Bracht, Kingsbury, and Rissel (1999) define community partnerships as a union of people that is focused on a collective action to achieve a common goal. A community partnership model for community development implies that the public health nurse works as an "equal" with the community. The community partnership model assumes that the public health nurse and community constituents will share responsibilities, decision making, and commitment to interventions and outcomes to improve the community's health.

Community partnership as a process consists of the public health nursing strategies used to actively engage community members as active participants in solving community problems. This process focuses on strengthening the community's competencies by building on its assets and capacities through active involvement in community development planning processes and engaging in the implementation of community-level interventions.

Community Organization Strategies _____

Public health nurses use several strategies to develop and organize community-level interventions. The major outcome of these measures centers on the development of community competence. The ultimate goal is the development of community members and groups that can identify and meet their community's needs. Community engagement, community mobilization, community empowerment, constituency development, capacity building, and coalition building will be discussed briefly.

Community Engagement

Community development is dependent on the public health nurse's ability to engage community members and organizations through collaborative efforts, coalitions, and partnerships. This process of involving community members is referred to as community engagement. Community engagement is defined by the CDC/ATSDR Committee on Community Engagement (1997) as the process of working collaboratively with groups of people who are affiliated by geographical proximity, special interest, or similar situations with respect to issues affecting their well-being. Social ecologists note that effective community engagement involves multiple levels of implementation. Community engagement should focus on individuals; social networks and support systems; various types of organizations in the community; community-based organizations; and public policy and regulations at the local, state, and national levels. Successful community engagement depends on the presence of several factors. Table 10.1 presents factors that contribute to successful community engagement.

Successful community engagement occurs through a shared vision and mission with the appropriate mix of community participation, leadership, management, and skills to address the key issues of relevance to the community. The community's ability to use its organizational capacities and community assets is critical to community development. The CDC/ATSDR Committee on Community Engagement (1997) has identified some principles of community engagement that can assist in the achievement of effective community engagement during community development. Table 10.2 outlines these nine principles of community engagement.

A crucial element of community engagement at these various levels is community participation. Community participation is important in developing a cohesive community group. A cohesive community group that has a "sense of community" will serve as the glue that keeps the community engaged in community development efforts. Other crucial concepts of community engagement that facilitate community development are community mobilization, community empowerment, capacity building, and coalition building.

Table 10.1 Factors for Successful Community Engagement

Environmental
- Community has history of collaboration or cooperation
- Collaborating group recognized as a leader in the community
- Favorable political and social climate

Membership
- Mutual respect and trust
- Representative cross-section of members
- Members view engagement as a part of their self-interest (benefits outweigh risks or cost)
- Ability to compromise

Process and Structure
- Community members are stakeholders in the process
- Decision making involves all levels of the organization
- Collaborating group is flexible
- Roles and guidelines are clear
- Sustainability during times of change

Communication
- Open channels of communication
- Informal and formal channels of communication

Purpose
- Clear and realistic goals for all community partners
- Shared vision
- Each entity is essential to the effort

Resources
- Fiscal resources
- Skilled human resources

Community Mobilization

Community development requires the active mobilization of community members and groups for action. Community mobilization means creating a sense of readiness or organization among community members or groups to engage in active community interventions. Community engagement gets the community ready for action and community mobilization gets it into action. Some key questions to consider in community mobilization efforts are as follows.

- Who are the community constituents and stakeholders?
- Is the community empowered to address the issues?
- Does the community have the necessary capacity?

Community Empowerment

Empowerment is the mobilization and organization of individuals, organizations, and institutions that makes it possible for them to influence

Table 10.2   CDC/ATSDR Committee on Community Engagement Principles of Community Engagement

Before Starting
- Have clear purposes or goals for the engagement effort and the populations or communities you want to engage.
- Be knowledgeable about the community's economic conditions, political structures, norms and values, demographic trends, and history and experience with engagement efforts. Be aware of the community's perceptions of those initiating the engagement activities.

Necessary Prerequisites
- Enter into the community to establish relationships, build trust, work with the formal and informal leadership, and seek commitment from community organizations and leaders to create a community mobilization process.
- Acknowledge and assume that community self-determination is the responsibility and right of all people who comprise a community. An external entity should not assume the ability to bestow on a community the power to act in its own self-interest.

For the Engagement to Succeed
- Partnering with the community is necessary for community-level change and health.
- The community engagement process must recognize and respect community diversity. Awareness of the diversity of the community's various cultures must be evident in the design and implementation of community engagement approaches.
- Community engagement is only sustained by identifying and mobilizing community assets and developing capacities and resources for community health decision making and action.
- An engaging organization or individual change agent must release control of actions or interventions and be flexible to meet the community's changing needs.
- Community collaboration requires long-term commitment through community engagement.

SOURCE: CDC/ATSDR Committee on Community Engagement (1997).

decision making and take action. Empowerment is defined as the ability to reach decisions that solve problems or produce desired outcomes (Rich, Edlestein, Hallman, & Wandersman, 1995). Rappaport (1984) simply defines empowerment as a process by which individuals, communities, and organizations gain mastery over their lives. Both definitions of empowerment imply a sense of ability or capability to control one's destination.

Empowerment is considered to exist on three levels (individual, group or organizational, and community) and requires active participation by community members and formal organizations, plus cooperative working relationships. Therefore, community empowerment consists of strategies that promote the participation of community members and groups or organizations within the community and the development of the community members', group's, or organization's skills or capacity to achieve community goals (Rich et al., 1995). An empowered community is a community that is powerful enough to take care of its own needs.

Constituency Development

In political terms, a constituency is a population of voters within a defined community. From a public health perspective, constituency is considered to be a group of public health supporters or consumers of public health services. The public health constituency is simply those community members who benefit from public health actions and the people who support public health services to improve the health of the community.

Constituency building is considered an art and a science. It is the process of establishing relationships among public health agencies and the population they serve, government bodies they represent, and other community-based organizations (Hatcher & Nicola, 2000). This process consists of public health nurses linking community members with various agencies and organizations within the community and cultivating the collaboration of these efforts. Constituency building is active relationship development focusing on community needs.

Inherent in constituency building is network development. Linking together community members, governmental agencies, and community-based organizations creates a powerful network of public health leaders. This network establishes a constituency alliance consisting of developed relationships, communication channels, and exchange systems as a measure to leverage, allocate, and distribute resources and power bases within a community to effect change (Hatcher & Nicola, 2000).

Capacity Building

Capacity building consists of providing community members or organizations with the skills that are needed to sustain community-level change over time. It differs from community empowerment in that capacity building provides skills and empowerment in the facilitation of active community member participation. Capacity building is sometimes considered the cumulative process of community organization strategies. Community capacity is the ability of community members and organizations to effect and sustain change over time and across different community issues.

Coalition Building

A coalition can consist of community members or of community organizations joining together as one entity. Coalition is defined as individuals or organizations grouping together because their collective interest converges on a central and shared objective even though individual members have separate agendas and interests of their own (Berkowitz & Wolff, 2000; Green & Kreuter, 1999). Community coalitions are unifying structures that

Table 10.3   Coalition-Building Principles

- Conduct individual and organizational capacity or assets assessments.
- Create a sense of interdependence and belonging.
- Promote a sense of collaboration.
- Establish a clear vision.
- Clearly articulate the mission or purpose and agenda of the coalition.
- Establish communication channels for information exchange.
- Legitimize the issue with research-based information.
- Develop membership guidelines and criteria—seek diversity in membership.
- Develop organizational structure and operating procedures.
- Determine leadership style—focus on leadership, not management.
- Agree on decision-making processes.
- Develop a plan of action or strategic plan.
- Establish trust among members.

can decrease duplication of services, reduce fragmentation of care, provide better coordination of services, assess community needs, advocate for the community, and evaluate the effectiveness and quality of services. Successful coalitions embrace strong leadership, emphasize community members' concerns, promote inclusiveness, and provide member support and ownership (Berkowitz & Wolff, 2000). Table 10.3 provides some principles for coalition building.

Community Change Models

Community development processes can be used in conjunction with models for community-level change. Community-level change models propose strategies to effect a change in the community dynamics as a means of achieving community competence that results in a healthy community. Three community change models will be presented: multilevel intervention, healthy cities, and social change.

The Multilevel Intervention Model

The multilevel intervention model assumes that an individual's personal environment and the larger environment are important determinants of health. As a result, to effect community-level change, interventions need to be developed based on individual and environmental assessment data. These interventions should target multiple levels within the community—community members (individual level), organizations and institutions (group level), and the environment—and encompass personal risk reduction strategies (individual level); capacity building (group level); and regulation, policy, and environmental control measures (environmental level).

Specifically, a program developed on the multilevel intervention model would have program objectives and interventions targeting each level, such as

- Individual level: health screenings, health education, medical care, counseling
- Group level: organizational capacity building, networking, coalition building, social action, networking
- Environmental level: policy and regulation development, public health laws, environmental controls (Simons-Morton, Simons-Morton, Parcel, & Bunker, 1988).

Healthy Cities

The Healthy Cities model is a global approach to community-focused health promotion and preventive health care initiated by the World Health Organization (WHO). This model is based in the belief that a community's health is influenced by its social and physical environments (Flynn, Ray, & Rider, 1994). To improve the health of the community, there must be multilevel change to improve the social and physical environments in which people live and work. Flynn (1992) labels these multiple levels as individual, subsystem, social connectedness, and community. The individual level focuses interventions on individual community members (personal risk reduction). The subsystem level consists of community groups and organizations. These first two levels are similar to the multilevel model presented earlier. Social connectedness emphasizes interventions that promote the development of interrelationships, communication channels, and networks among the groups and organizations at the subsystem level. This subsystem level is part of the public health system infrastructure development that will assist in promoting coordinated health-care services within the community. Lastly, community-level interventions (e.g., community mobilization, community empowerment, policy change, and mass media campaigns to promote community competence) target the entire community.

The Social Change Model

Bracht's (1990) social change model is based on systems theory. The community is considered to consist of multiple subsystems. In the model, these subsystems are considered to be interdependent social structures that are long-lasting, functional, and relatively stable. Change may be introduced at any level in the system. A change in one subsystem will effect a change in another subsystem because each of the subsystems is interdependent and related. Community-level change may occur over a long period of time, depending on the subsystem in which the change is implemented. Changes in the total community will occur over time due to changes in one

Table 10.4   Community Competence

Commitment	Community members are attached to their community with loyalty and pride
Self- and other awareness	Community members are aware of who they are and how they relate to others in the community and larger society
Effective communication	Community members know the channels of communication and feel informed on community issues
Conflict containment and accommodation	Community can effectively manage conflict and negotiate solutions
Management of relations with larger society	Community members are able to communicate with and secure allocation of resources from the larger society
Machinery for facilitating participant interaction and decision making	Governmental and public health infrastructure permits community member engagement and participation in decision making

or more subsystems. However, the public health nurse can use a multilevel intervention approach and target interventions at multiple subsystems to expedite total community-level change.

Community Competence

The goal of community development processes and measures is to develop a competent community. A competent community has the ability to engage in effective problem solving to meet the community's needs (Iscore, 1980). A competent community collaborates effectively in identifying community problems and needs, achieves a working consensus on community goals and priorities, agrees on strategies and interventions to meet goals, and effectively collaborates (Goeppinger & Baglioni, 1985). Cottrell (1976) identified eight conditions that are necessary for a community to be considered competent: (a) commitment, (b) self- and other awareness and clear definitions of situations, (c) articulateness, (d) effective communication, (e) conflict containment and accommodation, (f) community participation, (g) management of relations with the larger society, and (h) machinery for facilitating participant interaction and decision making. Table 10.4 further describes the essential conditions for community competence (Goeppinger, Lassiter, & Wilcox, 1982).

Community competence can influence the public health systems that exist in the community. To achieve the Healthy People 2010 objectives, communities are dependent on competence at multiple levels—individual, community, and within the public health system. Characteristics of a competent public health service system are (a) coordination, (b) holistic approach, (c) integrated multisector planning, (d) cooperation and collaboration, (e) accessible information, (f) empowered community, (g) advocacy,

(h) proactive, (i) preventive focus, (j) community participation and engagement, (k) ability to problem solve, (l) existence of community constituents and networks, and (m) effective community partnerships (Berkowitz & Wolff, 2000).

Summary

Key issues in community development key are as follows.

- The greatest assets of a community are the community members and groups that exist within the community.
- The current paradigm in public health is the promotion of assets building with a concentration on the mobilization of community members.
- The community-based paradigm promotes decentralization of public health decision making by engaging community members in all phases of public health assessment, program planning, implementation of interventions, and evaluation.
- Community members are identified as key stakeholders in the public health system.
- The ultimate goal of community development processes is the development of competent communities.
- Community organization involves a process that empowers and mobilizes individual community members and groups to achieve the community's identified goals.
- Organization of the community occurs through community engagement, community empowerment, capacity building, and coalition building.
- Four models used to effect community organization are social planning, local community development, social action, and community partnerships.
- Social planning is a top-down approach to community organization that emphasizes the need for an expert public health practitioner with technical skills to implement community-level change.
- Community development is a bottom-up or grassroots approach to community organization. In this approach, community members identify their issues, participate in decision-making processes, and determine the community-level interventions needed and strategies to be used to effect community-level change.
- Social action is the most politically focused model. It assumes that there is inequity or disparity in the power distribution within the community that is affecting the community's health.
- Community partnerships are a union of people focused on a collective action to achieve a common goal.
- Community engagement is defined as the process of working collaboratively with groups of people who are affiliated by geographical proximity, special interest, or similar situations with respect to issues affecting their well-being.

- A cohesive community group that has a sense of community will serve as the glue that keeps the community engaged in community development efforts.
- Community mobilization means creating a sense of readiness or organization among community members or groups to engage in active community interventions.
- Empowerment is defined as the ability to reach decisions that solve problems or produce desired outcomes.
- Empowerment consists of a sense of developing the ability or capability to control one's destination.
- Community empowerment consists of strategies that promote the participation of community members, groups, or organizations within the community and the development of the community members', group's, or organization's skills or capacity to achieve community goals.
- A public health constituency consists of those community members who benefit from public health actions and the people who support public health services to improve the health of the community.
- Constituency building is the process of establishing relationships among public health agencies and the population they serve, government bodies they represent, and other community-based organizations.
- Capacity building consists of providing community members or organizations with the skills that are needed to sustain community-level change over time.
- Community coalitions are unifying structures that can decrease duplication of services, reduce fragmentation of care, provide better coordination of services, assess community needs, advocate for the community, and evaluate the effectiveness and quality of services.
- Three community change models are multilevel intervention, healthy cities, and social change.
- Multilevel interventions target multiple levels within the community, such as community members (individual level), organizations and institutions (group level), and the environment.
- The healthy cities model is a global approach to community-focused health promotion and preventive health care that is based in the belief that a community's health is influenced by its social and physical environments.
- Community-level interventions target the entire community.
- The social change model consists of enhancing the longevity, functionality, and stability of multiple, interdependent social structures (community subsystems).
- The goal of community development processes and measures is to develop a competent community.
- A competent community has the ability to engage in effective problem solving to meet the community's needs.

- Eight conditions that are necessary for a community to be considered competent are commitment, self- and other awareness and clear definitions of situations, articulateness, effective communication, conflict containment and accommodation, community participation, management of relations with the larger society, and machinery for facilitating participant interaction and decision making.
- Competent public health service systems demonstrate coordination, holistic approach, integrated multisector planning, cooperation and collaboration, accessible information, empowered community, advocacy, proactive involvement, preventive focus, community participation and engagement, ability to problem solve, existence of community constituents and networks, and effective community partnership.

References

Berkowitz, B., & Wolff, T. (2000). *The spirit of the coalition*. Washington, DC: American Public Health Association.

Bracht, N. (1990). *Health promotion at the community level*. Newbury Park, CA: Sage.

Bracht, N., Kingsbury, L., & Rissel, C. (1999). A five-stage community organization model for health promotion: Empowerment and partnership strategies. In N. Bracht (Ed.), *Health promotion at the community level: New advances* (pp. 83-103). Thousand Oaks, CA: Sage.

Centers for Disease Control and Prevention/Agency for Toxic Substances and Disease Registry Committee on Community Engagement. (1997). *Principles of community engagement*. Atlanta, GA: Centers for Disease Control and Prevention Public Health Practice Program Office.

Cotrell, L. (1976). The competent community. In B. Kaplan, R. Wilson, & A. Leighton (Eds.), *Further explorations in social psychiatry*. New York: Basic Books.

Flynn, B. (1992). Healthy cities: A model of community change. *Family and Community Health, 15*(1), 13-23.

Flynn, B., Ray, D., & Rider, M. (1994). Empowering communities: Action research through healthy cities. *Health Education Quarterly, 21*(3), 395-405.

Goeppinger, J., & Baglioni, A. (1985). Community competence: A positive approach to needs assessment. *American Journal of Community Psychology, 13*(5), 507-523.

Goeppinger, J., Lassiter, P., & Wilcox, B. (1982). Community health is community competence. *Nursing Outlook, 30*(8), 464-467.

Green, L., & Kreuter, M. (1999). *Health promotion planning: An educational and ecological approach* (3rd ed.). London: Mayfield.

Hatcher, M., & Nicola, R. (2000). Building constituencies in public health. *Journal of Public Health Management and Practice, 6*(2), 1-10.

Iscore, I. (1980). Community psychology and the competent community. *American Psychologist, 29*, 607-613.

Rappaport, J. (1984). Studies in empowerment: Introduction to the issue. *Prevention in Human Services, 3*, 1-7.

Rich, R., Edlestein, M., Hallman, W., & Wandersman, A. (1995). Citizen participation and empowerment: The case of local environmental hazards. *American Journal of Community Psychology, 23*(5), 657-676.

Simons-Morton, D., Simons-Morton, B., Parcel, G., & Bunker, J. (1988). Influencing personal and environmental conditions for community health: A multilevel intervention model. *Family and Community Health, 11*(2), 25-35.

Swanson, J., & Albrecht, G. (1993). *Community health nursing: Promoting the health of aggregates.* Philadelphia, PA: W. B. Saunders.

United Nations International Children's Emergency Fund & World Health Organization Joint Committee on Health Policy. (1981). *National decision making for primary health care.* Geneva, Switzerland: WHO.

Veazie, M., Teufel-Shone, N., Silverman, G., Connolly, A., Warne, S., King, B., et al. (2001). Building community capacity in public health: The role of action-oriented partnerships. *Journal of Public Health Management Practice, 7*(2), 21-32.

11

Community-Level Interventions

Public health nurses engage in multiple interventions directed at the promotion and prevention, maintenance, and rehabilitation of public health conditions within a defined population. These interventions should be appropriately targeted at multiple levels: individual, family, aggregate, and entire community. This chapter focuses on defining community-level interventions; presenting community-level interventions, such as mass media campaigns, small print-media interventions, work-site programs, and school-based programs; and concludes with a description of intervention mapping.

Introduction

Attainment of the Healthy People 2010 goals to increase the quality and years of healthy life and eliminate health disparities requires the collaborative efforts of community members and public health nurses (DHHS, 2000). Public health outcomes related to the attainment of these goals are frequently the result of public health interventions that reduce a population's morbidity and mortality risk factors. An intervention is considered some action that occurs during some dynamic systematic process; it is an action that occurs between two events as a means of affecting the outcome of the second event (decreasing or eliminating the population's risk for morbidity or mortality). For example, an intervention may consist of immunizing a population that has recently been exposed to a communicable disease. The intervention occurs between the two events of population exposure and illness outbreak. The immunization, depending on the communicable disease, can alter the development of an outbreak of the illness within the existing community. Public health nurses conduct multilevel interventions at the individual, family, aggregate, and community levels. Public health interventions are actions implemented to improve, promote, maintain, or rehabilitate the public's health status. Public health interventions can consist of policies, regulations, statutes, or programs that affect multiple levels within the community—individuals, groups, or the entire community. The focus of this entire book is on interventions that are population based in a defined community and that use a multilevel approach (refer to chapter 10).

Community-Level Interventions Defined

Public health principles assume that individual- and population-level risks for morbidity and mortality exist on a continuum. Most people have an average risk of morbidity and mortality. Most public health interventions focus on reducing the risks for high-risk individuals rather than for the entire population within a defined community. A population-based approach to community-level interventions implies that a small decrease in risk in the larger population may have a greater community-level impact than larger decreases in risk among a smaller number of high-risk individuals (Cohen & Scribner, 2000; Cohen, Scribner, & Farley, 2000; Rose, 1992). A corollary to prevention principles is that the quality (or intensity) of an intervention is not as important as the quantity (or coverage) of an intervention within a community (Cohen et al., 2000; Rose, 1992).

The Public Health in America Vision of "Healthy People in Healthy Communities" is consistent with a population-based, community-level intervention approach to public health practice (Public Health Functions Steering Committee, 1995). Population-based care consists of community-level interventions that focus on health promotion and disease prevention activities that affect the community's overall health profile (DHHS, 1994). Community-level interventions are developed for a defined community and are consistent with a population-based care approach to public health. Community-level interventions are defined as interventions that target the majority of the population (at all levels of risk) and have a communitywide impact (Green & Kreuter, 1999). Community-level interventions are consistent with populationwide approaches that attempt to produce small changes in risk across a larger or entire population rather than focusing only on high-risk individuals or groups within a community. Community-level interventions can (a) develop or build community competence, (b) promote collaborative community partnerships, (c) develop community coalitions, and (d) develop individual and community capacity to promote health and prevent disease.

Community-level interventions should be distinguished from interventions in a community. Interventions in a community provide more intensive risk reduction within a defined subpopulation, usually within or from a specific community site such as workplaces or schools. This chapter will provide some examples of both approaches—community-level interventions and interventions in a community—that have not been presented elsewhere

Table 11.1   Principles of Media Communication

- Keep messages and language simple.
- The message should be culturally relevant to the audience.
- The message should be timely.
- The message should occur within the appropriate political and social contexts.
- Use multiple communication channels, with consistent messages and themes.
- Promote interactive dialogue with community—communicate the message, but also listen to community concerns. The message should be framed within the context of community concerns.

in this book. Community-level interventions that are presented throughout this book are coalition building, constituency building, public health law, public health policy, public health marketing, community leadership, and environmental interventions.

Mass Media Campaign

Communication is an essential intervention underlying most public health interventions. Hirano and Christensen (2001) suggest five roles for communication in public health practice: (a) increase service utilization, (b) promote healthier lifestyles, (c) improve organizational performance, (d) inform and support health policies, and (e) promote effective emergency management. These roles are based on principles of effective communication. Table 11.1 outlines the principles of effective communication (Hirano & Christensen, 2001). Effective communication occurs through media-related, community-level interventions. For our purposes, media may be defined as the channels or pathways by which a public health message reaches community members. These channels are merely the method or route by which the communication occurs—visual, auditory, or written. Media channels can be differentiated based on the following characteristics: (a) extent to which specific subpopulations are targeted, (b) senses affected, (c) size and characteristics of the populations reached, (d) ability of message to be repeated, (e) message length and duration, (f) opportunity for message feedback, (g) amount of control over receiver, (h) type of message coding, and (i) power of message preservation (McGuire, 1981; Schramm, 1982).

Mass media are communication channels designed to reach large segments of a population (Bracht, 1990). Mass media can serve as the primary intervention, complement other interventions, or serve as a collaborative strategy in the recruitment and promotion of services and programs. Mass media campaigns can be used to build community constituencies and promote public health program visibility. To integrate mass media interventions into a community-level intervention, Bracht proposes the following process:

Table 11.2   Media Collaboration Strategies

- Identify gatekeepers to communication channels.
- Match message with media priorities.
- Develop relationship with media gatekeeper.
- Involve media in message planning.
- Plan the use of multiple media communication channels over time using several departments in the media organization.
- Advocate with the media on priority health issues for the community.
- Educate the media about health information.
- Provide media personnel with access to background information on issues and policies.
- Monitor content of media message and provide feedback to media organization on mass media campaign.
- Provide media organization with an articulate and competent public health professional.

1. Conduct a media resource assessment.

2. Analyze the role of media organizations in the community.

3. Determine the role of mass media in public health programs.

4. Implement a mass media–based intervention.

5. Evaluate the mass media intervention.

The media resource assessment identifies existing communication opportunities in the community, media gatekeepers, and opportunities for opening new communication channels. Specific media resources assessed are news media, newspapers, television, radio, billboards, public forums, and local publications. Each media organization's mission, purpose, and media communication style should be assessed. Through this assessment, the mass media organization's role in public health programs should be determined. A determination of congruence between the mass media message and the appropriateness of the mass media organization is critical to releasing the message through the organization. Collaboration with mass media sources can be promoted through several measures. Table 11.2 proposes measures to increase media collaboration (Helvie, 1998). Interactions with the media are frequently intense and can create offensive or defensive reactions. Table 11.3 provides some basic media interaction guidelines (Hirano & Christensen, 2001).

The implementation of mass media messages through media organizations should be evaluated with both quantitative (number of individuals reached, number of times mass media message is implemented) and qualitative outcomes of satisfaction with working with media and message. McGuire's persuasion communication model is proposed as one method of evaluating mass media communication.

The Persuasion Communication Model

McGuire's (1985) persuasion communication model notes the following stages in reception of persuasive communications: (a) exposure to the

Table 11.3   Media Interaction Guidelines

- Ensure accuracy in message.
- Prepare for interaction with media.
- Be prompt to meeting.
- Answer questions completely.
- Provide relevant documents.
- Communicate honestly.
- Speak articulately and clearly.
- Admit any mistakes.
- Do not say "no comment."
- Avoid arrogance, an appearance of indifference, and incompetence.

message, (b) attention to the message, (c) comprehension of the arguments and conclusions, (d) acceptance of the arguments, (f) retention of the content resulting from content integration, and (g) changes in attitudes. McGuire proposes a persuasion communication matrix, shown in Table 11.4, in which media messages match with each step in successful communication (attention, comprehension, attitudes, social influences, self-efficacy, behavior, and maintenance). The message context, program audience, communication context, and the message source are chosen depending on which communication step is being addressed.

This matrix provides public health professionals with a framework they can use to identify the objectives of the mass media campaign that correspond with each respective stage of communication: attention, comprehension, attitudes, social influences, self-efficacy, behavior, and maintenance. Additionally, this matrix provides a framework that public health nurses can use to identify and correlate message content, program audience, communication context, and message source with communication objectives.

Small Print Media

Small print media consist mainly of flyers and brochures distributed to a subpopulation or an entire population, forming a communication channel that promotes the dissemination of health educational materials within the target audience. Small print media campaigns can be either community-level interventions or interventions in a community, depending on the population level reached.

The effectiveness of small print media is related to the quality of the educational material. Public health nurses are challenged with designing and critiquing the appropriateness of small print media for the target audience. Goldman and Schmalz (2001) provide criteria for assessing the appropriateness of educational materials that can be applied to small print media. Table 11.5 provides a framework for an educational material assessment. The readability assessment is critical to the effectiveness of small print

Table 11.4 Persuasion Communication Matrix

	Message Content	Audience	Communication Context	Message Source
Attention				
Comprehension				
Attitudes				
Social influences				
Self-efficacy				
Behavior				
Maintenance				

Table 11.5 Educational Material Assessment

- What is the intended audience?
- What is the purpose or objective of the material?
- What is the major theme or message?
- Will the material appeal to the intended audience?
- Is the information accurate?
- What approach will be used? Is it relevant?
- Is the material organized? Is the campaign organized?
- Is the material complete?
- Is the tone appropriate?
- Are there any indications of ableism, classism, homophobism, ageism, sexism, racism?
- Are the material's physical characteristics appropriate to the audience, to the campaign?
- Does the material have good graphic quality?
- Is the vocabulary appropriate for the target audience?
- Is the material readable?
- How much will the material cost? How much will the campaign cost?

media educational materials. Two formulas are frequently used to assess readability: SMOG and Flesch. In addition to the readability, the type, format, and language of the small print media should be culturally sensitive. Social marketing principles should be used to establish the readability and cultural appropriateness of the small print media.

SMOG Grade Formula

The SMOG (simplified measure of gobbledygook) grade formula involves using three samples from the educational material to be evaluated, each comprising 10 consecutive sentences. Each word in the 10 sentences selected that has 3 or more syllables is counted. The square root of this number is taken and rounded to the nearest perfect square. Three (3) is added to this perfect square number. This number is the readability grade (not the educational grade level). The readability grade is then translated into the educational grade level needed for reading and comprehension of the material. Grades 13 to 16 indicate a need for college education, 17 and 18 need graduate-level education, and 19 or greater indicates the need for professional qualifications (McLaughlin, 1969).

Flesch Formula

The Flesch formula uses a sample of 100 words from every other page of the material. Each sample starts at the beginning of a paragraph. Each syllable of each word within the sample is counted. The average sentence length for each sentence is then counted. From this, the Flesch reading ease (FRE) is calculated. The results are interpreted in terms of readability, using a scale of 0 to 100: 0 to 30 FRE is very difficult, 30 to 50 FRE is difficult, 50 to 60 FRE is fairly difficult, 60 to 70 FRE is standard, 70 to 80 FRE is fairly easy, 80 to 90 FRE is easy, and 90 to 100 FRE is very easy (Flesch, 1948).

Work-Site Programs

Work-site health programs are frequently referred to as community-level programs. However, according to the definitions provided earlier, work-site programs are interventions within a community. The work-site community is considered a "captive audience" for public health interventions. Work-site programs provide an excellent channel for providing targeted interventions. Bracht (1990) proposes the following steps to implementing a successful work-site health promotion program:

- Build work-site community support: Assess norms, culture, and activities and build a work-site advisory board.
- Assess the work site's culture and norms. Identify assets and barriers to a work-site program.
- Solicit administrative support for the work-site program.
- Use the employee constituency in the assessment, planning, and implementation of the program.
- Provide social and environmental support conducive to a work-site program
- Monitor and evaluate the program.

Implementation of work-site health programs provides the public health nurse with an opportunity of affecting a subpopulation with an existing community that is "captive." The impact on the subpopulation can influence changes within the larger community population. Work-site programs that extend benefits to family members and social networks can have a larger impact on a subpopulation of the community population. Work-site health programs frequently promote behavioral lifestyle changes to reduce health risks. Bracht

(1990) divides work-site interventions into three types: motivation or incentive, educational and skills training, and environmental or social social support.

Work-site interventions are motivation and incentive strategies, educational and skills training, and environmental and social support activities. Motivational and incentive strategies consist of health screenings, health-risk appraisals, and incentives for lifestyle behavioral changes. Educational and skills training consist of self-help literature, classroom education, and individual counseling. Environmental and support activities restructure the physical environment (vending machines with healthy food choices, nonsmoking areas) and foster social networks (buddy programs; Bracht, 1990).

School-Based Programs

Categorization of school-based programs as either community-level interventions or interventions in the community remains controversial. The ultimate determination is dependent on the type of community defined, the population considered within the community, and the type and scope of the interventions provided (interventions targeted at individuals in the school or at the school as an entire population). In this chapter, most school-based programs are categorized as interventions in the community unless the school population is considered the entire community of concern. The primary public health provider in school-based programs is the school nurse. A discussion of the historical origins of school-based programs and the evolution of the school nurse role follows.

Historical Perspective

The origins of school health nursing can be traced to the late 19th century in London. School health conditions were so deplorable that a school manager contacted a nursing association for services. The changes implemented by these nurses were so significant that other school districts in London began to contract for service arrangements with local nursing associations to improve the conditions in their schools. During this time period in the United States, it was not atypical for more than 20% of the children in a school to be absent on a given day due to infectious diseases. Medical inspections of schools were conducted primarily to exclude children from school, not to provide health-promoting or -maintenance services. Lillian Wald's Henry Street Settlement services were extended into the schools when Miss Wald agreed to place nurses in several schools as an experiment. The first school nurse, Linda Rogers, a resident of the Nurses' Settlement, provided nursing services for an hour each day in four downtown schools, treating communicable diseases such as ringworm, scabies, impetigo, inflamed eyes, and wound infections and teaching personal cleanliness. The work of the Henry Street Settlement nurses was so successful and the workload so demanding that more nurses were supplied to perform school nursing functions. This was the initial formative link that inextricably bound school health nursing with that of public health practice. The success of this experiment was repeated in the early 1900s in Los Angeles, Philadelphia, Baltimore, Boston, Chicago, and San Francisco; thus evolved the school nurse role and school-based programs as an intervention in the community (Hawkins, Hayes, & Corliss, 1994).

Historically, the school nurse role was aligned with that of physicians who conducted medical inspections of the schools and provided periodic examinations of children. Eventually, the physicians conducted only monthly medical inspections and the nurses assessed the health status of the children on a daily basis. Additionally, nurses began conducting after-school home visits to assess children who were absent from school. School nurses provided treatments using specific protocols and also provided health education. As the role expanded, school nurses continued to provide clinical services within the school but also initiated health education programs, taught home nursing, made home visits, conducted child health clinics, and became environmental activists who addressed issues such as the purification of drinking water (Hawkins et al., 1994).

After World War II, the role of the school health nurse evolved further. As communicable diseases were brought under control by the development of immunizations and improved economic conditions, the role of the school nurse began to focus on secondary preventive practices, such as hearing and vision screening. Health teaching in the classroom decreased the number of home visits. Home visits were then made for the sole purpose of assessing health and safety hazards. By the 1960s and 1970s, the growth of the school population and the increased number of culturally and educationally disadvantaged students contributed to another expansion of the school health nurse role. The expanded role reintroduced home visits and, in some parts of the country, primary care school health models were implemented. There was a return to teaching health concepts in the classroom, and nurse practitioners were integrated into school health programs. Today, school nursing continues to integrate models of coordinated school health programs that are comprehensive in scope. Nurse academicians are continuing to educate and prepare nurses to manage the current and ever-changing health problems experienced in school and work-site populations (Hawkins et al., 1994).

Centers for Disease Control and Prevention Coordinated School Health Model

Schools are challenged with educating our youth to meet communities' established educational goals. School administrators, teachers, and school health nurses are faced with the inextricable link between students' health status and their ability to learn. Smith (1996) postulates that students can only learn when they are healthy and emphasizes that health and learning potential are coexistent and inseparable. School initiatives, frequently referred to as school health programs, are designed to provide services that promote and maintain a student's health status. The CDC has proposed a model program, *coordinated school health*, which provides comprehensive and coordinated health-related programs based in the school's learning environment. The coordinated school health program consists of eight components: physical education; school health services; school nutrition services; school counseling, psychological, and social services; a healthy school environment, school-site health promotion for staff; family and community involvement in school health; and comprehensive school health education (McKenzie & Richmond, 1998).

Intervention Mapping

The immediate evidence of the effectiveness of an intervention is an alteration or change in the antecedents and determinants of a behavior or environmental condition. To ensure an appropriate evaluation that detects these changes, interventions must be constructed based on theoretical foundations and evidence- or research-based data. Intervention mapping is a framework designed to assist public health nurses with effective decision-making at each step in intervention planning, implementation, and evaluation (Bartholomew, Parcel, Kok, & Gottlieb, 2001). Therefore, intervention mapping serves as a blueprint for intervention design, implementation, and evaluation. There are five fundamental steps to the intervention mapping process.

- *Proximal program objective matrices.* Create matrices of proximal program objectives based on determinants of health, antecedents, and environmental conditions.
- *Theory-based methods and practical strategies.* Select theory-based intervention methods and practical strategies.
- *Program plan.* Translate methods into organized programs.
- *Adoption and implementation of plan.* Integrate adoption and implementation plans.
- *Evaluation plan.* Generate an evaluation plan (Bartholomew et al., 2001).

Each of these steps encompasses review and application of relevant theory, inclusion of empirical evidence, and revision with new qualitative and quantitative data obtained from interaction with the target population.

Table 11.6   Intervention Mapping Steps and Tasks

Proximal program objectives matrices	• State expected changes in behavior and environment • Specify performance objectives • Specify determinants • Create matrices
Theory-based methods and practical strategies	• Brainstorm methods • Translate methods into practical approaches • Organize methods for each ecological level
Program plan	• Operationalize strategies into plans • Develop design documents • Produce and pretest program materials
Adoption and implementation plan	• Develop linkage systems (partnerships) • Specify adoption and implementation objectives • Specify determinants • Create matrix or planning table • Write implementation plan
Evaluation plan	• Develop an evaluation model • Develop evaluation questions • Develop indicators and measures • Specify evaluation designs • Write evaluation plan

Table 11.6 outlines the tasks that correspond with each of these steps in the intervention mapping process. Following is a brief summary of each step. It is beyond the scope and ability of this book to present an in-depth summary of this process.

An ecological approach is used to develop the proximal program objectives. In the proximal program objectives matrices step, performance objectives for each ecological level are merged with determinants, antecedents, and environmental conditions. A series of performance objective matrices are constructed. Theory-based intervention methods that correspond with the proximal program objectives are developed in the theory-based methods and practical strategies step. During this step, intervention methods and strategies are produced. The program plan step includes a description of the scope and sequence of the interventions, completion of program materials, and development of protocols for implementation. The adoption and implementation step consists of juxtaposing the proximal program objectives with the matrix created for adoption and implementation to ensure concrete plans for adoption, implementation, and sustainability. The evaluation plan consists of data analysis to determine whether health and social problems have been reduced, changes in behavioral antecedents or behaviors, environmental changes, and attainment of the performance objectives (Bartholomew et al., 2001).

Summary

Key issues for community-level interventions are as follows.

- An intervention is considered an action that occurs during some dynamic systematic process involving two events as a means of affecting the outcome of these two events.
- Public health interventions are actions implemented to improve, promote, maintain, or rehabilitate the public's health status.
- A population-based approach to community-level interventions implies that a small decrease in risk in the larger population may have a greater community-level impact than larger decreases in risk among a smaller number of high-risk individuals.
- Population-based care is defined as community-level interventions that focus on health promotion and disease prevention activities that affect the community's overall health profile.
- Community-level interventions take place in a defined community and are consistent with a population-based care approach to public health.
- Community-level interventions are defined as interventions that target the majority of the population (at all levels of risk) and have a community-wide impact.
- Interventions in a community provide more intensive risk reduction within a defined subpopulation, usually within or from a specific community site.
- Five roles of communication in public health practice are increasing service utilization, promoting healthier lifestyles, improving organizational performance, informing and supporting health policies, and promoting effective emergency management.
- Media can be defined as the channels or pathways by which a public health message reaches the community members.
- Mass media are communication channels designed to reach large segments of a population.
- Integrating mass media interventions into a community-level intervention involves conducting a media resource assessment, analyzing the role of media organizations in the community, determining the role of mass media in public health programs, implementing a mass media–based intervention, and evaluating mass media interventions.
- Media resource assessment identifies existing communication opportunities in the community, media gatekeepers, and opportunities for opening new communication channels.
- Stages in the persuasion communication model consist of exposure to the message, attention to the message, comprehension of the arguments and conclusions, acceptance of the arguments, retention of the content resulting from content integration, and changes in attitudes.

- Small print media consist mainly of flyers and brochures distributed to the target audience.
- Two formulas are frequently used to assess readability: SMOG and Flesch.
- Steps to successfully implementing a successful work-site health promotion program are building work-site community support; assessing work-site culture and norms; soliciting administrative support for the work-site program; using the employee constituency in the program's assessment, planning, and implementation; providing social and environmental support conducive to a work-site program; and monitoring and evaluating work-site programs.
- Students can only learn when they are healthy. Health and learning potential are coexistent and inseparable.
- A coordinated school health program consists of eight components: physical education; school health services; school nutrition services; school counseling, psychological, and social services; a healthy school environment, school-site health promotion for staff; family and community involvement in school health; and comprehensive school health education.
- The immediate evidence of the effectiveness of an intervention is an alteration or change in the antecedents and determinants of a behavior or environmental condition.
- Intervention mapping is a framework designed to assist public health nurses with effective decision making at each step in intervention planning, implementation, and evaluation.

References

Bartholomew, L., Parcel, G., Kok, G., & Gottlieb, N. (2001). *Intervention mapping: Designing theory and evidence-based health promotion programs*. Mountain View, CA: Mayfield.

Bracht, N. (1990). *Health promotion at the community level*. Newbury Park, CA: Sage.

Cohen, D. A., & Scribner, R. A. (2000). An STD/HIV prevention intervention framework. *AIDS Patient Care*, 14(1), 37-45.

Cohen, D. A., Scribner, R. A., & Farley, T. A. (2000). A structural model of health behavior: A pragmatic approach to explain and influence behaviors at the population level. *Preventive Medicine*, 30, 146-154.

Department of Health and Human Services. (1994). *Consensus conference on the essentials of public health nursing practice and education: Report of the conference*. Rockville, MD: Author.

Department of Health and Human Services. (2000). *Healthy people 2010: Understanding and improving health*. Washington, DC: Author.

Flesch, R. (1948). A new readability yardstick. *Journal of Applied Psychology, 32,* 221-233.

Goldman, K., & Schmalz, K. (2001). Tool 1: Deja view: Criteria for previewing educational materials. *Health Promotion Practice*, 2(2), 109-111.

Green, L., & Kreuter, M. (1999). *Health promotion planning: An educational and ecological approach* (3rd ed.). London: Mayfield.

Hawkins, J., Hayes, E., & Corliss, P. (1994). School nursing in America—1902-1994: A return to public health nursing. *Public Health Nursing, 11*(6),416-425.

Helvie, C. (1998). *Advanced practice nursing in the community*. Thousand Oaks, CA: Sage.

Hirano, D., & Christensen, B. (2001). Communication and media relations. In L. Novick & G. Mays (Eds.), *Public health administration: Principles for population-based management* (pp. 457-473). Gaithersburg, MD: Aspen.

McGuire, W. (1981). Theoretical foundation of campaigns. In R. Rice & W. Paisley (Eds.), *Public communication campaigns* (pp. 41-70). Beverly Hills, CA: Sage.

McGuire, W. (1985). Attitudes and attitude change. In G. Lindzey & E. Aronson (Eds.), *The handbook of social psychology. Vol. 2. Special fields and applications* (3rd ed., pp. 223-346). New York: Knopf.

McKenzie, F., & Richmond, J. (1998). Linking health and learning: An overview of coordinated school health programs. In E. Marx & S. Wooley (Eds.), *Health is academic: A guide to coordinated school health programs*. New York: Teachers College Columbia University.

McLaughlin, G. (1969). SMOG grading: A new reliability formula. *Journal of Reading, 5*, 639-646.

Public Health Functions Steering Committee. (1995). *Public health in America*. Washington, DC: Public Health Services.

Rose, G. (1992). *The strategy of preventive medicine*. New York: Oxford University Press.

Schram, W. (1982). Channels and audiences. In G. Gumpert & R. Cathcart (Eds.), *Inter/Media: Interpersonal communication in a media world* (pp. 78-92). New York: Oxford University Press.

Smith, D. (1996). *Healthy children are prepared to learn: School health programs in action*. Austin: Texas Department of Health.

12

Public Health and Community Health Program Planning

Comprehensive public health programs directed at population-based community health needs must be strategically planned. Public health nurses influence the success of program interventions through effective program planning strategies. This chapter focuses on program planning models and program planning processes.

Introduction

Population-based assessments provide the supporting data to conduct program planning. A multilevel intervention approach to community assessment and intervention development can provide a framework from which to integrate population-based activities at multiple levels into a comprehensive program that expands community assets or ameliorates community needs.

A program is defined as a collection of interventions, activities, or projects designed to produce a particular result (Dignan & Carr, 1992). Population-based program planning focuses on "upstream programming" rather than "downstream programming." Programming is defined as the program planning process. It consists of all the processes that are conducted in sequence or simultaneously to develop a program. Upstream programming takes into consideration the societal and environmental context in which the public health issue exists and in which the public health program must be developed. In contrast, downstream programming focuses on individual-level interventions designed to reduce individual-level risk factors (Butterfield, 1990; Steingraber, 1997).

Program Planning Models

Various models offer a framework that may be used to guide program planning. Some of these models provide a philosophical and methodological basis for population-based program planning at the community level. Chapter 10 described community organization models that can be used to guide program planning activities: social planning, local community development and community development, and social action. In addition to these models, the "creating strategic planning" method, the McLaughlin model of health planning, and the four-step planning process will be presented as other models that can guide the program planning process.

The Creating Strategic Planning Method

The creating strategic planning method provides a structure and process that can be used to promote organizational growth and change through program planning. Piercy (1996) proposed this process-oriented method as a way of focusing on the opportunities that exist during organizational transition periods. The approach emphasizes working with rather than reacting to transitional forces that affect an organization during a period of organizational change or transition. The creating strategic planning method attempts to

- Create a vision and priorities
- Build on an organization's assets and strengths
- Determine strategies to maximize opportunities
- Apply entrepreneurial energy and leadership to challenges
- Decide on actions necessary to attain goals
- Create plans that are reflective of the community and constituents' needs and external environmental and internal organizational priorities
- Build consensus and acceptance by the community and constituents (Piercy, 1996).

This model demonstrates a program planning process that occurs in four phases: creative energy, confusion, clarity, and creative action. Creative energy is the phase of program planning in which enthusiasm builds and potential options are generated. The confusion phase begins with the development of multiple complex challenges that emerge during the program planning process. The multiplicity of challenges and solutions creates a hectic and confused period of time when multiple challenges and activities occur simultaneously. Expression of this confusion eventually leads to a breakthrough. This breakthrough is the beginning of the clarity phase. During the clarity stage, the public health organization decides what and how actions will be planned, leading into the action phase. From this phase, the creative action phase emerges when the public health organization adopts a strategic plan to act on an issue (Ervin, 2002; Piercy, 1996).

Piercy (1996) states that the creative model is in direct contrast to the reacting model. Reacting is considered a negative organizational state, driven by fear, with actions that are limited to blaming, idolizing, "should-ing," and assuming. The creative model focuses the organization on opportunities; the reacting model focuses the organization on problems and limitations facing the public health organization during program planning. The creative model focuses on public health organizational processes that result in the development of documents that articulate a vision, goals, and measurable objectives through which the organization can attain its vision. This creative strategic planning method supports program planning as a continual spiral that is an ongoing process (Ervin, 2002). The model uses times of organizational transition as an opportunity to make creative changes.

The McLaughlin Program Planning Model

The McLaughlin (1982) program planning model is outcome oriented. McLaughlin (1982) compartmentalizes populations into groups that cluster on one of the four quadrants formed by the intersection of two axes. The horizontal axis portrays a perceived wellness continuum. The vertical axis shows a continuum of perceived psychological readiness to act on health benefits based on the intention to act. The intersection of these two axes forms four quadrants. Figure 12.1 diagrams these two axes. The four quadrants are used to define community health interventions to be included in the program planning process to affect the population's health status. McLaughlin asserts that the placement of groups within the four quadrants assists in determining the cues to action that need to be included in program planning to affect the population's health.

The Four-Step Planning Process

The four-step planning process is an organized response to opportunities, challenges, or needs facing an individual, organization, or community. This model uses four interdependent steps as the core of program planning: defining, analyzing, choosing, and mapping (Ervin, 2002). Prior to the initiation of these four interdependent steps, the vision is created.

Following the creation of a vision, the defining stage consists of gathering and organizing data from multiple types of assessments (behavioral, public health organizational, environmental, and community). During program planning, new data and data about past responses to the same or similar needs are collected. In the defining stage, preliminary outcome goals are developed, based on desired results by the public health organization or community. The analyzing stage consists of critically evaluating the various data sources to reveal the problem, need, or challenge. The program planner analyzes possible programmatic or policy responses, barriers, and

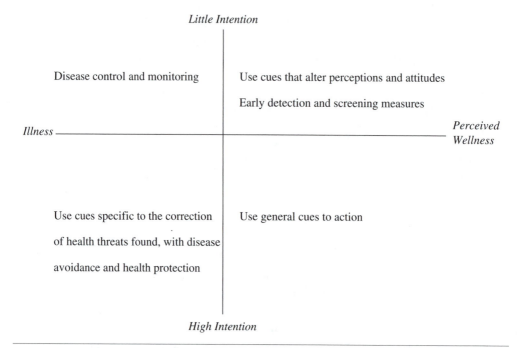

Figure 12.1 McLaughlin Model of Program Planning

resources available and needed. Alternative responses to address the defined problem are evaluated for effectiveness in producing the desired outcomes. Choosing consists of selecting the programmatic activities that will yield the most cost-effective outcomes. The outcome goals are finalized. A time-linked action plan is developed during the mapping stage in which each step for implementing the program is mapped out, with resources and evaluation criteria identified. Figure 12.2 outlines the four-step planning process (Ervin, 2002).

The Program Planning
Process (Programming)

Program planning uses data from behavioral, public health, environmental, and community assessments to determine the current situation and the desired situation for the future based on current, population-based assets and needs. The program planning process proposed here consists of the following steps: need determination, formulation of a vision and mission, program hypothesis, formulation of goals and objectives, program strategy

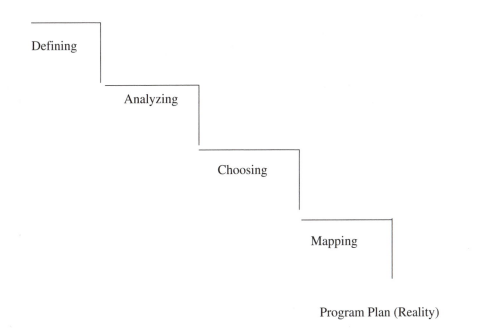

Vision

Defining

Analyzing

Choosing

Mapping

Program Plan (Reality)

Figure 12.2 The Four-Step Planning Process

identification and planning, resource allocation, and evaluation. The program planning process begins with the determination of a need.

Need Determination

Needs are determined through an analysis of behavioral, public health, environmental, and community assessment data. Kettner, Moroney, and Martin (1999) describe four perspectives of needs that drive program planning efforts: normative, perceived, expressed, and relative. Normative needs permit program planners to generate objective targets. Normative needs are determined from predetermined standards, norms, or criteria. Perceived needs are determined based on what community constituents think or feel their needs are. Perceived needs can change with each community constituent encountered. Expressed needs are based on "demand statistics." Demand statistics provide program planners with estimates regarding the number of community constituents who have sought certain types of program activities. Expressed needs are demonstrated through the accurate documentation of people's requests for assistance. Relative need is based on the gap in program activities or level of services provided in one community when compared to the level of similar services provided in other communities in the same geographic area or in comparable communities (Kettner et al., 1999).

Formulation of Vision and Mission

Vision and mission statements are two components of a strategic planning framework used for organizational development or program planning. This framework is commonly known as VMOSA: vision, mission, objectives, strategies, and actions. Simply defined, strategic planning is a process of determining how an organization or program can move from its current state to where it wants to be in the future. The VMOSA framework consists of

- Vision: the desired state or dream
- Mission: the purpose
- Objectives: measurable outcomes
- Strategies: broad initiatives with which to address the mission
- Action plans: the specific actions that will be done, by whom, when, and at what cost

Further explanations of vision and mission statements follow. Goals and objectives will be addressed separately.

Vision and mission statements provide the overarching foundation for program planning. The vision and mission statements of the public health organization can serve as the foundation of the program, or these statements can be developed specifically for the program. Vision and mission statements developed specifically for a public health program should be in alignment with the vision and mission statements of the public health agency and community.

Vision and mission statements define the future directions and common purpose of the program. The vision statement is the desired state or dream for the organization or program. Vision statements provide the "big picture" of the way public health ought to be. A vision statement should inspire motivation and teamwork; stimulate hope; and provide a basis for the mission statement, objectives, and other strategic planning activities. Vision and mission statements are essential to public health leadership (Hesselbein, Goldsmith, & Beckhard, 1996; Nanus, 1992). An example of a vision statement for an HIV prevention program might be "A community united in eliminating HIV infection."

Mission statements describe the organization or program's purpose. The mission statement should describe what the organization or program will achieve and why. The mission statement should be written, preferably in one sentence, as a broad goal that is general and flexible but outcome oriented (Hesselbein et al., 1996; Nanus, 1992). The mission statement should be achievable, motivating, and specific. The public health market (population) should be the focus of public health mission statements rather than products. A key feature of mission statements is their external focus. The external focus targets the broad class of needs that the public health organization or program is attempting to satisfy rather than the product or service that is currently being provided (which would be an internal focus; Donnelly, Gibson, & Ivancevich, 1997). An example of a mission statement for an HIV prevention program would be "To provide community members with comprehensive, holistic, and culturally competent HIV prevention programs."

Program Hypothesis Development

The program hypothesis functions to assist in developing the goals, objectives, program design, and evaluation criteria. The program hypothesis assists the program planner in identifying meaningful objectives and structuring the objectives in hierarchical statements. A hypothesis is considered an "if-then" statement that proposes a relationship between an independent variable (a program or activities within a program) and some dependent variable (the desired outcome of the program or program activities). Program hypotheses are relational statements that link the need to program activities and an outcome that also provides direction for program monitoring and evaluation. An example of a hypothesis for an HIV prevention program would be "If we can identify behavioral antecedents to unsafe sexual practices, and if we can develop interventions to alter these antecedents, then the rate of HIV infection can be reduced."

Formulation of Goals and Objectives

The next step in the program planning process is the formulation of goals and objectives. Goals and objectives should be consistent with the vision and mission and in alignment with the program hypothesis. The program hypothesis provides direction for the establishment of goals and objectives or may link community interventions to the program's broader vision and mission. Goals and objectives are the initial operationalization components of the program planning process.

Goals are broad statements of the expected outcomes of a future situation, condition, or status. Goals are stated in terms that do not have to be measurable but are usually attainable at some time in the future. Goals should be statements of a program's expected long-range accomplishments. Goals should be ambitious and idealistic but feasible (Ervin, 2002; Kettner et al., 1999). Goals are frequently written beginning with an action verb, such as to provide, to establish, to develop, to improve, and to increase. An example of a goal statement might be "To reduce the HIV transmission rate among heterosexual women in the community."

In contrast to goal statements, objectives are statements of expected outcomes that are measurable, time limited, and behavioral in nature. Kettner et al. (1999) state that a "good objective is clear, specific, measurable, time

Table 12.1   Alignment: Vision, Mission, Hypothesis, Goals, and Objectives

Vision

"A community united in eliminating HIV infection."

Mission

"To provide community members with comprehensive, holistic, and culturally competent HIV prevention programs."

Hypothesis

"If we can identify behavioral antecedents to unsafe sexual practices and if we can develop interventions to alter these antecedents, then the rate of HIV infection can be reduced."

Goals

"To reduce the HIV transmission rate among heterosexual women in the community."

Objectives

Outcome Objectives

"By [date], to reduce by 75% the number of heterosexual women 19 to 44 years old in [city] who report unprotected sexual intercourse during their last sexual encounter"

"By [date], to increase condom self-efficacy of at least 100 heterosexual women 19 to 44 years old in [city], as measured by the Condom Self-Efficacy Scale"

Process Objective

"To distribute at least 5,000 male and 5,000 female condoms with educational pamphlets to local venues frequented by heterosexual women 19 to 44 years old in [city] by [date]"

"To recruit at least 100 heterosexual women 19 to 44 years old in [city] by [date] into a condom skills–building workshop"

limited, and realistic and represents a commitment" (p. 97). Objectives should focus on what is expected to change (in behavioral terms) in a population as a result of the public health program. Clearly written objectives assist with program evaluation. Objectives can be of two differing types, outcome or process. The specific results or end expectations of a program are referred to as the outcome objectives. Process objectives are specifications of services provided or means by which outcome objectives will be achieved (Kettner et al., 1999).

Writing program objectives is a challenge for the program planner. Objectives are best written in behavioral terms. Behavioral objectives should include (a) action verbs, (b) a description of the expected behavior, (c) identification of who performs what actions under what conditions, (d) a description of the expected results and how they will be measured, and (e) a timeline (Ervin, 2002; Green & Kreuter, 1999; Kettner et al., 1999). Kettner et al. note specific elements that should be included in program objectives: clarity, a time frame, the target of change, products (process) or results (outcomes) to be achieved, criteria by which the products or results will be documented or measured, and responsibility for implementing and measuring achievement of the objectives. An example of outcome and process objectives is provided in Table 12.1.

In summary, program objectives, both outcome and process, should have a clear alignment with the program's goals, mission, and vision. Figure 12.3 depicts this alignment, and Table 12.1 provides examples. Objectives should also be analyzed for measurability. The following questions can be posed to evaluate an objective's measurability:

- Is the objective specific? What is to be achieved? By how much? Who is to be affected?
- Is the objective measurable?
- Is the objective achievable?
- Is the objective relevant to the program's goals, mission, and vision?
- Is the objective time limited?
- Is the objective challenging?

Program Strategy Identification and Planning

After goals and objectives are established, the next step is to identify strategies and actions with which to achieve program goals and objectives. Objectives provide the overall aim and strategies provide the means to accomplish objectives. Each objective is broken down into specific strategies. Strategies are general statements about how the objectives will be accomplished. These statements are further refined into action plans. Action plans describe the actual activities that have to occur to achieve the objectives (Kettner et al., 1999). The best strategies and activities are generated with inclusion of the community constituents in the program planning. Several techniques are used to generate strategies and actions to achieve program objectives.

Program Planning Techniques to Generate Strategies and Activities

Engagement of community constituents in program planning increases the identification of multiple strategies and activities and promotes program endorsement by community constituents. Program planners use multiple techniques to generate program strategies. Some program planning techniques are reviewed as follows.

Brainstorming. Brainstorming uses a small group of community constituents to provide a large number of strategies. In a brainstorming session, community constituents are encouraged to either verbalize or write down numerous strategies without any inhibitions. Members are initially instructed as to the purpose and structure of the brainstorming process. The purpose of a brainstorming session is to generate numerous potential strategies that can later be evaluated for applicable integration into the program.

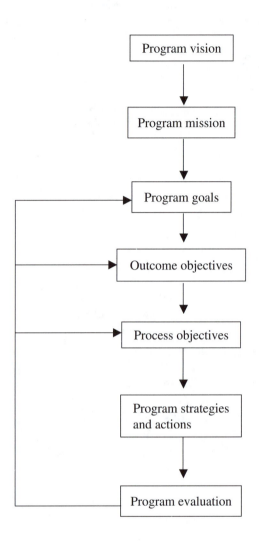

Figure 12.3 Alignment of Public and Community Health Programs

Members are encouraged to recommend as many strategies as possible, without concern for resources, and are also encouraged during this session not to criticize any recommendations, no matter how far-fetched. Brainstorming promotes free-flowing thinking to generate innovative and creative ideas for program strategies.

Nominal Group Technique. Nominal group technique (NGT) uses a small group of 6 to 10 community constituents. The main purpose of NGT is to generate a large number of program strategies in a short period of time. NGT is conducted in the following manner:

1. Community constituents are welcomed and group structure is explained.

2. Program objectives are briefly explained, and silent brainstorming begins.

3. The group forms a semicircle or circle.

4. The group facilitator moves around the group in a round-robin format, asking each member, one at a time, for strategies.

5. Strategies are recorded in summary form during this process on a board, and the number of members who identified the same strategy is recorded next to the idea.

6. The round-robin generation of ideas and voting continues until no new strategies are identified.

7. Any unclear statements are clarified.

8. Each member votes on the posted items, either by rank-ordering them or by selecting the top three.

9. Members are given a break while the voting is tallied.

10. The group is reconvened, and the results are disseminated.

11. The floor is opened for discussion and further prioritization of strategies (Witkin & Altschuld, 1995).

Delphi Process. The Delphi process is a set of procedures that uses an iterative survey over time with the same panel of experts to generate ideas or strategies. This process is also used in research to generate consensus from a group of national experts, frequently on research priorities. The process can be used to generate recommendations for program strategies from experts who are knowledgeable about the current state of science regarding the respective community need. The Delphi process consists of (a) determining the purpose of the Delphi process; (b) identifying a panel of experts; (c) contacting the experts to solicit participation; (d) developing a survey that requests program strategies to be identified that are consistent with the program vision, mission, goals, and objectives; (e) sending the survey to the expert panel (round 1); (f) collecting surveys and analyzing data from round 1; (g) structuring a scaled survey based on recommended strategies identified from the round 1 survey results; (h) sending the scaled survey to the expert panel (round 2); (i) collecting surveys and analyzing data from round 2; and (j) continuing the process of structuring scaled surveys and surveying the expert panel until the recommended strategies are repeated (iterated) by the panel of experts (Witkin & Altschuld, 1995).

Focus Groups. Focus groups consist of a group of 8 to 12 community constituents among whom semistructured to structured interviews are conducted. The purpose of a focus group is to generate in-depth information regarding program strategies. Consensus attainment is not a goal of focus groups. A trained facilitator leads the group through the interview process, focusing the discussion and probing to gain a depth of information regarding recommended program strategies. Focus group interactions are frequently audiorecorded. The audiotape is transcribed and the narrative text is subjected to a qualitative data analysis to generate program strategies. Clarification regarding recommended program strategies can be accomplished through follow-up one-on-one interviews or through a follow-up focus group process (Krueger, 1988; Witkin & Altschuld, 1995).

For each activity identified, there should be a target date for completion; a responsible individual identified; and identification of material, human, and other fiscal resources. Figure 12.4 proposes a suggested format with which to summarize activities' alignments with program objectives and goals.

Resource Allocation

Resources for achieving the program plan should be sought both within and outside of the community. Assets within the community should be promoted to ensure self-sustainability of the program. The program planner should not be conservative in planning the needed resources to accomplish the program's goals and objectives. The program must have adequate resources to achieve each strategy and activity. Approval of program goals, objectives, and activities should be made with full disclosure of the material, human, and fiscal resources needed to achieve the program's goals and objectives. Fiscal and human resource budgeting and management will be explored further in chapter 20.

Evaluation

Program evaluation is a process in which the performance of the program is assessed in regard to its alignment with the established goals and objectives. Program evaluation data are used to measure the achievement of the program's goals and objectives (see Figure 12.3). Program evaluation can be formative, summative, process, impact, or outcome oriented. These types of evaluation methods will be further explored in chapter 13.

Goal: _____

Objective: _____

Action	Time Period or Month												Responsible Person	Resources
	1	2	3	4	5	6	7	8	9	10	11	12		

Figure 12.4 Program Activity Table

Summary

Key issues in public health community health program planning are as follows.

- A program is defined as a collection of interventions, activities, or projects designed to produce a particular result.
- Programming is defined as the program planning process.
- The creating strategic planning method provides a structure and process with which to promote organizational growth and change through program planning.
- The creating strategic planning method assumes that the program planning process occurs in four phases: creative energy, confusion, clarity, and creative action.
- The McLaughlin program planning model is outcome oriented and compartmentalizes populations into groups that cluster in one of the four quadrants formed by the intersection of two axes (intention, from little to high, and health, from illness to perceived wellness).
- The four-step planning process is an organized response to opportunities, challenges, or needs facing an individual, organization, or community through four interdependent steps that are the core of program planning: defining, analyzing, choosing, and mapping.
- The program planning process proposed here consists of the following steps: need determination, formulation of a vision and mission, program hypothesis, formulation of goals and objectives, program strategy identification and planning, resource allocation, and evaluation.
- Normative needs are determined from predetermined standards, norms, or criteria.
- Perceived needs are determined based on what community constituents think or feel their needs are.
- Expressed needs are based on demand statistics.
- Relative need is based on the gap in program activities or level of services provided in one community when compared to the level of similar services provided in other communities in the same geographic area or in comparable communities.
- Strategic planning is a process of determining how an organization or program can move from its current state to where it wants to be in the future.
- The VMOSA framework consists of vision, mission, objectives, strategies, and action plans.
- A vision statement puts into words the desired state or dream for the organization or program.
- The mission statement describes the organization or program's purpose.
- The mission statement should be achievable, motivating, and specific.

- The program hypothesis assists the program planner in identifying meaningful objectives and structuring program objectives in hierarchical statements.
- Program hypotheses are relational statements that link the need to program activities and the program outcome. Program hypotheses also provide direction for program monitoring and evaluation.
- Goals are broad statements of the expected and desired outcomes of a program.
- Objectives are statements of expected outcomes that are measurable, time limited, and behavioral in nature.
- Process objectives are the specific services that will be provided or the means by which the outcome objectives will be achieved.
- Outcome objectives are the specific results or end expectations of the program.
- Behavioral objectives should include an action verb, a description of the expected behavior, identification of who performs what actions under what conditions, a description of the expected results and how results will be measured, and a timeline.
- Program objectives, both outcome and process, should have a clear alignment with the program's goals, mission, and vision.
- Strategies are described in general statements about how the objectives will be accomplished.
- Action plans describe the actual activities that have to occur to achieve the objectives.
- Brainstorming uses a small group of community constituents to provide a large number of strategies.
- NGT uses a small group of 6 to 10 community constituents to generate a large number of program strategies in a short period of time.
- The Delphi process is a set of procedures that uses an iterative survey over time with the same panel of experts to generate ideas or strategies.
- Focus groups consist of a group of 8 to 12 community constituents among whom semistructured to structured interviews are conducted so that in-depth information about program strategies may be gained.
- Program evaluation is a process used to assess the performance of the program in relation to the established goals and objectives.

References

Butterfield, P. (1990). Thinking upstream: Nurturing a conceptual understanding of the social context of health behavior. *Advances in Nursing Science, 12*(2), 1-8.

Dignan, M., & Carr, P. (1992). *Program planning for health education and promotion* (2nd ed.). Philadelphia, PA: Lea & Febiger.

Donnelly, J., Gibson, J., & Ivancevich, J. (1997). *Fundamentals of management* (10th ed.). Boston, MA: Richard D. Irwin.

Ervin, N. (2002). *Advanced community health nursing practice: Population-focused care.* Upper Saddle River, NJ: Prentice Hall.

Finnegan, L. & Ervin, N. (1989). An epidemiological approach to community assessment. *Public Health Nursing,* 6(3):147-151.

Green, L., & Kreuter, M. (1999). *Health promotion planning: An educational and ecological approach* (3rd ed.). London: Mayfield.

Hesselbein, F., Goldsmith, M., & Beckhard, R. (1996). *The leader of the future: New visions, strategies and practices for the next era.* San Francisco: Jossey-Bass.

Kettner, P., Moroney, R., & Martin, L. (1999). *Designing and managing programs: An effectiveness-based approach* (2nd ed.). Thousand Oaks, CA: Sage.

Krueger, R. (1988). *Focus groups: A practical guide for applied research.* Newbury Park, CA: Sage.

McLaughlin, J. (1982). Toward a theoretical model for community health programs. *Advances in Nursing Science, 5*(1), 7-28.

Nanus, B. (1992). *Visionary leadership.* San Francisco: Jossey-Bass.

Piercy, D. (1996). *Day's strategic planning manual for non-profit organizations.* Chicago: CreateNet.

Steingraber, S. (1997). *Living downstream: An ecologist's look at cancer and the environment.* Menlo Park, CA: Addison-Wesley.

Witkin, B., & Altschuld, J. (1995). *Planning and conducting needs assessments: A practical guide.* Thousand Oaks, CA: Sage.

Part IV

Public Health Monitoring, Evaluation, Quality Improvement, Outcome Measures, and Evidence-Based Practice

13

Program Monitoring and Evaluation

Effective program management is dependent on program monitoring and evaluation activities to ensure that program implementation occurs as planned. Program monitoring and evaluation data are used to correct program implementation problems and improve the program implementation to ensure that program goals and objectives are achieved. This chapter focuses on definitions of program monitoring and evaluation; proposes evaluation designs, measurements, and approaches; and describes evaluation models and processes.

Introduction

Monitoring and evaluation of public health interventions and programs are high priority for public health organizations. Public health nurses are increasingly being held accountable to their constituency for their actions and implementation of public health programs. Monitoring and evaluation of public health interventions and programs document the level of effectiveness and achievement of an intervention or program's mission, goals, and objectives.

Local, state, and national public health agencies are mandated to increase accountability and engage in performance-based management through the use of monitoring and evaluation plans. Mandates for increased accountability and performance-based management have resulted in a greater focus on results and outcomes in evaluating program effectiveness and measuring progress toward achieving national goals and objectives such as Healthy People 2010.

Evaluation processes provide data that document the influence and effectiveness of public health interventions on population-based community health problems. These data are also used to measure achievements in the Healthy People 2010 agenda. Additionally, evaluation data are used by multiple constituents in decision-making processes regarding the allocation of resources for and implementation of public health interventions and programs. Green and Kreuter (1999) identify three reasons for program evaluation: (a) to provide elected officials with evaluation data so that they can demonstrate program accomplishments and prove that legislative mandates or administrative policy requirements have been met; (b) to guide program decisions; and (c) to determine improvements in health outcomes that can be linked to a specific public health program, intervention, or behavior change. Soto (2001) adds that evaluation data supports evidence-based decision making. Rossi, Freeman, and Lipsey (1999) state that the purposes of evaluation are to improve programs, ensure accountability, generate knowledge, and maintain and promote political issues or public relations.

Performance Monitoring and Evaluation Defined

Performance monitoring and evaluation processes assist public health agencies to measure the accomplishment of their mission, goals, and objectives; establish performance indicators or targets; and explain a program's successes and deficits. Performance monitoring and evaluation are not mutually exclusive concepts or processes. Performance monitoring should be included as an essential element in the evaluation plan because it provides continual feedback about the program for evaluation. Performance monitoring is an ongoing measurement, providing information about program accomplishments and progress toward the pre-established goals and objectives consistent with the final evaluation process. Performance monitoring can consist of process, output, or outcome measures and processes. Rossi et al. (1999) define program monitoring as "the systematic documentation of key aspects of program performance that are indicative of whether the program is functioning as intended or according to some appropriate standard" (p. 192). Program monitoring involves measurements of service utilization, program organization, and outcomes.

Ongoing program monitoring facilitates the evaluation process. Evaluation can be defined in terms of a process, method, or conceptual approach to data management (Soto, 2001). Evaluation is defined as a process that uses multiple conceptual approaches to determine the effectiveness of public health programs and judge their worth. Evaluation consists of comparing the point of interest (the program goal or objective) against a predetermined standard of acceptability (Green & Kreuter, 1999; Soto, 2001). Rossi et al. (1999) define program evaluation as the use of social research methods to systematically investigate the effectiveness of programs. Patton (1997) gives this working definition of program evaluation: "The systematic collection of information about the activities, characteristics, and outcomes of programs to make judgments about the program, improve program effectiveness, and/or inform decisions about future programming" (p. 23).

Table 13.1   Evaluation Standards Framework: Four Criteria

Utility	Evaluation provides practical information uses for the stakeholders
Feasibility	Evaluation is realistic, prudent, diplomatic, and frugal
Propriety	Evaluation is conducted in a legal and ethical manner with regard for the welfare of those individuals involved in and affected by the process
Accuracy	Evaluation process yields adequate information to determine the effectiveness or worth of a program

SOURCE: CDC (1999) and Patton (1997).

Evaluations Standards Framework

In 1981, a joint committee was formed, consisting of a 17-member committee appointed by 12 professional organizations, to develop evaluation standards. In 1994, the standards were revised after an extensive review. From the individual standards, an overarching framework was developed that consisted of four criteria: utility, feasibility, propriety, and accuracy (Joint Committee on Standards for Educational Evaluation, 1994; Patton, 1997). Table 13.1 defines each of the criteria (Patton, 1997).

Evaluation Stakeholders

A primary objective of the evaluation process is to produce evaluative data that can be used by someone. A person who uses evaluation data and maintains a vested interest in the evaluation process is considered an evaluation stakeholder. The evaluator managing the evaluation process is challenged with engaging the evaluation stakeholders early in the evaluation process, at the stage when the evaluation plan is written. Rossi et al. (1999) identify evaluation stakeholders as program consumers, granting sources or funding agencies, program planners, and individuals implementing the program. Table 13.2 lists and describes potential evaluation stakeholders that public health professionals should include throughout the evaluation process.

Evaluation Standards of Acceptability

Evaluation consists of comparing the data obtained to some predetermined standard. These standards of acceptability define how the point of interest in the evaluation process measures up to the expected standard. The standards provide information regarding the targets that define whether an objective has been effectively achieved. Green and Kreuter (1999) have identified seven types of acceptability standards: (a) arbitrary, (b) scientific,

Table 13.2   Stakeholders

Policy makers and decision makers	Individuals who make decisions regarding the program's implementation, revision, and elimination
Program sponsors	Individuals or organizations that fund the program
Evaluation sponsors	Individuals or organizations that fund the evaluation process
Target participants	Individuals, groups, or communities that receive the intervention or services being evaluated
Program managers	Program personnel responsible for the implementation and administration of the program
Program staff	Program personnel responsible for delivering the program services
Program competitors	Individuals, groups, or organizations that compete for the program's resources
Contextual stakeholders	Individuals, groups, or organizations that are in the program's immediate environment and that are concerned with the program's goals, objectives, and activities
Evaluation and research community	Academicians and program evaluators who critique the technical quality and credibility of the evaluation process

(c) historical, (d) normative, (e) compromise, (f) case example, and (g) model. Table 13.3 provides a definition of each type of acceptability.

Evaluation Designs

Evaluation methods and designs determine the blueprint and method of data collection that will be used during the evaluation process. These evaluation methods and designs will be described briefly. A further description of these methods and designs is provided in chapter 15. Evaluation methods and designs should adequately measure whether a program has been as effective as planned.

Experimental Designs

Experimental designs use the highest level of research design to evaluate a program. Experimental designs compare the results achieved between two or more groups. Three essential elements of an experimental design are manipulation of an independent variable, use of a control group, and randomization. There are many different kinds of research designs that are classified as experimental.

Quasiexperimental Designs

A quasiexperimental design resembles an experimental design with one of the three essential elements not present. Quasiexperimental designs frequently lack random assignment of target participants into one of the

Table 13.3   Evaluation Acceptability Standards

Arbitrary	Program planners or evaluators declare what amount of change is expected (extreme opposite of scientific or best practices)
Scientific or best practices	Research or evidence-based data are used to determine the level of change expected
Historical	Historical performance data are used to determine the level of change expected
Normative	Standards are established based on achievement data of similar programs
Compromise	Standards are developed based on consensus of administrators, researchers, evaluators, practitioners, and stakeholders
Case example	Uses a combination of other types of acceptability standards to study a specific case. From this case analysis, new standards are established
Model	Representatives from multiple agencies or from local, state, and national organizations collaborate on the best practices to determine some model standard based on the best available evaluation data

program's intervention groups. Quasiexperimental designs are not as powerful as experimental designs.

Nonexperimental Designs

There are multiple nonexperimental designs that will be discussed in chapter 15. Nonexperimental designs are typically descriptive, exploratory, comparative, or correlative in nature. Anecdotal reports used in evaluation provide a wealth of information that can be used in nonexperimental designs.

Case Study

Case study involves an in-depth analysis of one specific case. Data are generated through structured or unstructured interviews with program participants or through case histories.

Efficiency Assessment

Efficiency assessments are designs that are planned to measure the cost-effectiveness of implementing a program in relation to some monetary value or in relation to the changes produced (Rossi et al., 1999; Soto, 2001).

Evaluation Measurement

Evaluation measurement is the process of assigning a numerical value to some attribute being evaluated to determine if an acceptable level or standard has been achieved. Program evaluators are challenged with locating instruments that adequately measure the point of interest. Instruments that collect data must be reliable and valid. Reliability is the ability of an instrument to consistently produce the same measure of a specific attribute under investigation (Green & Kreuter, 1999). Reliability is also referred to as the stability of the instrument in measuring an attribute. An instrument is determined to be valid if it yields an accurate or true measure of what it is designed or supposed to measure.

Evaluation measurement produces various types of data: nominal, ordinal, interval, or ratio. Nominal measurement assigns a numerical value to an attribute that is categorized into a mutually exclusive category that cannot be ordered or added, such as yes or no, male or female. Ordinal measurement assigns a numerical value to attributes that are rank ordered in mutually exclusive and exhaustive categories, such as excellent, good, and bad. Interval measurement assigns a numerical value to categories that are of equal distance on a scale that represents equal amounts of the attribute being measured. Ratio measurement assigns a numerical value to categories that are of an equal distance on a scale that represents equal amounts of the attribute being measured, like interval measurement, but unlike interval measurement, ratio measurement can have a value of absolute zero.

Green and Kreuter (1999) note that the final analysis of evaluation measurements determines changes in population concerns or economics. Changes in population concerns or economics are frequently used as measures to assess whether a program has achieved planned goals and objectives.

Evaluation of population concerns could consist of a change in need, reach, coverage, impact, efficacy, or effectiveness resulting from the program. Need refers to a change in the number of individuals in a defined population who need specific program activities. Reach is the number of individuals contacted through the program. Coverage is the percentage of people reached of those in need of the program's services. Impact refers to the immediate or short-term effects of the program. Efficacy is a measure of the impact of the program for those people who acquired program services. Effectiveness measures the proportion of people who received program services for whom the outcome was the intended result of the program services (Green & Kreuter, 1999).

The evaluation of program economics consists of program cost, efficiency, cost effectiveness, benefits, cost-benefit, income, and net gain or loss measures. Program cost is the estimated measure of the total expenditures incurred to implement the program, excluding program evaluation cost. Efficiency measures the cost incurred for each person who attended the program and is also called the unit cost for service delivery. Cost effectiveness measures the cost per unit of impact, or how much it costs to achieve a desired effect. Benefits are described as the general gains to the community, society, organization, or sponsor that result from the program. Cost-benefit analysis is the ratio of program expenditures to benefits derived from the program. Income is the amount of revenue generated from implementing the program. Net gain or loss is the difference between the income generated by the program and the cost of the program (Green & Kreuter, 1999).

Evaluation Approaches

Evaluation approaches define evaluation methodologies for data collection. There are multiple approaches to conducting program evaluation; which is employed depends on the evaluation model and framework used in the evaluation process.

Structure, Process, and Outcome

Donabedian (1996) provides a management framework that can be used to organize the evaluation process. Structure assesses the environment in which the public health program is implemented. Structure evaluation measures the organizational structure; resources and resource allocation; management and staff qualifications; and adherence to policy, procedures, and legal requirements. Process measures the manner in which the program is implemented. Process evaluation measures whether the program is implemented according to the implementation plan and includes the monitoring of program activities in regard to the proposed timeline for implementation. Outcome evaluation measures the level to which the program's goals and objectives are achieved and frequently measures changes in the population's health determinants. Other common measures of program outcomes are changes in knowledge, attitudes, behaviors or skills, morbidity and mortality statistics, and quality of life (Helvie, 1997; Patton, 1997; Rossi et al., 1999).

Impact Objective Measurement and Impact Theory

Impact evaluation assesses the immediate effect of the program on the target population. Impact measurements frequently correspond to the short-term objectives written in the program plan. Impact objective measurement differs from program impact theory. Program impact theory is a causal theory that measures the cause-and-effect relationship between the sequence of events in the program activities and the resultant changes in the target population (Rossi et al., 1999).

Formative and Summative Evaluation

Formative and summative evaluation implies an evaluation process with a temporal element. Formative evaluation is the ongoing evaluation of the

Table 13.4 Participatory Evaluation Principles

- The evaluation process involves participants in learning evaluation logic and skills.
- Participants own the evaluation process through focus and design decisions and drawing conclusions.
- Participants focus the evaluation process on outcomes and processes they consider important and to which they are committed.
- Participants work together as a group, with the evaluator facilitating the group process, cohesion, and collective inquiry.
- All evaluation aspects are understandable to the evaluation participants.
- Internal, self-accountability and a "community first" attitude is valued.
- The evaluator serves as a facilitator, collaborator, and learning resource. The participants are the decision makers and evaluators.
- The evaluator recognizes and respects the participant's perspectives and expertise. The evaluator also encourages participants to recognize their own value and expertise.
- Status differences between evaluators and participants are kept to a minimum.

daily activities of the program. Formative evaluation data should provide a foundation for the summative evaluation. Formative evaluation processes provide data for immediate program improvements on a continual and ongoing basis. For summative evaluation, data are collected with the purpose of making a judgment as to whether the program objective was achieved as planned. Summative evaluation activities are associated with the program's long-term objectives. Summative evaluation measures are similar to the outcome evaluation approach proposed by Donabedian (Helvie, 1997).

Evaluation Models

Several program evaluation models can be used to guide the evaluation process. Three program evaluation models will be reviewed as exemplars. These models were selected based on their congruence with the current evaluation paradigm for community and public health practice. These models are referred to as collaborative and participatory models because they involve the evaluation stakeholders in the evaluation process. Collaborative evaluation models are determined based on three criteria: control of the evaluation process, stakeholder selection for participation in the process, and depth of stakeholder participation in the process (Butterfoss, Francisco, & Capwell, 2001). Participatory evaluation suggests that evaluators collaborate with individuals, groups, or community constituents who have some stake in the program being evaluated (Butterfoss et al., 2001). Table 13.4 presents some principles of participatory evaluation.

Utilization-Focused Evaluation

A basic premise of utilization-focused evaluation is that evaluation processes should be based on their utility and actual use. Therefore, in this

Table 13.5   Evaluators' Guiding Principles

Systematic inquiry	Conduct systematic data-based inquiries
Competence	Stakeholders receive competent performance by evaluator
Integrity and honesty	Honesty and integrity of the evaluation process maintained
Respect for people	Respect the security, dignity, and self-worth of respondents, program participants, clients, and other stakeholders
Responsibilities for general and public welfare	Consider the diversity of interest and values related to the general and public welfare during the evaluation process

evaluation model, program evaluators must take into consideration the use of the evaluation information produced during the development of the evaluation plan, from beginning to end. A primary focus of the utilization-focused evaluation process is on the intended use of the evaluation data by the intended users (Patton, 1997).

Utilization-focused evaluation embraces the guiding principles for evaluators developed by the American Evaluation Association. Table 13.5 lists and describes each of these guiding principles (Patton, 1997; Shadish, Newman, Scheirer, & Wye, 1995). Utilization-focused evaluation does not advocate any evaluation process, method, or model: The evaluation model used is determined by the program evaluator. Utilization-focused evaluation does, however, propose a framework from which to approach the evaluation process. The first challenge the program evaluator encounters with utilization-focused evaluation is engendering the support and commitment to the evaluation process and use of the evaluation data by the identified stakeholders (Patton, 1997).

Utilization-focused evaluation is inherently collaborative and participatory in nature. Fourteen fundamental premises of utilization-focused evaluation are presented in Table 13.6 (Patton, 1997).

Empowerment Evaluation

Empowerment forms the basis for the empowerment evaluation model. Empowerment is defined as "both a psychological sense of personal control or influence and concern with actual social influence, political power, and legal rights" (Rappaport, 1987, p. 121). Empowerment evaluation is defined as the use of "evaluation concepts, techniques, and findings to foster improvement and self-determination" (Fetterman, Kaftarian, & Wandersman, 1996, p. 4). Empowerment evaluation embraces both qualitative and quantitative data collection methods. This evaluation model can be used at multiple levels—for individuals, groups, aggregates, and communities. The model focuses on processes designed to empower individuals, groups, aggregates, and communities and on the resultant outcomes.

Empowerment evaluation is flexible and collaborative and focuses on program improvement (Butterfoss et al., 2001). This evaluation model is

Table 13.6   Premises of Utilization-Focused Evaluation

- The driving force in the evaluation process is the intended use by the intended users.
- The evaluator is continually strategizing about the use of evaluation data, from the beginning to the end of the process.
- Personal factors, personal interest, and commitments contribute significantly to evaluation data use.
- A stakeholder analysis should identify primary intended users of evaluation data.
- Evaluations must be focused on intended users.
- Focusing on intended users requires deliberate and thoughtful choices.
- Useful evaluations are designed and adapted to specific situations.
- The commitment of intended users is nurtured and enhanced by including them in the decision-making process.
- High-quality participation is preferred as the goal rather than high-quantity participation.
- High-quality involvement of intended users will result in high-quality, useful evaluation data.
- The evaluator's credibility and integrity are always at risk. The evaluator should be active, reactive, and adaptive during the evaluation process.
- The evaluator's commitment to increasing the use of evaluation data means that the evaluator will train the evaluation data users.
- Evaluation data use is different from merely reporting and disseminating the results of the evaluation.
- A commitment to use of evaluation data requires output of money and time.

designed to help people help themselves and to ultimately improve their programs. This is accomplished through self-evaluation and reflection (Fetterman et al., 1996).

The evaluation process of empowerment uses a collaborative group effort to assist people to empower themselves through assistance and coaching activities. This evaluation process is developed on fundamental democratic principles that invite all stakeholders to participate in an examination of issues of concern to the entire community. The examination process frequently occurs in an open-forum atmosphere. The key facets of empowerment evaluation are training, facilitation, advocacy, illumination, and liberation (Fetterman et al., 1996).

The training facet demystifies the evaluation process. Stakeholders are educated in the process so that they can conduct their own self-evaluations. This eventually will promote evaluation as an ongoing process. Empowerment evaluators coach the stakeholders as group facilitators during the evaluation process, assisting stakeholders in conducting the self-evaluation. As a facilitator, the empowerment evaluator keeps the stakeholders in charge of their own evaluation activities. In some groups of stakeholders, it is necessary for the empowerment evaluator to conduct an evaluation of the group. Through advocacy, the empowerment evaluator may have the individual or group conduct a self-evaluation, then meet with the individual or group to arrive at a consensus of the findings of the self-evaluation and the empowerment evaluator's evaluation of the individual or group. In this manner, the self-evaluation performed by the individual and the empowerment evaluator becomes an advocacy tool. The self-evaluation process becomes an eye-opening, revealing, and enlightening experience that provides the individual with new insight into or understanding of the roles, structures, processes, and dynamics of the program. Liberation is defined as "being freed or freeing oneself from preexisting roles and constraints" (Fetterman et al., 1996, p. 16). This involves a new conceptualization of oneself or the program, which occurs through the self-evaluation process. This generation of liberated feelings further promotes individual, group, or community empowerment (Fetterman et al., 1996).

Program Evaluation in Public Health (CDC Framework)

The CDC developed the "program evaluation in public health" framework as a continuing commitment to improving the overall health of communities. The CDC considers effective program evaluation to be a systematic method of improving public health accountability through procedures that are useful, feasible, ethical, and accurate. This framework provides public health professionals with essential elements of program evaluation in a practical, nonprescriptive manner (CDC, 1999). Figure 13.1 provides a visual version of the framework.

The CDC framework consists of six steps: (a) engaging the stakeholders, (b) describing the program, (c) focusing the evaluation design, (d) gathering credible evidence, (e) justifying conclusions, and (f) ensuring the use and sharing of lessons learned (CDC, 1999). This framework builds on the four evaluation standards of utility, feasibility, propriety, and accuracy.

Engaging Stakeholders

Program stakeholders must be engaged in the inquiry process to ensure that their perspectives are included in the evaluation process. It is critical to include three principle stakeholder groups in the evaluation process: those involved in program operations, the constituents served or affected by the program, and the primary users of the evaluation data (CDC, 1999).

Describing the Program

Program descriptions include the mission, goals, and objectives of the program being evaluated. Comprehensive program descriptions provide the program evaluator with measures to use when comparing similar programs. A comprehensive program description should include the need, expected effects, activities, resources, stage of development, context, and model logic (CDC, 1999).

Focusing the Evaluation Design

The evaluation design must be focused to address the program stakeholders' major areas of concern and commitment. The evaluation plan

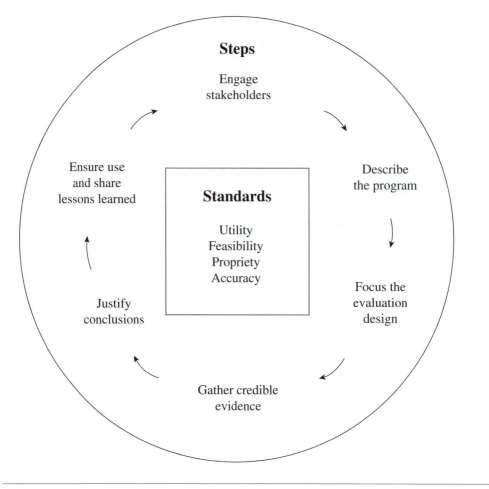

Figure 13.1 CDC Framework for Program Evaluation

takes into consideration the intended uses of the evaluation data and creates evaluation strategies that produce results that are useful, feasible, ethical, and accurate. The evaluation design must consider the evaluation purpose, users, uses, questions, methods, and agreements. The purposes of public health evaluations are generally to gain insight, change practice, assess effects, and affect participants. The users are the individuals who receive the evaluation results and data analysis. Uses are the ways in which the evaluation data will be applied. Questions define the program evaluation boundaries by describing what aspects of the program will be evaluated. Methods consist of scientific research designs and data collection methods. Agreements clarify the roles and responsibilities among all individuals involved in the evaluation process (CDC, 1999).

Gathering Credible Evidence

The evidence that is collected must be credible to the stakeholders. Credible evidence strengthens the evaluation judgments. Participation by stakeholders is also considered a method of producing credible evidence. Indicators, sources, quality, quantity, and logistics influence the credibility of data. Indicators are the program attributes that pertain to the evaluation's focus and questions. The indicators reflect those aspects of the program that have been identified as meaningful for monitoring. Sources of evidence are persons, documents, and observations. Quality of the evidence refers to the appropriateness and integrity of the information (reliable and valid data). Quantity is the amount of evaluation evidence gathered. Logistics are the methods, timing, and physical infrastructure for collecting and managing evaluation evidence (CDC, 1999).

Justifying Conclusions

Evaluation conclusions are justified through their linkage with the credible evaluation evidence collected during the evaluation process. Justifying conclusions consists of application of standards, analysis and synthesis, interpretation, judgments, and recommendations. Standards should reflect the values of the stakeholders. Analysis and synthesis consist of detecting patterns in the data, isolating important findings (analysis), and combining sources of information to reach an understanding of the data (synthesis). Interpretation is the assignment of meaning to the evidence. Judgments are statements regarding the merit, worth, or significance of the evaluation data to the program. Recommendations means consideration of whether certain actions may improve the evaluation process or the program (CDC, 1999).

Ensuring Use and Sharing Lessons Learned

Use of evaluation data is not ensured without strategic measures in place to provide opportunities to share the lessons learned. Planning to ensure use and sharing of the lessons learned must take into consideration the design, preparation, feedback mechanisms, follow-up, and dissemination methods selected during the evaluation planning process (CDC, 1999).

Evaluation Process

In summary, an evaluation process is proposed here based on concepts presented in this chapter. This evaluation process integrates several fundamental concepts and premises of the evaluation information provided.

- Step 1: Engage program stakeholders
  - Program staff
  - Program constituents
  - Funding agencies
  - Community members

- Step 2: Define and clarify the goals and purposes of the evaluation process

- Step 3: Describe the program to be evaluated
  - Program need
  - Program goals and objectives
  - Program activities
  - Program timeline
  - Program resources

- Step 4: Design evaluation plan
  - Select and describe the evaluation approach or model to be used
  - Refine the goals and purposes of the evaluation process
  - Describe the method of evaluating each program objective and identify the concepts to be measured with each program objective
  - Differentiate the program monitoring and program evaluation activities and discern their relationship to each other
  - Select or develop reliable and valid data collection tools
  - Determine who will be responsible for evaluating each program objective
  - Determine the timeline for evaluation of each program objective
  - Define the evaluation standards of acceptability for each objective
  - Determine evaluation outcomes: process, impact, output, and outcome

- Step 5: Collect evaluation data
  - Pilot and evaluate the data collection tools
  - Collect data

- Step 6: Evaluation data analysis and synthesis
  - Analyze data
  - Synthesize the findings

- Step 7: Draw evaluation conclusions and recommendations for program improvement

- Step 8: Disseminate findings
  - Written report
  - Oral presentations
  - Scholarly publication

Summary

Key issues in program monitoring and evaluation are as follows.

- Three reasons for program evaluation are providing elected officials with evaluation data that can demonstrate program accomplishments and meet legislative mandates or administrative policy requirements, guiding program decisions, and determining improvements in health outcomes that can be linked to the public health program, intervention, or behavior change.
- Performance monitoring and evaluation processes assist public health agencies to measure the accomplishment of their mission, goals, and objectives; establish performance indicators or targets; and explain a program's successes and deficits.
- Performance monitoring is an ongoing process of measuring and reporting program accomplishments and progress toward preestablished goals and objectives that are consistent with the final evaluation process.
- Evaluation is defined as a process that uses multiple conceptual approaches to determine the effectiveness of public health programs and judge their worth.
- Four criteria of adequate evaluation are utility, feasibility, propriety, and accuracy.
- A person who uses evaluation data and maintains a vested interested in the evaluation process is considered an evaluation stakeholder.
- Seven types of acceptability standards are arbitrary, scientific, historical, normative, compromise, case example, and model.
- Evaluation methods and designs determine the blueprint and method of data collection that will be used during the evaluation process.
- Three essential elements of an experimental design are manipulation of an independent variable, presence of a control group, and randomization.
- Quasiexperimental designs frequently lack random assignment of the target participants.
- Nonexperimental designs are typically descriptive, exploratory, comparative, or correlative in nature.
- Case study involves an in-depth analysis of one specific case.
- Efficiency assessments are designs that are planned to measure the cost effectiveness of implementing a program.
- Evaluation measurement is the process of assigning a numerical value to a specific attribute.
- Reliability is the ability of an instrument to consistently produce the same measure of an attribute under investigation.

- An instrument is determined to be valid if it yields an accurate or true measure of what it is supposed to measure.
- Changes in population concerns or economics are frequently used as measures to assess whether a program has achieved its planned goals and objectives.
- Evaluation of population's concerns could consist of a change in need, reach, coverage, impact, efficacy, or effectiveness resulting from the program.
- The evaluation of program economics consists of program cost, efficiency, cost effectiveness, benefits, cost:benefit, income, and net gain or loss measures.
- Structure evaluation measures the organizational structure; resources and resource allocation; management and staff qualifications; and adherence to policy, procedures, and legal requirements.
- Process evaluation measures whether the program is implemented according to the implementation plan and includes the monitoring of program activities in accordance with the proposed timeline for implementation.
- Outcome evaluation measures the level of achievement of the program's goals and objectives and frequently measures changes in the population's health determinants.
- Impact evaluation assesses the immediate effect of the program on the target population.
- Program impact theory measures the cause and effect relationship between the sequence of events in the program activities and the resultant changes in the target population.
- Formative evaluation is the ongoing evaluation of the daily activities of the program.
- For summative evaluation, data is collected so that judgment may be made as to whether the program objective was achieved as planned.
- A basic premise of utilization-focused evaluation is that evaluation processes should be based on their utility and actual use.
- A primary focus of utilization-focused evaluation is on the intended use of the evaluation data by the intended users.
- Empowerment evaluation is defined as the use of evaluation concepts, techniques, and findings to foster improvement and self-determination.
- The six steps of the CDC framework are engaging the stakeholders, describing the program, focusing the evaluation design, gathering credible evidence, justifying conclusions, and ensuring the use and sharing of lessons learned.

References

Butterfoss, F., Francisco, V., & Capwell, E. (2001). Stakeholder participation in evaluation. *Health Promotion Practice, 2*(2), 114-119.

Centers for Disease Control and Prevention. (1999). Framework for program evaluation in public health. *Morbidity and Mortality Weekly Report, 48*(RR-11), 1-40.

Donabedian, A. (1996). Evaluating the quality of medical care. *Milbank Quarterly, 44,* 166-204.

Fetterman, D., Kaftarian, S., & Wandersman, A. (1996). *Empowerment evaluation: Knowledge and tools for self-assessment and accountability.* Thousand Oaks, CA: Sage.

Green, L., & Kreuter, M. (1999). *Health promotion planning: An educational and ecological approach* (3rd ed.). London: Mayfield.

Helvie, C. (1997). *Advanced practice nursing in the community.* Thousand Oaks, CA: Sage.

Joint Committee on Standards for Educational Evaluation. (1994). *The program evaluation standards.* Thousand Oaks, CA: Sage.

Patton, M. (1997). *Utilization-focused evaluation: The new century text* (3rd ed.). Thousand Oaks, CA: Sage.

Rappaport, J. (1987). Terms of empowerment/exemplars of prevention: Toward a theory of community psychology. *American Journal of Community Psychology, 15,* 121-148.

Rossi, P., Freeman, H., & Lipsey, M. (1999). *Evaluation: A systematic approach* (6th ed.). Thousand Oaks, CA: Sage.

Shadish, W., Newman, D., Scheirer, M., & Wye, C. (1995). Guiding principles for evaluators. San Francisco, CA: Jossey-Bass.

Soto, M. (2001). Evaluation of public health interventions. In L. Novick & G. Mays (Eds.), *Public health administration: Principles for population-based management* (pp. 324-358). Gaithersburg, MD: Aspen.

14

Performance Measurement and Improvement

Community members are demanding increased accountability and access to quality public health programs. Therefore, it is critical for public health nurses to be familiar with the monitoring and evaluation methods covered in chapter 13. Additionally, public health nurses must be familiar with methods used to measure performance and improve the quality of public health services delivered in the community. This chapter focuses on the dimensions of quality; reviews several approaches, such as quality control, quality assurance, and total quality management; quality improvement measurements and data charts are reviewed; and performance standards are described.

Introduction

The IOM's declaration that public health practice was in a state of disarray in 1988 challenged public health nurses to improve the provision of public health services, albeit with limited resources. The public health system faces multiple challenges to improve the provision of public health services that transcend multiple levels—public health professionals, programs, agencies, and interorganizational collaborations and partnerships (Turnock & Handler, 2001). To meet such challenges, public health nurses must use management tools to effectively and systematically improve the quality of care. This improvement in the quality of public health services must be documented using performance measurements that provide data on the effectiveness of the systematic changes implemented. To ensure that the desired effects are achieved, public health nurses conduct performance measurements to determine the quality of public health services.

Public health adopted the principles and concepts of continuous quality improvement as a management philosophy in the 1990s to address these issues of quality. Quality improvement and measurement in public health practice focuses on *doing the right things right* and *making continuous improvements* (Dever, 1997). Some public health assessment processes that are also quality improvement management tools are APEXPH and PATCH.

Both of these processes were discussed in chapter 6. The current paradigm for improving public health practice is continuous quality improvement and measurement. This paradigm developed from the original processes of quality assurance and quality control, both of which are reviewed briefly. The primary focus for this chapter, however, is on the current paradigm for public health improvement, continuous quality improvement.

Dimensions of Quality

Quality can be an elusive concept. Several management leaders have attempted to provide defining attributes of quality from the managerial perspective. Quality per se has not been defined, but the attributes or characteristics that have been used to identify or measure quality can be described.

Structure, Process, and Outcome

Donabedian (1980) identifies three aspects of quality—structure, process, and outcome—that are necessary to evaluate the quality of public health services. Structure is the organizational structure and resources available to provide quality services. Process is the actual implementation of activities according to an expected standard and plan. Outcome is the eventual change in specific criteria, the expected result of the process.

Fourteen Quality Points

Deming (1982) has identified 14 points of quality:

1. Constancy—creating constancy of purpose toward improving quality by having a plan

2. Philosophy—adopting a quality improvement philosophy

3. Statistical data—decisions are data driven

4. Price—if the need is for quality service, price cannot be the central focus

5. Problem solving—find the problem and continually work on the system

6. Personnel training

7. Supervision—adequate delegation balanced with control

8. Fear—fear of reprisal for negative events that occur must be decreased

9. Barriers—systems should alleviate interdepartmental or interagency barriers

10. Methods—goals are defined by methods of achievement

11. Quotas—eliminate numerical quotas

12. Pride

13. Education

14. Management—support from top management to enforce the previous 13 points

Quality Trilogy

Joseph Juran (Juran & Godfrey, 1998) proposed a trilogy of quality. The quality trilogy consists of quality planning, quality control, and quality improvement. The particular aspect of quality in any given situation is dependent on which component of the trilogy is being followed at the respective time.

The quality planning aspect of the trilogy consists of identifying customers, determining their needs, developing product or service features to address those needs, establishing quality goals, developing a process to achieve the quality goals, and proving process capability. The quality control component consists of selecting which aspect to control, selecting the units of measurement, establishing the measurement methods, establishing the standards for quality performance, measuring the actual performance, analyzing the data, and making data-driven decisions. The quality improvement component consists of proving the need for improvement, identifying the projects for improvement, organizing the quality improvement project, conducting a causal analysis, identifying the causes, taking corrective actions, proving that the corrective actions are effective (evaluation), and providing controls to maintain the effective corrective action (Juran & Godfrey, 1998).

Quality Control

Quality control is conceptually different from quality assurance and continuous quality improvement. Quality control primarily focuses on problem identification and problem solving. The quality control process involves identifying a problem, correcting the problem, and returning the state of affairs back to the status prior to the occurrence of the problem. Quality control merely rectifies a problem without focusing on the improvement of the systems that may have caused the problem (Dever, 1997) or changing the system so that its status is higher or better than before.

Quality Assurance

A premise of quality assurance is that an appropriate public health practice is known. The quality assurance process focuses on identifying any departures from the standards of this known, appropriate, public health practice and correcting the deviations (Bellin & Dubler, 2001). From a health promotion planning perspective, Green and Kreuter (1999) describe quality assurance as the systematic application of audits, checks, and corrections to ensure that the strategies and methods applied, relative to program objectives, reflect the highest possible quality.

In the quality assurance paradigm, the purpose is to improve the quality of care through retrospective assessments of outcomes. The actions of quality assurance are directed at people involved in public health practice. The aims of quality assurance are to solve problems and identify individuals whose outcomes are outside the identified threshold of acceptable limits. Some methods of data collection in the quality assurance paradigm are audits, nominal group technique, hypothesis testing, and indicator measurement (Dever, 1997).

Quality assurance consists of monitoring for deviations from the standard established indicator levels. Quality assurance is an event-based assessment that frequently causes defensive posturing among those public health professionals identified as outliers in the quality assurance assessment (Dever, 1997). An outlier is a value that is outside of the expected range of values or deviates from the expected standard level of indicators.

Total Quality Management: The Continuous Quality Improvement Paradigm

Deming (1986) proposed the idea of total quality management. Deming's management principles for total quality management proposed a flexible, dynamic system that involves all personnel in the production of services that are designed to meet the client's needs, perform as they are designed to, are effective every time, and are constantly being improved (Deming, 1986; McLaughlin & Kaluzny, 1999). The basic principles of total quality management as outlined by Deming are (a) a customer focus, (b) obsession with continuous improvement of quality, (c) continual improvement of systems (focus not on individuals, as with quality assurance, but on the problems in the system that affect quality), (d) unity of purpose, (e) teamwork, (f) employee involvement throughout the process, (g) education and training, (h) scientific approach to measurement, and (i) long-term commitment to quality (Deming, 1982, 1986). Deming also proposed 14 beneficial points and seven deadly sins of total quality management. Table 14.1 outlines these beneficial points and deadly sins.

Table 14.1 Deming's 14 Points and Seven Deadly Sins of TQM

14 Beneficial Points
- Create constancy of purpose toward improvement
- Adopt the TQM philosophy
- Build in quality from the beginning, don't rely on inspection
- Stop awarding contracts based on monetary bids
- Improve the system continuously
- Institute training
- Institute leadership
- Drive out individual-level fear
- Break down interdepartmental or interagency barriers
- Eliminate slogans, exhortations, and workforce targets
- Eliminate quotas and management by objectives, substitute leadership
- Remove barriers to personnel pride
- Institute programs of education and self-improvement
- Make quality everyone's job

7 Deadly Sins
- Lack of constancy in purpose
- Emphasis on short-term profits or short-term thinking
- Management by objectives
- Managerial job hopping
- Using only visible data with little consideration for what is known or felt
- Excessive medical expenditures
- Excessive liability cost

From the total quality management philosophy evolved a paradigm shift from quality assurance to continuous quality improvement. Continuous quality improvement recognizes that the process is one of a continued endeavor to improve (Bellin & Dubler, 2001). The paradigm shift of continuous quality improvement is to continual improvement, whereas the focus of quality control and quality assurance are on fixed goals and corrective actions to return to the fixed goals or previous level of functioning. Chowanec (1994) describes continuous quality improvement as a philosophy and a set of techniques for managing the quality of services. Both the philosophy and the techniques are based in the application of quantitative measures of quality-focused outcomes. Public health nurses must shift their thinking to focus on continually improving public health services to meet the client's needs.

Continuous quality improvement attempts to improve client services directed at public health needs through actions directed at systems processes, not individuals. The aim is to improve public health services continually, even if no problems are identified. The focus of continuous quality improvement is on why something happened, not who caused it to happen, as in quality assurance. Some data collection methods for the continuous quality improvement paradigm are brainstorming, nominal group technique, force-field analysis, flowcharting, histogram, pareto chart, run and control charts, and benchmarking.

Table 14.2 Modified PDCA Cycle

- Identify customers—Who matters?
- Identify customer expectations and professional standards—What do they require?
- Translate customer expectations and professional standards into process and operational requirements—What do they need to fulfill their requirements?
- Decide on measures of both outcome and process—How will we know how we are doing?
- Measure performance using indicators—How are we doing?
- Report results clearly—Share the results!
- Engage staff in drawing conclusions from the data—So what? What are the quality improvement opportunities?
- Pursue quality improvements—Implement PDCA cycle
  - Plan—plan the improved service
  - Do—implement improvements
  - Check—Determine results, evaluate the implementation of the improvement
  - Act—standardize the improvement to maintain quality
  - Analyze—analyze how the improved service is received in terms of quality, cost, and so on
- Repeat cycle

The PDCA Cycle

Deming (1982, 1986) proposed the PDCA (plan, do, check, act) cycle as a process for performing continuous quality improvement. Dever (1997) has prefaced the PDCA cycle with four steps that elaborate on Deming's model. These four steps and the PDCA cycle are summarized in Table 14.2.

The MAPP Model

Mobilizing for action through planning and partnerships (MAPP) is a community-wide strategic planning tool designed to improve the quality of a community's health. MAPP is a quality improvement tool that can be used by public health nurses to prioritize public health issues and identify needed resources (NACCHO, 2002). MAPP is based on broad community participation, collective thinking, and community ownership, and is proposed here as a community-level, population-based, quality improvement process. Table 14.3 outlines the MAPP process.

The MAPP process begins with a lead community agency assuming the leadership role to implement MAPP. During this time, the lead community agency develops collaborative partnerships. This phase consists of a planning process that builds commitment and engages participants to develop a plan. This phase is known as organizing for success and partnership development. The steps of this phase are (a) determine the need for the MAPP process, (b) identify and organize participants, (c) design the planning process, (d) assess resources and secure commitments in memoranda of agreement and understanding, (e) conduct a readiness assessment, and (f) manage the process (e.g., with calendars, meeting agendas; NACCHO, 2002).

Table 14.3 The MAPP Process

- Organize for success and develop partnerships
- Visioning
- Four MAPP assessments
  - Community themes and strengths assessment
  - Local public health system assessment
  - Community health status assessment
  - Forces for change assessment
- Identify strategic issues
- Formulate goals and strategies
- Action
  - Plan
  - Implement
  - Evaluate

Note: MAPP = mobilizing for action through planning and partnerships.

The next phase of MAPP is "visioning." Visioning consists of developing a shared community vision for continuous improvement and identifying shared community values. The vision developed here is the community's vision with respect to quality improvement and not necessarily the direct outcome of the process. The steps of visioning are (a) identify other visioning efforts and integrate all into a coherent vision statement, (b) design the visioning process and select a facilitator, (c) conduct the visioning process, (d) formulate vision and value statements, and (e) keep the vision and values alive throughout the MAPP process (NACCHO, 2002).

Four MAPP assessments are the next phase. The key issues addressed by these assessments are community themes and strengths, the local public health system, the community's health status, and the "forces of change." Community themes and strengths are assessed to identify community members' thoughts, opinions, and concerns and create a sense of ownership. The local public health system assessment focuses on how the 10 essential public health services are provided to the community. The community health status assessment collects population-based data on the community's health status and morbidity and mortality statistics. The forces of change assessment attempts to identify specific threats or opportunities that are present in the community in relation to continuous community improvement projects (NACCHO, 2002). After conducting the four MAPP assessments, the community members should have a good picture of the driving and restraining forces present in the community that facilitate or serve as barriers to continuous improvement.

The next phase is to identify strategic issues: the most important issues facing the community, as identified by community members. The steps of this phase are (a) brainstorm about potential strategic issues, (b) develop an understanding of these issues, (c) determine the potential negative implications of not addressing an issue, (d) merge overlapping or related issues, and (e) arrange issues into a prioritized listing (NACCHO, 2002).

Goals and strategies are formulated based on the prioritized list. The steps for this process are (a) develop goals related to the vision and strategic issues, (b) generate a listing of potential strategies, (c) consider barriers to implementation, (d) define the implementation plan, (e) select and adopt the strategies, and (f) draft a report of the planned goals and strategies (NACCHO, 2002).

The next phase, the action cycle, resembles the continuous quality improvement process. The action cycle consists of planning, implementing, and evaluating. The steps for this process are as follows:

- Planning
- Organize for action
- Develop objectives and establish accountability
- Develop action plans
- Implementation
- Review action plans for opportunities to coordinate and collaborate
- Implement action plans
- Evaluation
- Prepare for evaluation
- Develop evaluation design
- Gather valid and reliable data (evidence)
- Share lessons learned and celebrate successes of improvement (NACCHO, 2002)

Quality Improvement Measurements

Continuous quality improvement is a concept that is consistent with public health evidence-based or research-based practice that is data driven. Continuous quality improvement decision-making is based in the generation of data from performance improvement measurements. Performance improvement uses multiple methods to conduct performance measurements such as epidemiological measurement (chapter 3), measures of central location and dispersion (mean, median, mode, range, and standard deviation calculations), assessment (chapters 5, 6, 7, and 8), program monitoring and evaluation (chapter 13), and public health research (chapter 15). These methods use a variety of problem identification tools, such as surveys, log sheets, checklists, focus groups, brainstorming, nominal groups, and flowcharts, to identify problems for quality improvement and generate the data to be analyzed. These data are extracted from the various tools and analyzed. The data are frequently presented in various data displays and charts, to be discussed later, and compared to an identified standard through a process known as benchmarking.

Benchmarking

Benchmarking identifies the best public health practice in relation to a specific practice and uses this best practice as a standard by which to measure and compare the same or similar practices in the evaluator's own public health institution (Buswell, 2000). There are several definitions in the literature to further explain the process of benchmarking. Naylor (1996) defines benchmarking as the practice of recognizing and examining the best industrial and commercial practices in an industry or in the world and using this knowledge as the basis for an improvement in all aspects of the business. Johnson and Scholes (1993) define benchmarks as key performance targets that should be met in the execution of public health activities. Both definitions provide a method with which to identify best public health practices for use in comparisons.

Benchmarking is an active process of analyzing and comparing a public health institution's data in relation to another agency or competitor. The activity or element benchmarked must be measurable. Yurk et al. (2001) identified some simple steps for benchmarking: (a) define the benchmark and population for comparison, (b) identify the benchmark point of reference (the benchmark from which comparisons will be conducted), (c) identify performance indicators, (d) identify measurement instruments and tools, and (e) interpret benchmark results. Benchmarking is an essential process in the continuous monitoring of performance indicators and continuous quality improvement. A key to benchmarking is understanding the composition of the benchmark and the referent population of the benchmark (McKeon, 1996). Many agencies have selected external agencies or standards from which benchmarking is conducted. The benchmark will change over time as both agencies continually strive for improvement in the delivery of public health services.

Quality Improvement Data Charts

The method of data presentation can affect the level of attention given to the quality improvement data. The data charts selected depend on the purpose of the data presentation, type of data present, and method of conducting comparative benchmarking. Some common quality improvement data charts are histograms, pareto charts, run charts, scatter diagrams, and control charts (Dever, 1997).

Histogram

A histogram is a frequency distribution with the vertical bars on the x-axis and the frequency of the item analyzed on the y-axis (Figure 14.1).

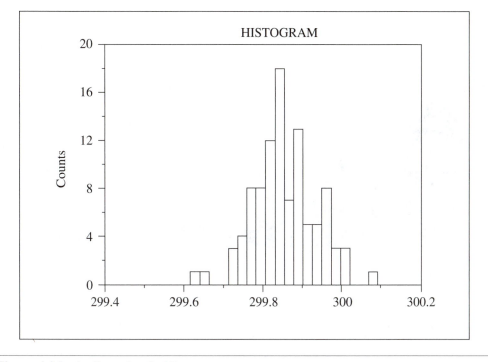

Figure 14.1 An Example of a Histogram

The x-axis usually represents some categorization of the variable under investigation. A histogram could be constructed to compare, for example, cancer-related mortality by age. In such a histogram, the age groups would be on the x-axis and the mortality rate for each age category would be on the y-axis (Dever, 1997).

Pareto Chart

A pareto chart is a special bar graph that presents the frequency of events in descending order (Figure 14.2). The x-axis presents some categorization of the variable under investigation and the y-axis represents the frequency of the item analyzed. The x-axis categories are arranged in descending order (Dever, 1997).

Run Chart

Run charts are a type of line graph. Surveillance data is frequently plotted using a run chart. Run charts present data organized in a time sequence (Figure 14.3). The data are plotted in the time sequence using a line graph.

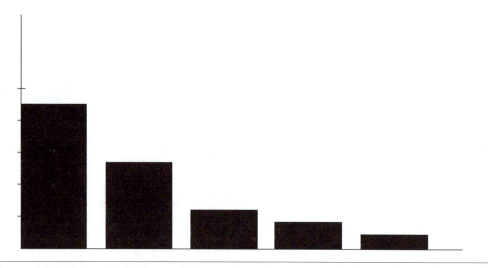

Figure 14.2 Example of a Pareto Chart

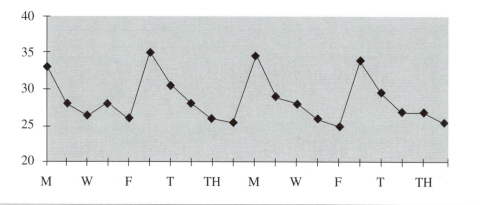

Figure 14.3 Example of a Run Chart

These charts are used when it is necessary to understand the temporal association of events, monitor changes, and detect changes (Dever, 1997).

Scatter Diagram

A scatter diagram graphs the relationship of one variable to another, making it possible to visually examine any relationships that may exist (Figure 14.4). A scatter diagram uses the x-axis to represent one variable and the y-axis another variable so that they may be graphed against each other. From scatter diagrams, the data plotted can visually appear as a positive correlation, negative correlation, or no correlation (Dever, 1997).

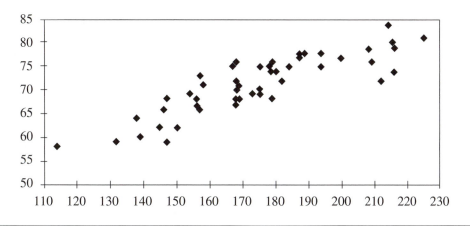

Figure 14.4 Example of a Scatter Diagram

Control Chart

A control chart is a run chart that has a statistically determined upper and lower limit drawn on either side of the data. This provides a visual presentation of what data are within the limits established as upper (upper control limits) and lower (lower control limits) and what data fall outside the limits (outliers; see Figure 14.5). Some control charts also include a center line that may mark the expected midpoint of the data (Dever, 1997).

Performance Standards

The National Public Health Performance Standards Program (NPHPSP) is a collaborative effort to enhance and improve the nation's public health system. Multiple agencies have partnered to develop clear and measurable performance standards for state and local public health systems, to provide guidance for improvement and ensure the accomplishment of essential public health services. The goals of the NPHPSP are to create tools for public health professionals to use in continuous quality improvement, to strengthen local and public health system mechanisms for accountability, and to enhance decision making based on evidence (NPHPSP, 2001a).

Three of the NPHPSP instruments will be discussed: the local, state, and governance instrument. The local public health instrument is designed to measure the public health system performance and capacity on a local level. The local instrument focuses on the local public health system from a broad system perspective rather than from the perspective of a single organization. Local public health systems include all public, private, and voluntary agencies that deliver public health services to a specific community (NPHPSP,

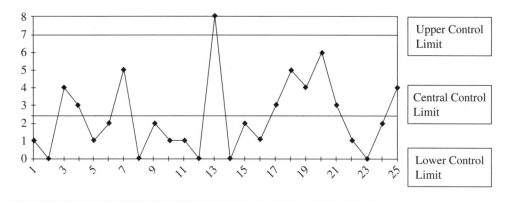

Figure 14.5 Example of a Control Chart

2001b). The state instrument focuses on improvements in the public health system at the state level. This instrument can be used to measure and improve a state's capacity to perform essential public health services, identify the strengths and weaknesses in state public health systems, promote effective communication, and build partnerships (NPHPSP, 2001c). The governance instrument is designed to assist governing bodies, such as boards of health at local and state levels, to evaluate themselves, compare strategic planning initiatives, and compare the effectiveness of the governing body with similar entities. The governance instrument focuses on five core responsibilities: ensuring authority, ensuring resources, policy development, ensuring continuous evaluation and improvement, and ensuring collaboration (NPHPSP, 2001d).

Summary

Key issues in performance measurement and improvement are as follows.

- Public health practice focuses on doing the right things right and making continuous improvements.
- Donabedian (1980) identifies three aspects of quality as structure, process, and outcome.
- Deming (1982, 1986) identifies 14 points of quality: constancy, philosophy, statistical data, price, problem solving, personnel training, supervision, fear, barriers, methods, quotas, pride, education, and managerial support.
- The quality trilogy consists of quality planning, quality control, and quality improvement.
- Quality control primarily focuses on problem identification and problem solving.

- The quality control process involves identifying a problem, correcting the problem, and returning the state of affairs back to the status prior to the occurrence of the problem.
- The quality assurance process focuses on identifying any departures from known, appropriate standards for a particular public health practice and correcting the deviations.
- Quality assurance is the systematic application of audits, checks, and corrections to ensure that the strategies and methods applied, relative to program objectives, reflect the highest quality possible.
- Deming's (1982, 1986) basic principles of total quality management are a focus on the customer, obsession with continuous improvement in quality, continual improvement of systems, unity of purpose, teamwork, employee involvement throughout the process, education and training, scientific approach to measurement, and long-term commitment to quality.
- Continuous quality improvement recognizes that the process is one of a continued endeavor to improve.
- PDCA stands for plan, do, check, and act and analyze.
- Mobilizing for action through planning and partnerships (MAPP) is a communitywide strategic planning tool designed to improve the quality of a community's health.
- In benchmarking, the best public health practice in relation to a specific practice is identified and used as a standard by which to measure and compare other practices.
- Benchmarking involves defining the benchmark and population for comparison, identifying the benchmark point of reference, identifying performance indicators, identifying measurement instruments and tools, and interpreting benchmark results.
- The data charting method selected depends on the purpose of the data presentation, type of data present, and method of conducting comparative benchmarking.
- A histogram is a frequency distribution with vertical bars on the x-axis and the frequency of the item analyzed on the y-axis.
- A pareto chart is a special bar graph that presents the frequency of events in descending order.
- Run charts present data organized in a time sequence.
- A scatter diagram graphs the relationship of one variable to another so that any relationships that exist may be visually examined.
- A control chart is a run chart that has a statistically determined upper and lower limit drawn on either side of the data.
- The NPHPSP is a collaborative effort to enhance and improve the nation's public health system.
- Three of the instruments used by the NPHPSP are local, state, and governance.

References

Bellin, E., & Dubler, N. (2001). The quality improvement–research divide and the need for external oversight. *American Journal of Public Health, 91*(9), 1512-1517.

Buswell, C. (2000). Benchmarking in nursing: Learning from industry. *Journal of Community Nursing, 14*(5):28, 30.

Chowanec, G. (1994). Continuous quality improvement: conceptual foundations and application to mental health care. *Hospital and Community Psychiatry, 45*(8), 789-793.

Deming, E. (1982). *Quality, productivity, and competitive position.* Cambridge, MA: Massachusetts Institute of Technology.

Deming, E. (1986). *Out of the crisis.* Cambridge, MA: Massachusetts Institute of Technology.

Dever, G. (1997). *Improving outcomes in public health practice: Strategies and methods.* Gaithersburg, MD: Aspen.

Donabedian, A. (1980). *The definition of quality and approaches to its assessment.* Ann Arbor, MI: Health Administration Press.

Green, L., & Kreuter, M. (1999). *Health promotion planning: An educational and ecological approach* (3rd ed.). London: Mayfield.

Johnson, G., & Scholes, K. (1993). *Exploring corporate strategy* (3rd ed.). London: Prentice Hall.

Juran, J., & Godfrey, A. (1998). *Juran's quality handbook* (5th ed.). New York: McGraw-Hill Professional.

McKeon, T. (1996). Benchmarks and performance indicators: Two tools for evaluating organizational results and continuous quality improvement efforts. *Journal of Nursing Care Quality, 10*(3), 12-17.

McLaughlin, C., & Kaluzny, A. (1999). *Continuous quality improvement in health care: Theory, implementation, and applications* (2nd ed.). Gaithersburg, MD: Aspen.

National Association of County and City Health Officials. (2002). *A strategic approach to community health improvement. MAPP: Mobilizing for action through planning and partnerships.* Retrieved June 19, 2003, from http://mapp.naccho.org/MAPP_Home.asp

National Public Health Performance Standards Program. (2001a). Retrieved June 19, 2003, from http://www.phppo.cdc.gov/nphpsp/index.asp

National Public Health Performance Standards Program. (2001b). *Local national public health performance standards.* Retrieved June 19, 2003, from http://www.phppo.cdc.gov/nphpsp/Documents/Local_v_1_OMB_0920-0555.pdf

National Public Health Performance Standards Program. (2001c). *State national public health performance standards.* Retrieved June 19, 2003, from http://www.phppo.cdc.gov/nphpsp/Documents/State_v_1_OMB_0920-0557.pdf

National Public Health Performance Standards Program. (2001d). *Governance instrument.* Retrieved June 19, 2003, from http://www.phppo.cdc.gov/nphpsp/Documents/Governance_Final.pdf

Naylor, J. (1996). Operations management. London: Financial Times Pitman Publishing.

Turnock, B., & Handler, A. (2001). Performance measurement and improvement. In L. Novick & G. Mays (Eds.), *Public health administration: Principles for population-based management* (pp. 431-456). Gaithersburg, MD: Aspen.

Yurk, R., Jenckes, M., Stuart, M., Shaffer, T., Lockwood, R., Das, A., et al. (2001). Benchmarking applications: Linking state strategic planning, quality improvement, and consumer reporting. *Journal of Public Health Management and Practice, 7*(3), 47-58.

15

Public Health Research

Nursing research consists of scientific inquiry that uses either qualitative or quantitative methods to answer relevant questions regarding public health nursing practice. Public health nursing research involves the investigation of nursing phenomena that pose a threat to public health and safety. This chapter focuses on defining public health research, identifying public health nursing research priorities, and describing the research process and community-based research partnerships and concludes with a discussion on institutional review boards and grants.

Introduction

The public health research paradigm has expanded from a primarily epidemiological orientation to one that incorporates research methods from other sciences, such as the behavioral and social sciences (Daly, Kellehear, & Gliksman, 1997). Research methods are integrated into community assessments, program monitoring and evaluation, and performance measurement and improvement. In fact, some public health professionals consider evaluation as a type or form of research. However, most professionals view public health research as beyond program monitoring and evaluation (Gadomski, 2001). Public health research often focuses on health promotion and disease prevention to ensure the health of populations. A key element in public health research is defining what public health interventions or programs work most effectively to generate a positive, population-level change in public health.

Public Health Research Defined

Research is often defined as the systematic search for and validation of knowledge about issues of importance to a specific discipline (Polit &

Hungler, 2001). Research is a means of generating new knowledge and providing information that can help to develop interventions directed at improving a population's health. Public health research is viewed as a vehicle for bridging gaps, such as those between basic research and public health practice, between prevention and treatment, and between academic institutions and public health practitioners (Gadomski, 2001). For the purposes of this book, public health research is defined as systematic inquiry or investigation done with the purpose of generating new public health knowledge or validating and refining existing public health knowledge through rigorous and systematic data collection and analysis, using either quantitative or qualitative methods.

Public health researchers engage in both basic and applied research. Basic public health research is undertaken to accumulate information, develop a theory, or refine a theory. The primary premise of basic public health research is the development of a knowledge base for the discipline of public health. In contrast, applied public health research focuses on identifying the effectiveness of interventions to solve a problem or improve public health practice (Polit & Hungler, 2001).

Public Health Research Priorities

Research priorities are identified by an authoritative body or organization as areas on which to focus to advance some defined larger public health agenda. In addition, funding agencies establish lists of research priorities that facilitate the achievement of their specific vision and mission. Traditional public health research priorities have focused on health promotion, health education, disease prevention, behavior modification, and risk reduction (Gadomski, 2001). A move to more interdisciplinary and collaborative research, along with technological and scientific advances, has promoted public health research to integrate basic, clinical, and population approaches with multiple public health practices from different disciplines that focus on specific public health research priorities. Gadomski has identified 12 areas of public health research. Table 15.1 outlines these public health research areas. Community health and public health nursing, as specific disciplines within the public health field, have developed discipline-specific research priorities. These priorities are unique in that they focus on areas of phenomenological inquiry relevant to public health nursing practice.

Association of Community Health Nurse Educators Public Health Nursing Research Priorities

The Association of Community Health Nurse Educators (ACHNE) charged the Research Committee/Task Force on Research Priorities for

Table 15.1   Public Health Research Areas

- Policy analysis
- Disease prevention
- Health promotion
- Social determinants of health
- Behavioral determinants of health
- Bioterrorism
- Health services
- Multilevel interventions (individual, group, and community)
- Environmental
- Communication, including risk communication
- Public health workforce
- Economic development and evaluation (cost effectiveness and cost:benefit)
- Community and population methodologies
- Research sustainability and dissemination

Community/Public Health Nursing with the responsibility to identify a broad set of priorities for methods, topics, and populations believed to be of relevance to public health nursing practice. These priorities are intended for the use of public health nurse researchers, practitioners, educators, students, nursing colleagues in other specialties, funding agencies, and policy makers. The purpose of the priorities is to (a) guide researchers to increase the body of public health knowledge; (b) identify research domains relevant to public health nursing; (c) target interventions to vulnerable, high-risk ethnic minority or underserved populations; (d) support the initiation of programs of research; (e) articulate the unique contributions of public health nursing research; (f) facilitate interdisciplinary collaboration; (g) foster dissemination and application of research findings; and (h) influence policy in service and funding agencies (ACHNE, 2000).

A major focus of research for ACHNE at this time is to explicate and refine research methods for studying aggregates and populations within the topical domains of public health nursing science. The ACHNE research priorities were categorized as methodological research priorities that cut across all topical areas, as well as being topical research priorities. Table 15.2 summarizes the ACHNE research priorities.

In addition to established public health research priorities, public health nurses generate researchable questions from public health practice. Other sources of research are practice experience, existing gaps in research or the need for research replication, theoretical development or empirical testing, and external bodies (governmental bodies or agencies; Playle, 2000a).

The Research Process

Public health nurses engage in the complete research process, which extends from posing a research question to finding the answer to the research question.

Table 15.2   ACHNE Public Health Nursing Research Priorities

Methodological Priorities
- Develop new and interpret existing middle-range theories or models for application to a community-as-client perspective
- Design and test instruments for measuring community-level phenomena and outcomes
- Refine and apply research methodologies for population-focused research
- Examine multifocal and multilevel targeted interventions in ethnic minority, vulnerable, underserved, and disenfranchised populations who are at high risk for health problems

Topical Priorities
- Culturally appropriate lifestyle interventions for health promotion, primary and secondary prevention, risk reduction, and health-seeking behaviors across the lifespan
- Systematic health-care service interventions
- Community strategies to reduce health risks
- Global and environmental health issues
- Violence
- Family care, caregiving, and preventive mental health
- Decreasing disparity in health status across minority or socioeconomic status and other vulnerable aggregates

The research process provides a logical and scientific sequence of events for the researcher to use so that the scientific rigor of inquiry is maintained (Playle, 2000b). Research is classified according to levels, depending on the nature and purpose of the research. Playle describes the levels of research as

- Descriptive—identifying, defining, and describing a phenomenon
- Exploratory—identifying significant trends in data and relationships between or among research variables
- Explanatory (correlative)—examining relationships between variables in a controlled manner
- Testing—testing and predicting relationships in a controlled manner
- Generalization—development of general rules to change public health practice

Public health nurses use multiple theoretical and conceptual frameworks to answer public health research questions and guide the design of public health research. Public health research can be either quantitative or qualitative in nature. The nature of the research process is dictated by which design is most appropriate to use in answering the public health research question. The research process differs for quantitative and qualitative research.

Quantitative research is the kind of investigation of public health phenomena that lends itself to precise measurement and quantification (Polit & Hungler, 2001). Public health researchers have traditionally relied on quantitative research to answer questions about public health phenomena. The research process for quantitative research is summarized in Table 15.3.

Table 15.3   Quantitative Public Health Research Process

- Identify the public health problem
- Conduct a comprehensive review of the literature
- Formulate a public health research question
- Define or develop a theoretical or conceptual framework
- Refine the public health research question
- Formulate testable research hypotheses
- Develop the research design
  - Identify population
  - Specify measurement methods
  - Design sampling plan
  - Conduct pilot study
  - Refine research design
- Collect data
- Prepare data for analysis
- Analyze data
- Interpret findings and results
- Provide recommendations for practice
- Disseminate research findings
- Put findings to use

Qualitative research is the kind of investigation of public health phenomena that lends itself to nonnumeric data; its purpose is to discover important underlying dimensions and patterns in the phenomena (Polit & Hungler, 2001). Qualitative research focuses on individuals' interpretations and assigned meanings of their own experiences to understand the behavioral and social reality of individuals, groups, and cultures (Holloway, 1997). Qualitative research was integrated into public health research when public health practice connected with the social and behavioral sciences. The qualitative research process is not a linear process like the quantitative research process. Qualitative research depends on which qualitative methodology (and its associated philosophical underpinnings) is selected for use. The qualitative methodology could be phenomenological, ethnographic, or grounded theory, with the research process differing for each methodology. Table 15.4 provides a general outline of qualitative research processes (Polit & Hungler, 2001).

Community-Based Research Partnerships

Community members representing the population under investigation have increasingly voiced dissatisfaction with the focus of community research (Sullivan et al., 2001). Community members have voiced several concerns regarding research conducted "on" communities, such as lack of cultural appropriateness and relevance, power imbalances, lack of trust, and

Table 15.4   Qualitative Public Health Research Process

- Choose a broad research area of study
- Use self-reflection and discussion to narrow the research area
- Conduct a cursory review of the literature (or not, depending on the research question and method selected)
- Select philosophical underpinnings
- Design research study
- Identify data collection site and setting
- Conduct study
  - Sampling, data collection, data analysis, and interpretation are typically an iterative process
- Disseminate research findings
- Make use of findings

communication difficulties (Sullivan et al., 2001). Community-based research proposes to address some of these concerns by including community members as active participants in the research process.

Community-based research is research conducted "with" the community, not "on" the community. Community-based research partnerships focus on developing a common research agenda and vision, with the purpose of building trust (Brownson, Baker, & Kreuter, 2001). Community-based research promotes a collaborative research approach with community members to promote equality among partners in the research process (Caldwell, Zimmerman, & Isichei, 2001). Researchers engaging in community-based research must understand the needs and dynamics of the populations within the community and the community as a whole when engaging the community members in the research process. The development of community-based research ensures that research applies, represents, and responds in a culturally appropriate manner to the diversity of community members present.

The development of a community-based research partnership is dependent on three critical elements to build the community base of support. The three critical elements to building a community base for community research partnerships are (a) the presence, influence, and insight of socially committed researchers; (b) participation of skilled, knowledge-oriented community activists; and (c) attention to an issue or problem of critical interest to the community members, community institutions and agencies, and the public health researcher (Schensul, 2001). Three driving forces that will support the maintenance of a community research partnership are (a) a compelling commitment to the public health issue, (b) recognition that a joint community effort is necessary to address the public health issue comprehensively, and (c) a shared belief that the information obtained from the research process is critical and relevant (Schensul, 2001). An outcome of community-based research is the integration of the resulting public health intervention into the community.

Sustaining Research Interventions in the Community

An important goal of community-based research is the maintenance of the community intervention in the community, provided the intervention was determined to be significantly beneficial to the population's health. Collaboration between the public health researcher and community leaders is essential for intervention maintenance. This maintenance is frequently referred to as sustainability. Sustainability is defined as the infrastructure that remains in place with the community after the research project ends to ensure that interventions are continued, organizations modify their actions, and individuals gain and retain the knowledge and skills acquired (Altman, 1995). An outcome of sustainability is the exchange of knowledge and resources between the researcher and community organizations and members.

Altman (1995) described phases of a community-based research framework intended to promote sustainability of interventions researched in the community. Altman states that the goal is to have the community adapt, use, and sustain effective interventions in the community. This occurs as a process that slowly passes the ownership of the researched intervention from the researcher to the community members and agencies.

The phases of the framework are research, transfer, transition, regeneration, empowerment, and sustainability. The research phase consists of developing the research design and implementing the community-based research interventions. Community processes during this phase consist of education, community development, and policy change to secure outcomes in behaviors and health status. Transferring consists of moving a project from a purely research base to a community base. Transferring is accomplished through community communication, collaboration, and coordination to achieve the outcome of diffusing the research project throughout the community. Transition consists of replication of the community intervention researched, adaptation of the research-generated interventions, or the development of innovative community interventions that are consistent with or go beyond the intervention investigated. The phase of transition is accomplished through training of community members, provision of technical assistance, and education for the outcomes of replication, adaptation, or innovation. Regeneration occurs when community organizations replicate, adapt, or develop new innovations based on the interventions researched and the sharing of new insights and experiences with researchers. Once the researched intervention is integrated into the community, the resultant outcomes are new research questions and change strategies that are provided as feedback to the research team. Empowerment results from the exchange between the researchers and community members during and throughout the community-based research process. Empowerment outcomes are ownership of the researched intervention and resource acquisition by the community. Sustainability is achieved

Table 15.5	IRB Review

- Risk to subjects is minimal
- Risk to subjects is reasonable in relation to anticipated benefits
- Subject selection is equitable
- Informed consent has been obtained and documented
- Research plan is scientifically meritorious and risk to subjects is minimized
- Subjects' privacy and confidentiality are protected
- Additional safeguards are provided for vulnerable populations

when the research infrastructure remains in place, making it possible to continually conduct research and implement the researched intervention (Altman, 1995).

Institutional Review Boards

Public health agencies are familiar with the protection of individuals and populations. The conduct of research involves special protective measures to ensure ethical practice. The protection of human subjects continues to evolve as research methods, technology, and science continue to evolve. The protection of human subjects involves key practices such as informed consent, subject selection, vulnerable population safeguards, and privacy and confidentiality assurances (MacCubbin, Gordon, & Prentice, 2001).

Federal regulations have mandated the development of institutional review boards (IRBs) as a measure to protect human subjects. A human subject is defined as a living individual about whom an investigator conducting research obtains data through an intervention or interaction or receives identifiable private information (MacCubbin et al., 2001). Federal regulations require that an IRB be composed of at least five members who possess sufficient experience and knowledge to review scientific research. Of these IRB members, one should be a community member who functions independently of the organization or institution supporting the functions of the IRB.

An IRB conducts a scientific review of the research proposal as a measure to facilitate the protection of human subjects. An IRB review consists of assessing the research proposal for critical elements. Table 15.5 outlines the critical elements of an IRB review (MacCubbin et al., 2001). Some research proposals are exempt from a full IRB review, but the same assurances for the protection of human subjects are maintained. It is not the sole responsibility of the IRB to protect human subjects. It is the responsibility of the public health nurse researcher to actually ensure that human subjects are protected during the research process.

Vulnerable populations are groups of individuals defined according to federal regulations as requiring special protections against risks posed by

Table 15.6   Elements of Informed Consent

- Study is identified as research
- Purpose of research explained
- Description of study provided
- All foreseeable risks or discomforts described
- Potential benefits described
- Appropriate alternatives to participation in study disclosed
- Extent to which information will be maintained as private and confidential described
- Cost and compensation described
- Access provided to researcher in case of questions
- Statement provided regarding voluntary participation and the right to refuse participation or withdraw from the study without reprisal
- Appropriate signature lines

human-subject research. Some vulnerable populations identified are pregnant women, children, and prisoners.

Informed consent is intended to ensure that human research subjects are fully aware of what the research consists of, their level of risk, and their ability to refuse or withdraw from participation without reprisal at any time (MacCubbin et al., 2001). The *Belmont Report*, developed by the National Commission for the Protection of Human Subjects of Biomedical and Behavioral Research (1979), established three fundamental ethical principles relevant to informed consent: respect for person, beneficence, and justice. Table 15.6 describes the elements of informed consent. Strauss et al. (2001) proposed the use of a community advisory board (CAB) to facilitate research by providing advice about the informed consent process and to design and implement research. The CAB can assist in developing a partnership between researchers and the community. A CAB should be composed of community members who share a common identity, history, language, and culture. The primary function of the CAB is to serve as a liaison between researchers and community members who are research subjects.

Grants

Grants can provide funding to support programs or research. Grants are of two general types: program grants or research grants. Program grants provide funding for the development of public health programs that provide services. Research grants provide funding for public health projects that generate knowledge or discover new information. Grants by private and public agencies, private foundations, associations, and other agencies may be conferred to support the national health-care agenda (Healthy People 2010) or to meet its mission.

Public health nurses should actively search for funding opportunities through contact with private and public agencies, private foundations,

Table 15.7 Major Components of a Grant Request for Proposal

- Application page
- Abstract
- Background
  - Need
  - Rationale or justification
  - Literature review integrated throughout background and entire proposal
- Institutional or organizational description
- Pilot data or previous program services delivered
- Research plan or program methodology
  - Goals and objectives
  - For research grants, research hypothesis, design, measurements, data collection process, data analysis
  - For program grants, a description of the services to be delivered, by who, when, and outcome measures for each goal and corresponding objective
  - Responsible individuals for each phase of the research plan or implementation of the program
  - Description of partnerships or linkages
  - Timeline
  - For research grants, human subjects protection
- Budget
  - Budget narrative with justification of requested funds
  - Budget spreadsheet with all income, expenditures, in-kind or matching funds described
- Evaluation plan
- Sustainability plan
- Dissemination or utilization plan
- References
- Biographical sketch of primary investigators
- Letters of support

associations, or other agencies. Additionally, there are computerized services that search and alert public health professionals to grant opportunities as they arise. Grant-writing skills are a necessity for public health professionals. Funding agencies release a request for proposal (RFP) that delineates the scope of the funding opportunity and the guidelines and requirements for writing the grant. Public health professionals should comply with all guidelines and requirements of the RFP to remain competitive during the grant review process. Table 15.7 outlines the general format of an RFP.

Summary

Key issues in public health research are as follows.

- A key element of public health research is defining which public health interventions or programs work most effectively to generate a positive, population-level change in public health.

- Public health research is defined as systematic inquiry or investigation to generate new public health knowledge or to validate and refine existing public health knowledge through rigorous and systematic data collection and analysis, using either quantitative or qualitative methods.
- The primary premise of basic public health research is the development of a knowledge base for the discipline of public health.
- Applied public health research focuses on identifying the effectiveness of interventions in solving a problem or improving public health practice.
- Research priorities are identified by an authoritative body or organization as areas on which to focus to advance some defined larger public health agenda.
- ACHNE nursing research priorities are meant to guide public health nurse researchers, practitioners, educators, students, nursing colleagues in other specialties, funding agencies, and policy makers in building the body of public health knowledge; identifying domains of research problems relevant to public health nursing; targeting interventions to vulnerable, high-risk, ethnic minority or underserved populations; supporting the initiation of programs of research; articulating the unique contributions of public health nursing research; facilitating interdisciplinary collaboration; fostering dissemination and application of research findings; and influencing policy in service and funding agencies.
- The research process provides a logical and scientific sequence of events for the researcher to use so that the scientific rigor of inquiry is maintained.
- Research is classified according to levels that depend on the nature and purpose of the research: descriptive, exploratory, explanatory, testing, or generalizing.
- The nature of the research process is dictated by which design is most appropriate to answer the public health research question.
- Quantitative research is the kind of investigation of public health phenomena that lends itself to precise measurement and quantification.
- Qualitative research is the kind of investigation of public health phenomena that lends itself to nonnumeric data, with the purpose of discovering important underlying dimensions and patterns in the phenomena.
- Community-based research promotes collaboration with community members to promote equality and partnership in the research process.
- The three critical elements to building a community base for community research partnerships are the presence, influence, and insight of socially committed researchers; participation of skilled, knowledge-oriented community activists; and attention to an issue or problem of critical interest to the community members, community institutions and agencies, and the public health researcher.

- Three driving forces that will support the maintenance of a community research partnership are a compelling commitment to the public health issue, recognition that a joint community effort is necessary to address the public health issue comprehensively, and a shared belief that the information obtained from the research process is critical and relevant.
- Collaboration between the public health researcher and community leaders is essential for intervention maintenance, often referred to as sustainability.
- Sustainability is defined as the infrastructure that remains in place with the community after the research project ends, ensuring that interventions are continued, organizations modify their actions, and individuals gain and retain the knowledge and skills they have acquired.
- Community research sustainability phases are research, transfer, transition, regeneration, empowerment, and sustainability.
- The protection of human subjects involves key practices such as informed consent, subject selection, vulnerable population safeguards, and privacy and confidentiality assurances.
- Federal regulations have mandated the development of IRBs as a measure to protect human subjects.
- Vulnerable populations are groups of individuals identified as requiring special protections against risks posed by human-subject research.
- Informed consent is intended to ensure that human research subjects are fully aware of what the research consists of, their level of risk, and their ability to refuse or withdraw from participation without reprisal at any time.
- The *Belmont Report* established three fundamental ethical principles relevant to informed consent: respect for person, beneficence, and justice.
- The primary function of a CAB is to serve as a liaison between researchers and community members who are research subjects.
- Grants can provide funding to support programs or research.
- Program grants provide funding for the development of public health programs that provide services.
- Research grants provide funding for public health projects that generate knowledge or discover new information.

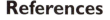

References

Altman, D. (1995). Sustaining interventions in community systems: On the relationship between researchers and communities. *Health Psychology, 14*(6), 526-536.

Association of Community Health Nurse Educators Research Committee. (2000). *Research priorities for public health nursing: 2000.* Pensacola, FL: Author.

Brownson, R., Baker, E., & Kreuter, M. (2001). Prevention research partnerships in community settings: What are we learning? *Journal of Public Health Management and Practice, 7,* vii-ix.

Caldwell, C., Zimmerman, M., & Isichei, P. (2001). Forging collaborative partnerships to enhance family health: An assessment of strengths and challenges in conducting community-based research. *Journal of Public Health Management and Practice, 7*(2), 1-9.

Daly, J., Kellehear, A., & Gliksman, M. (1997). *The public health researcher: A methodological guide.* New York: Oxford University Press.

Gadomski, A. (2001). Public health research. In L. Novick & G. Mays (Eds.), *Public health administration: Principles for population-based management* (pp. 359-373). Gaithersburg, MD: Aspen.

Holloway, I. (1997). *Basic concepts for qualitative research.* Oxford: Blackwell Scientific.

MacCubbin, P., Gordon, B., & Prentice, E. (2001). Protecting human subjects in public health research. In L. Novick & G. Mays (Eds.), *Public health administration: Principles for population-based management* (pp. 374-394). Gaithersburg, MD: Aspen.

National Commission for the Protection of Human Subjects of Biomedical and Behavioral Research. (1979). *The Belmont report: Ethical principles and guidelines for the protection of human subjects of research.* Retrieved June 20, 2003, from http://www.tarleton.edu/~grants/BelmontReport.pdf

Playle, J. (2000a). Developing research questions and searching the literature. *Journal of Community Nursing Online, 14*(2). Retrieved June 20, 2003, from http://www.jcn.co.uk/journal.asp?MonthNum=02&YearNum=2000&Type=backissue&ArticleID=211

Playle, J. (2000b). The nature of research. *Journal of Community Nursing Online, 14*(1). Retrieved June 20, 2003, from http://www.jcn.co.uk/journal.asp?MonthNum=01 &YearNum=2000&Type=backissue&ArticleID=304

Polit, D., & Hungler, B. (2001). *Nursing research: Principles and methods* (6th ed.). Philadelphia, PA: Lippincott.

Schensul, J. (2001). *The development and maintenance of community research partnerships.* Retrieved June 26, 2003, from http://www.mapcruzin.com/community-research/schensul1.htm

Strauss, R., Sengupta, S., Quinn, S., Goeppinger, J., Spaulding, C., Kegeles, S., et al. (2001). The role of the community advisory boards: Involving communities in the informed consent process. *American Journal of Public Health, 91*(12), 1938-1943.

Sullivan, M., Kone, A., Senturia, K., Chrisman, N., Ciske, S., & Krieger, J. (2001). Researcher and researched-community perspectives: Toward bridging the gap. *Health Education and Behavior, 28*(2), 130-149.

16

Evidence-Based Public Health Practice

Evidence-based practice is a common term that is used but often misunderstood in the medical arena. The nursing profession has historically focused on the use of research findings to improve practice, which has, historically, been referred to as research utilization. This chapter focuses on describing processes of research utilization, defining research-based and evidence-based practice, and providing an evidence-based, public health framework and an evidence hierarchy.

Introduction

Public health nurses are responsible for developing public health interventions and programs that are appropriate for, accountable to, and that generate effective results in the population. There remains a considerable gap between public health practice and the large amounts of data generated through community assessments, public health evaluations, public health research, or performance measurements and improvement activities. There is also an increasing demand by the public for the delivery of effective public health care services that are cost effective, cost efficient, and of quality.

A consistent and recurring message is that public health nurses must make sound decisions that are based on evidence or research data. Public health policies, programs, and practice guidelines must be based on evidence or research data that meet the rigors of scientific merit. This can be accomplished through the practice of research-based or evidence-based practice. Research- and evidence-based practice are considered synonymous terms by some professionals and different concepts by others. There is also a lack of commonality in the definitions and defining characteristics of each term. These terms will be differentiated for the purpose of this book. Neither term can be sufficiently discussed without a discussion of research utilization. This chapter will primarily focus on evidence-based practice, the broader perspective of using data for decision making.

Research Utilization

Research utilization is considered to provide the foundational framework for both research- and evidence-based practice. Polit and Hungler (2001) define research utilization as the "use of some aspect of a scientific investigation in an application that is unrelated to original research" (p. 645). Prior to the 1970s, nursing research was primarily focused on conducting nursing research and publishing the findings. In the 1970s, nursing research began focusing on research utilization and the activities necessary to incorporate research findings into clinical nursing practice. Today, the nursing research cycle has expanded to focus on the conduct of nursing research, publication of nursing research findings, utilization of nursing research in clinical practice, and the publication of information about the research utilization. Figure 16.1 presents the current nursing research utilization cycle (Goode, 2000).

Several projects were initiated to stimulate the implementation of nursing research utilization. The two most well known, the Western Interstate Commission for Higher Education (WICHE) Project and the Conduct and Utilization of Research in Nursing (CURN) Project, are briefly introduced here.

The WICHE Project

The WICHE Project is the very first nursing research utilization project initiated in the world by the Western Interstate Commission for Higher Education (Goode, 2000). WICHE had three major goals: (a) collaborative, nontargeted research (bringing together nurses from academia and practice to work on clinical problems), (b) collaborative, targeted research (multiple studies designed to study the same problem in multiple settings), and (c) research utilization. The WICHE Project linked nurse clinicians with nurse researchers to identify a clinical problem, retrieve and critique studies related to the problem, develop and implement a research-based plan of care, and evaluate the outcomes from using the research data from the studies reviewed (Goode, 2000). The major problems encountered in the WICHE Project had to do with identifying scientifically sound, reliable nursing research with clear implications for nursing practice (Polit & Hungler, 2001).

The CURN Project

The CURN Project was designed to increase the use of research findings in daily nursing practice. Additionally, the CURN Project wanted to stimulate the conduct of nursing research in practice. The CURN Project considered

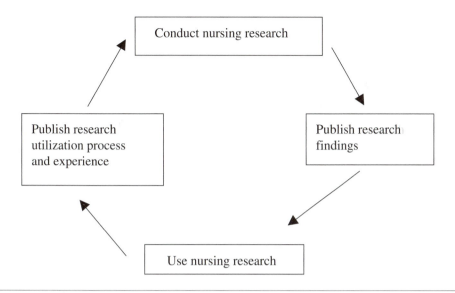

Figure 16.1 Research Utilization Cycle

that research utilization was primarily an organizational process that needed to occur. Organizational support was considered a prerequisite to nursing research utilization (Goode, 2000; Polit & Hungler, 2001).

The CURN Project disseminated current research findings, facilitated organizational change for the implementation of practice based on research findings, and encouraged the collaborative conduct of research. From the CURN Project, six phases of the research utilization process were identified:

- Identification of clinical practice problems
- Evaluation of the relevance of research to the identified clinical problem, the organization's values and current policies, and the cost-benefit ratio
- Design of nursing interventions based on the research
- Conduct of clinical trial and evaluation of the intervention
- Decision to adopt, revise, or reject the intervention developed based on the research
- Development of strategies to extend the intervention to other settings (Polit & Hungler, 2001).

Fostering Research Utilization

To bridge the gap between public health research and practice, research utilization must be considered a significant component and intent of the nursing research process. Public health researchers engaged in public health research are responsible for the utilization of their research findings. The following strategies are recommended to facilitate the timely utilization of research findings:

- Conduct high-quality, scientifically meritorious research.
- Conduct relevant outcomes research.
- Replicate studies in various populations and settings.
- Collaborate with other practitioners and disciplines.
- Disseminate findings aggressively and broadly.
- Communicate findings clearly.
- Provide recommendations for clinical implementation based on findings.
- Read widely and critically.
- Attend professional conferences.
- Seek environments that support research.
- Promote a climate of intellectual curiosity.
- Reward research utilization efforts.
- Collaborate with a nursing mentor who values nursing research (Polit & Hungler, 2001).

In addition, Day (1997) indicates other activities that can promote the use of research findings. Day proposes (a) the formation of research committees, research groups, or task forces; (b) an increase in the availability of professional literature in the public health environment; (c) continuing education programs on research; (d) coordinating research conferences; (e) disseminating a research newsletter; (f) monthly journal clubs to review research articles; and (g) the formation of multiagency community research groups.

Closing the gap between public health research and practice requires that public health leaders deliver a consistent message regarding the use of research findings. Pressures to implement research findings will continually challenge the public health system as public expectations of accountability increase and resources decrease. Haines and Donald (1998) propose the following steps to promote research utilization from a systems communication perspective:

- Define the gap between research and practice.
- Define the message to be communicated about the gap.
- Decide what processes need altering.
- Involve key stakeholders.
- Identify barriers to research utilization and develop plans to overcome barriers.
- Decide the method of promoting change.
- Identify existing mechanisms or processes through which to diffuse the research utilization.
- Monitor the research utilization project to determine if the desired outcome is achieved.

Research Utilization Criteria

Three broad criteria for research utilization have been proposed that should be considered regardless of the model or framework for research utilization: clinical relevance, scientific merit, and implementation potential (Polit & Hungler, 2001). Clinical relevance is determined based on the significance of the problem identified to the practice of community and public health nursing. Questions that should be asked to determine clinical relevance are (a) Does the research have the potential to solve problems currently faced by practitioners? (b) Does the research have the potential to affect decision making regarding risks, complications, or selection of the appropriate intervention? (c) Is the research based on or testing theoretical propositions? (d) Does the intervention have potential for implementation into practice? (e) Is the intervention within the scope of community and public health nursing? and (f) Can the research measures be used in clinical practice? Scientific merit is based on the researcher's critique of the research design and methods used to conduct the research. Implementation potential consists of the extent to which the research findings can actually be implemented in practice. To determine implementation potential, assessment must be made of the transferability of the findings to practice, the feasibility of implementing the findings, and the cost-benefit ratio of implementing the findings.

Research-Based Public Health Practice Defined

Research-based public health practice is closely related to and consistent with research utilization. The term *research-based practice* is frequently used interchangeably with *evidence-based practice*. Research-based public health practice is defined separately in this book but is considered a component and source of the evidence used in evidence-based practice. Research-based public health practice is defined as the systematic process of conducting public health research, appraising public health research findings, and using these research findings as the basis for public health decision making. Based on this definition, the distinguishing element between research-based public health practice and evidence-based public health practice is that the only evidence used in research-based practice is that data derived solely from research. Other sources of data, such as expert opinion, are not included in research-based public health practice (Rimer, Glanz, & Rasband, 2001).

Evidence-Based Public Health Practice Defined

The evidence-based practice movement began in England during the 1990s. This movement resulted from the increasing need to base practice on sound

Table 16.1   Evidence-Based Practice, Evidence-Based Medicine, and Nursing Practice
Definitions

Evidence-Based Practice

- Uses research findings derived chiefly from randomized controlled clinical trials or other experimental designs to evaluate specific interventions (Gerrish & Clayton, 1998, p. 58)
- Evidence-based clinical practice involves the synthesis of knowledge from research, retrospective or concurrent chart review, quality improvement and risk data, international, national, and local standards, infection control data, pathophysiology, cost effectiveness analysis, benchmarking data, patient preferences, and clinical expertise (Goode & Piedalue, 1999, p. 15)

Evidence-Based Medicine

- Evidence-based medicine de-emphasizes intuition, unsystematic clinical experience, and pathophysiologic rationale as sufficient grounds for clinical decision making and stresses the examination of evidence from clinical research (Evidence-Based Practice Working Group, 1992, p. 2420)
- Evidence-based medicine is the conscientious, explicit, and judicious use of current best evidence in making decisions about the care of individual patients. The practice of evidence-based medicine means integrating individual clinical expertise with the best available external clinical evidence from systematic research (Sackett, Rosenberg, Gray, Hayes, & Richardson, 1996, p. 71)

Evidence-Based Nursing

- Evidence-based nursing is defined as the incorporation of evidence from research, clinical expertise and patient preferences into decisions about the health care of individual patients (Mulhall, 1998)
- Evidence-based nursing practice is the conscientious, explicit, and judicious use of theory-derived, research-based information in making decisions about care delivery to individuals or groups of patients and in consideration of individuals' needs and preferences (Ingersoll, 2000, p. 151)

evidence through a critical appraisal of research, expert practice, and expert opinion. Evidence-based practice extends research-based practice through the inclusion of additional information such as patient preferences, cost and clinical knowledge, and practitioner expertise (Goode, 2000). The purpose of the evidence-based practice movement in England was to provide clinically effective health care with the resources available (Coyler & Kamath, 1999). The evidence-based nursing movement also began in England (Goode, 2000).

The literature abounds with multiple definitions of evidence-based practice. Most definitions of evidence-based practice are based on the synthesis of research, use of research, and the inclusion of expertise as valid sources of evidence for decision making. Disciplines have begun to define evidence-based practice from the perspective of their scope of practice. Table 16.1 provides some definitions of evidence-based medicine and evidence-based nursing practice found in the literature.

In addition to disciplines' specifically defining the characteristics of evidence-based practice, some groups are delineating what evidence constitutes inclusion into their definition of evidence-based practice. The Evidence-Based Practice Working Group (1992) deemphasizes intuition, unsystematic clinical experience, and pathophysiological rationales as sufficient evidence for evidence-based decision making in medical practice. Evidence-based nursing practice deemphasizes ritual, isolated, and unsystematic clinical experience and ungrounded opinions and traditions as a basis for evidence-based decision making in nursing practice (Stetler, Brunell, et al., 1998).

The literature lacks a clear definition of evidence-based public health practice. For the purposes of this book, evidence-based public health practice is defined as the conscientious, explicit, and judicious use of the current best evidence in making decisions about population-based public health practice, including the use of evidence from epidemiological and surveillance data, expert public health practice, monitoring and evaluation data, and performance improvement data. Various evidence-based practice frameworks provide the structure from which to guide the selection and use of such evidence.

Evidence-Based Public Health Practice Framework

The evidence-based practice framework for public health consists of five basic elements. The five elements are lifelong learning, setting priorities, setting guidelines, measuring performance, and improving performance (Dever, 1997). Evidence-based practice is considered to exist within the context of lifelong learning. Public health nurses must first *determine the level of importance* of the problem under consideration. This is accomplished through priority setting. The next step involves answering the question, "How should the problem be managed?" This step, *setting guidelines*, answers this question based on evidence. *Measuring performance* consists of the systematic collection of quality performance data regarding the changes implemented in public health based on the guidelines determined from the evidence. The data derived from the performance measure add additional evidence from which to continually improve public health practice; hence the last step, *improving performance*. This framework focuses on the use of one type of data, quality improvement data. Other types of data are used based on their strength (Dever, 1997).

Evidence Hierarchy

Evidence can consist of research data, expert opinions, facts, experience, patient views, and practitioner views (Hek, 2000). Evidence to be used in decision making is ranked according to evidence hierarchies. The purpose of evidence hierarchies is to evaluate the strength of the evidence according to its reliability, validity, generalizability, and feasibility.

Table 16.2 Evidence Hierarchy Summary

Strength of Evidence Hierarchy (Gill, 2000)
- Evidence from a systematic review of multiple, well-designed, randomized, controlled trials
- Evidence from one or more well-designed, randomized, controlled trials
- Evidence from trials without randomization; a single group before and after; cohort studies; time series studies; matched, case-controlled studies; or observational studies
- Evidence from well-designed descriptive studies or qualitative research
- Opinion from expert committees or respected authorities that is based on clinical evidence
- Personal, professional, or peer expertise and experience

Agency for Healthcare Research and Quality Hierarchy (Agency for Health Care Policy and Research, 1994)

Ia. Meta-analysis of randomized controlled trials

Ib. One randomized controlled trial

IIa. One well-designed controlled study without randomization

IIb. One well-designed quasiexperimental study

III. Well-designed nonexperimental study (of comparative, correlative, or descriptive design)

IV. Expert committee reports, expert opinion, consensus statements, expert judgment

Stetler et al. (1998) Hierarchy

I. Meta-analysis of multiple controlled studies

II. Individual experimental study

III. Quasiexperimental study

IV. Nonexperimental study

V. Systematically obtained, verifiable, quality improvement program evaluation or case report data

VI. Opinions of national authorities based on clinical experience or opinion of expert committee; regulatory or legal opinions

Chulay (1998) Hierarchy

I. Manufacturers' recommendation only

II. Theory-based evidence without research data; recommendations from expert group

III. Laboratory data without supporting clinical data

IV. Limited clinical studies

V. Clinical studies in more than one population or situation

VI. Clinical studies in a variety of populations and situations

The evidence is critically appraised. The decision made based on the evidence appraised is given a hierarchical notation. Table 16.2 provides several common evidence hierarchies used in evidence-based practice. These hierarchical notations designate the strength of the practice recommendation

Table 16.3   Practice Guideline Recommendations

- Guidelines should be feasible, based on scientific evidence and other empirical information
- Potential benefits of guidelines are immediate and far reaching
- Guidelines have a circumscribed scope
- Guidelines are flexible rather than prescriptive
- Guidelines are dynamic
- Major stakeholders involved in guideline development
- Critical questions structure the evidence-collection process
- Database search conducted for scientific studies
- Other sources of documentary evidence systematically evaluated
- Empiric evidence from local, state, and national programs sought, evaluated, and incorporated as appropriate
- Guidelines stimulate needed research
- Guidelines are pilot-tested before dissemination and then continuously evaluated

based on the strength of the evidence used in the decision-making process. The Council on Linkages between Academia and Public Health Practice (1995) recommends that evidence should be appraised prior to developing public health practice guidelines. In addition to the evidence hierarchies described in Table 16.2, evidence should be appraised in regard to its availability, applicability, and utility. The council also provides practice guidelines developed from an evidence-based practice framework. Table 16.3 summarizes these recommendations.

Summary

Key issues of research utilization and evidence-based public health practice are as follows.

- Public health nurses must make sound decisions that are based on evidence or research data.
- Research utilization is defined as the use of some aspect of a scientific investigation in an application that is unrelated to original research.
- The three major goals of WICHE were collaborative, nontargeted research; collaborative targeted research; and research utilization.
- The CURN Project was designed to increase the use of research findings in daily nursing practice.
- Strategies to facilitate research utilization are conducting high-quality, scientifically meritorious research; conducting relevant outcomes research; replicating studies in various populations and settings; collaborating with other practitioners and disciplines; disseminating findings aggressively and broadly; communicating findings clearly; providing recommendations for clinical implementation based on

findings; reading widely and critically; attending professional conferences; seeking environments that support research; promoting a climate of intellectual curiosity; rewarding research utilization efforts; and collaborating with a nursing mentor who values nursing research.

- Other activities to promote research utilization are the formation of research committees, research groups, or task forces; increasing the availability of professional literature in the public health environment; continuing education programs on research; coordinating research conferences; disseminating a research newsletter; monthly journal clubs to review research articles; and the formation of multiagency community research groups.
- Research utilization criteria are clinical relevance, scientific merit, and implementation potential.
- Research-based public health practice is defined as the systematic process of conducting public health research, appraising public health research findings, and using these research findings as the basis for public health decision making.
- Evidence-based practice extends research-based practice through the inclusion of additional information, such as patient preferences, cost and clinical knowledge, and practitioner expertise.
- Evidence-based public health practice is defined as the conscientious, explicit, and judicious use of the current best evidence in making decisions about population-based public health practice, including the use of evidence from epidemiological and surveillance data, expert public health practice, monitoring and evaluation data, and performance improvement data.
- The evidence-based practice framework for public health consists of five basic elements: lifelong learning, setting priorities, setting guidelines, measuring performance, and improving performance.
- The purpose of evidence hierarchies is to evaluate the strength of the evidence according to its reliability, validity, generalizability, and feasibility.

References

Agency for Health Care Policy and Research. (1994). Clinical practice guidelines: Number 9. Management of cancer pain (AHCPR Publication No. 94-0592). Rockville, MD: Department of Health and Human Services.

Chulay, M. (1998). Information for contributors. *AACN protocols for practice.* Aliso Viejo, CA: American Association of Critical-Care Nurses.

Council on Linkages between Academia and Public Health Practice. (1995). *Practice guidelines for public health: Assessment of scientific evidence, feasibility, and benefits.* Albany, NY: University at Albany School of Public Health.

Coyler, H., Kamath, P. (1999). Evidence-based practice: A philosophical and political analysis. Some matters for consideration by professional practitioners. *Journal of Advanced Nursing, 29*(1), 188-193.

Day, D. (1997). Promoting research utilization in the community hospital setting. *Kansas Nurse, 72*(4), 2-3.

Dever, G. (1997). *Improving outcomes in public health practice: Strategies and methods.* Gaithersburg, MD: Aspen.

Evidence-Based Practice Working Group. (1992). A new approach to teaching the practice of medicine. *Journal of the American Medical Association, 268,* 2420-2425.

Gerrish, K., & Clayton, J. (1998). Improving clinical effectiveness through an evidence-based approach: Meeting the challenge for nursing in the United Kingdom. *Nursing Administration Quarterly, 22*(4), 55-65.

Goode, C. (2000). Building on a legacy of excellence in nursing research: Evidence-based practice. *Communicating Nursing Research, 33*(8), 3-11.

Goode, C., & Piedalue, F. (1999). Evidence-based clinical practice. *Journal of Nursing Administration, 29*(6), 15-21.

Haines, A., & Donald, A. (1998). Getting research findings into practice: Making better use of research findings. *British Medical Journal, 317*(7150), 72-75.

Hek, G. (2000). Research: Evidence-based practice: Finding the evidence. *Journal of Community Nursing, 14*(11), 19-20, 22.

Ingersoll, G. (2000). Evidence based nursing: What it is and what it isn't. *Nursing Outlook, 48*(4), 151-152.

Mulhall, A. (1998). Nursing, research and the evidence. *Evidence Based Nursing, 1,* 4-6.

Polit, D., & Hungler, B. (2001). *Nursing research: Principles and methods* (6th ed.). Philadelphia, PA: Lippincott.

Rimer, B., Glanz, K., & Rasband, G. (2001). Searching for evidence about health education and health behavior interventions. *Health Education and Behavior, 28*(2), 231-248.

Sackett, D., Rosenburg, W., Gray, J., Hayes, R., & Richardson, W. (1996). Evidence-based medicine: What it is and what it isn't. *British Medical Journal, 312,* 71-72.

Stetler, C., Brunell, M., Giuliano, K., Morsi, D., Prince, L., & Newell-Stokes, V. (1998). Evidence-based practice and the role of nursing leadership. *Journal of Nursing Administration, 28*(7/8), 45-53.

Stetler, C., Morsi, D., Rucki, S., Broughton, S., Corrigan, B., Fitzgerald, J., et al. (1998). Utilization-focused integrative reviews in nursing service. *Applied Nursing Research, 11*(4), 195-206.

Part V

Public Health–Community Health Leadership and Administration

17

Public Health–Community Health Leadership

Leadership is the ability to influence a group to move forward toward a mutually agreed-upon community goal. Leaders are focused on moving the public health agenda forward toward a healthier nation. Public health nursing leadership requires a desire, commitment, and the adequate public health preparation and experience to effectively lead. This chapter focuses on defining leadership; describing power; differentiating the concepts of administration, management, and leadership; providing leadership principles and styles; and how in the future, public health nursing will provide leadership in change.

Introduction

Public health nurses are challenged with ensuring the provision of public health services in an environment of change that requires adequate preparation in the discipline of public health and the leadership ability to mobilize communities. In addition, public health nurses need the necessary leadership skills to guide public health practitioners forward during times of uncertainty and to ensure that the public health needs of various and diverse populations are met. This is validated by Boedigheimer and Gebbie (2001) in their exploration of the adequacy of public health administrators' preparation. These authors identified several critical skills that are indicative of public health leadership (see Table 17.1). This chapter focuses on the necessary leadership skills required of public health nurses serving in leadership and administrative roles. The leadership skills presented in this chapter formulate the basis of other critical leadership skills identified by Boedigheimer and Gebbie.

Leadership Defined

Leadership is considered an essential element that is critical to the success of individuals, organizations, institutions, and communities. Therefore, a

Table 17.1   Leadership Skills Critical for Public Health Administrators

- Communication
- Informatics
- Experience in public health practice
- Understanding of public health values, history, and methods
- Cultural competence
- Visioning and strategic planning
- Coalition building and mobilization
- Organizational management
- Personal development and assessment
- Negotiation skills
- Systems thinking
- Change management
- Quality assurance and performance improvement
- Public health emergency decision-making abilities

SOURCE: Boedigheimer and Gebbie (2001).

considerable amount of energy has been consumed in identifying what makes a good leader. Some suggested characteristics of a good leader are (a) controls subordinates in a bureaucratic manner; (b) certain personal characteristics or attributes, such as honesty, integrity, respect; (c) ability to maintain communication; (d) the knack of adapting their own behavior to a situation, thus fostering the growth and development of others and moving forward; (d) charisma; (e) an ability to envision the future and inspire and excite others; and (f) political astuteness (Morton, 1999). Morton identified factors that were considered to be important as a leadership model for community health nurses. Morton's qualitative analysis determined that community health nurses felt that nursing leadership consisted of being an expert, a planner, autonomous, a good communicator, focusing on achievement, and being supportive. Coaching, mentoring, and training were considered essential to develop the leadership ability of other community health nurses. Negative characteristics were identified that leaders should not possess: being self-opinionated, overconfident, and rigid and establishing unrealistic and unattainable goals. Morton summarizes the characterization of a leader as someone who has skills and attributes that are encompassed in being credible, having technical skills, possessing democratic behavior, being an excellent communicator, setting goals, being supportive, teaching, coaching, and mentoring. From these qualities evolves the concept of nursing leadership.

Kotter (1996) defines leadership as "a set of processes that creates organizations in the first place or adapts them to significantly changing circumstances . . . defines what the future should look like, aligns people with that vision, and inspires them to make it happen despite the obstacles" (p. 25). Donnelly, Gibson, and Ivancevich (1997) define leadership as "the ability to persuade others to enthusiastically pursue mutual goals and objectives. . . . it is the human factor that binds a group together toward mutual goals and objectives." Leadership is considered a process in which one exerts influence over another. For the purposes of this book, leadership is defined as a process that aligns a diverse population of individuals with a vision as a means of enthusiastically pursuing mutually defined community goals and objectives.

The influence that leaders exert over others is considered *power*. The term power frequently is associated with negative images in leadership theory. Therefore, some leadership authors have coined other positive terms to describe power. Lee (1997) defined principle-centered power as "the power that inspires loyalty and devotion and that transcends time and place" (p. 2). Principle-centered power is based on values such as trust and respect for an individual; therefore, principle-centered power is "based on honor extended to you from others and by you to others" (p. 16). Lee recognizes several types of power but considers power to be of two primary types: coercive and utility.

Types of Coercive and Utility Power

Coercive power relies on control of other individuals and uses fear as its instrument (Donnelly et al., 1997; Lee, 1997). Coercive power is considered to result in feelings of fear and only a temporary, reactive control of other individuals. Coercive power is considered primarily self-centered rather than principle centered. Based on fear of the leader, coercive power instills feelings in the followers of negative control, resistance, and desire to sabotage.

Utility power is based on principles of negotiation. Utility power considers the possibility of exchange between the leader and followers, with fairness as a foundation. Fairness is considered to exist in win-win situations (Lee, 1997). Lee identifies 10 types of utility power:

- Reward—provide incentives to others who act in alignment with goals and objectives
- Positional or legitimate—influence ascribed to an individual by virtue of their position in the organization or title
- Expert—influence related to the individual's expertise, skills, or knowledge
- Charisma or natural leadership—personal traits portrayed by a leader that draw others to follow up
- Informational—influence exerted by having specialized knowledge that others need
- Opportunity—the ability to influence others by assuming a leadership role in a time of emergency or crisis
- Resource—influence through the control of persons, commodities, goods, and other services

- Instrumental—the ability to get things done and mobilize others
- Appraisal—the ability to give informative and constructive corrective feedback to others
- Relational—the existence of an association with someone who is considered to be powerful

Public health nurses use multiple types of power in their leadership roles. Public health nurses typically do not subscribe to only one power type; rather, the type of power public health nurses use is matched to their values, experience, administrative position, and the professional situation requiring the use of such power.

In addition to employing different types of power, public health nurses engage in community interventions that require the sharing of power with community members. Romig (2001) points out that the sharing of power by the leader increases mutual commitment to the desired interventions by all parties involved in the process. The three levels of power sharing are (a) constituents or stakeholders providing ideas to the leader, (b) constituents or stakeholders participating in the decision-making process through exercises such as brainstorming, and (c) an equal sharing of power in decision making between the leader and the constituents or stakeholders.

Differentiation of Administration, Management, and Leadership

Administration, management, and leadership are frequently considered or referred to as interchangeable terms. Each of these has distinct characteristics that are different but not always exclusive. For example, administrators are considered managers, but managers may or may not be considered leaders. An informal leader may not have administrative or management responsibilities. This section will differentiate the underlying meanings of administration, management, and leadership (also, see Table 17.2).

Administration is considered an umbrella term for management and leadership (all leaders do not occupy an administrative or managerial position). Administration is the performance of executive duties as identified by the public health nurse's position description within an organization. The simple execution of ascribed duties by virtue of the public health nurse's position is considered the performance of administrative duties.

Management is considered both an act and art. Management is a process used by public health nurses to conduct, supervise, or coordinate the activities of multiple individuals (other nurses or community members) to achieve defined goals and objectives that are not achievable by one individual alone (Donnelly et al., 1997). Planning, organizing, and controlling are basic management functions. Managers use the planning function to assist

Table 17.2   Comparison of Management and Leadership

Management	Leadership
Position allocated through organizational chart, influence through organizational position	Ascribed by virtue of organizational position or accomplishments in the organization, influences the organization regardless of position in the organization
Planning and budgeting—develops detailed steps, timelines, and allocates resources	Establishes a direction through visioning, creates new resources
Organizing and staffing—develops structures, policies and procedures, and systems	Alignment of people—builds teams and coalitions to strategically achieve the mission
Controlling and problem solving—continual monitoring of results, identification of variances, solving problems	Motivating and inspiring—energizes people, is politically active
Improves efficiency	Improves effectiveness

SOURCE: Kotter (1996)and Romig (2001).

their organization to define and meet its goals and objectives. The organizing function uses leadership principles to implement the organization's plan. The assurance that the organization conforms to planned activities occurs through the controlling function (Donnelly et al., 1997).

Leadership Principles

Public health nursing professionals aspire to be leaders in their profession and within the community. Leadership requires a positive attitude and a healthy, balanced perspective on life (Magee, 2000). Dedication to the following leadership principles will facilitate achieving respect and recognition as a public health nursing leader.

- Self-appreciation
- Self-awareness of strengths and weaknesses
- Maintains optimism and confidence
- Confronts adversity with confidence and persistence
- Visualizes the ultimate goal (write specific goals)
- Shoulders responsibility for decision making
- Maintains a positive attitude
- Commits to active listening
- Listens to conscience (values are voiced in your conscience) and maintains values
- Communicates effectively (Mays, 1997)
- Gains social capital
- Uses power judiciously (share your power)

- Practices "wholism" (groups can achieve much) and promotes teamwork (Magee, 2000)
- Builds positive relationships
- Surrounds self with excellence
- Fails successfully
- Displays flexibility
- Maintains the mission
- Acts for the right reasons
- Provides followers with win-win situations
- Role-models and promotes integrity
- Mentors the next generation in leadership (Maxwell, 2001).

Mentoring

Mentoring is a leadership function. A mentoring relationship is considered an excellent mechanism with which to ensure professional development (Goldman & Schmalz, 2001). Mentoring and mentorship are terms that are frequently used interchangeably. However, a distinction between these terms is important. Mentorship is an intense relationship that promotes the personal, professional, and scholarly development of a novice nurse. Mentoring is the process that evolves from the formal and informal mentorship relationship and promotes the mentee's (protégé's) development. The mentor is typically an older, wiser, experienced nurse who guides, nurtures, and facilitates the personal, professional, and scholarly development of the novice nurse (Glanville & Porche, 2000).

Nursing mentoring is defined as a process of teaching and learning that takes place within a long-term personal, professional, and reciprocal relationship between two nurses who are different in relation to level of experience and expertise, age, personality, and credentials (Smith, McAllister, & Crawford, 2001). Benefits of mentoring are growth and development of nurses, enhanced thinking, increased risk taking, self-esteem development, professional development, job enrichment, clinical competence, political savvy, empowerment, job satisfaction, and preservation of a legacy (Goldman & Schmalz, 2001; Madison, 1994; Smith et al., 2001).

The mentor's characteristics are self-assurance, confidence, competence, acceptance, knowledge, and sensitivity. Mentors are supportive, caring, and giving. In comparison, the protégé's characteristics are commitment to learning, loyalty to the mentor, sincerity, honesty, and warmth (Smith et al., 2001). The responsibilities of mentor and protégé should be identified and negotiated early in the development of their mentoring relationship. Table 17.3 compares mentor and protégé responsibilities during the mentoring process.

The mentoring process occurs within a supportive relationship where there is mutual respect and trust, described as a patron system (Table 17.4). Each stage of the patron system has specific behaviors that promote the

Table 17.3   Mentor and Protégé Responsibilities Compared

Mentor	Protégé
Explains political and social barriers	Respects mentor's personal and social space
Shares values and vision	Appreciates people and resources
Provides trusting and caring relationship	Appreciates mentoring
Advocates for protégé	Asks for assistance
Career advisement	Is receptive to assistance
Provides challenging opportunities	Critically self-evaluates
Coaches and counsels	Open disclosure with mentor
Conceptualizes the "big picture" for protégé	Develops professional bond with mentor
Discusses problems and solutions	Recognizes problems and seeks solutions
Empowers, inspires, and encourages	Listens and learns
Provides focus and friendship	Spends time with mentor
Provides autonomy	Strives for excellence
Provides opportunities for collaboration	Seizes opportunities
Protects and sponsors	Dedication to mentoring experience
Role modeling and socialization	Time and energy
Structured goal setting and evaluation	Mentors others
Time, energy, and knowledge	Acts on information provided by mentor
Creates a supportive learning environment	
Balances praise and criticism	
Nurtures independence	
Commitment to mentoring process	
Assesses self and protégé's learning needs	

SOURCE: Goldman and Schmalz (2001) and Smith et al. (2001).

mentoring and development of the protégé. Successful mentorship will facilitate the development of a more collegial mentor-protégé relationship.

Delegation

Delegation is considered a management skill; however, most successful leaders can effectively delegate. Delegation is the allocation of jobs and responsibilities to other individuals or teams (Roebuck, 1998). Effective delegation assigns the right task to the right individual with the right amount of authority and responsibility to effectively achieve the goal. Effective delegation requires skill recognition, time management, and team motivation. Benefits of effective delegation are resource maximization, effective use of experts, building teams, providing individuals with an opportunity to develop skills, motivating teams, enhancing the leader's role, and the improving leadership skills of the leader and the followers.

The leader's delegation style (controller, coach, consultant, or coordinator-facilitator) must be matched to the individual who is being delegated. The four styles of individuals who are delegated to are beginner, learner, regular, and performer (Roebuck, 1998). Beginners are highly motivated and committed but have little experience in the task. The learner is not a

Table 17.4   Patron System

Stage	Relationship Status
Peer Pal	A colleague that shares a similar professional level with equal professional status. This relationship is the collegial sharing of support and information to assist each member of the partnership in achieving a new level.
Guide	A colleague who is not at the same collegial level but who assists the protégé in understanding the organizational structure and politics of the system.
Sponsor	A colleague of higher professional status who promotes the recognition of the protégé's accomplishments by individuals of their peer level.
Patron	A colleague of higher professional status who uses his or her power base to advance the protégé's career.
Mentor	A colleague who engages in a paternalistic relationship that crosses personal and professional boundaries. This person advocates, teaches, guides, provides expert and experiential advice, and promotes the development of the protégé's career. The mentor exhibits a caring nature on a personal and professional level.

SOURCE: Glanville and Porche (2000).

full expert but has some experience with the task. Learners have medium levels of knowledge and motivation. Regulars have medium to high knowledge regarding the task at hand, with medium motivation. At the highest end of the spectrum is the performer. The performer has high motivation and high knowledge regarding the task at hand.

Table 17.5 outlines the match between the leader's delegation style and the person delegated to. The controller provides specific instructions and closely supervises the task delegated. Coaches closely supervise but have a less directive approach. Coaches offer advice and support throughout the task. Consultants outline the task in general details and provide the person with more freedom to implement the task. Consultant delegators are available to provide help and support but are not directive in their supervision. The coordinator-facilitator gives an overall direction but leaves any specifics to the individual. The coordinator-facilitator provides the maximum level of autonomy in achieving the task but does define time intervals at which the individual must report on progress.

Delegation is considered a process that requires the leader to monitor the delegated task, assume responsibility for the task, and still provide the delegate with enough autonomy to achieve the desired results. Heller (1998) defines the process of delegation as encompassing five stages: analysis, appointment, briefing, control, and appraisal.

Analysis consists of deciding which tasks can be or should be delegated. Analysis consists of the leader assessing his or her time, the delegate's time, and the priority level of the task (Heller, 1998).

Table 17.5 Delegation Style Matching

Person Delegating Style	Style of Person Delegated to
Controller	Beginner
Coach	Learner
Consultant	Regular
Coordinator-facilitator	Performer

SOURCE: Roebuck (1998).

Appointment is the assignment of the right person to the right task. A careful assessment of the person's knowledge, experience, and specific abilities are required in relation to the task prior to appointment (Heller, 1998).

Briefing is the disclosure of the task to the delegate. The most important part of briefing is to clearly define the objective of the task (Heller, 1998). Roebuck (1998) defines the briefing format as including (a) background information on why the task is being done and why the individual has been chosen; (b) objectives of what needs to be achieved; (c) general tasks outlining the overall plan to achieve the objectives; (d) specific task details outlining how the general outline is to be achieved and what each team member is required to do; (e) administrative information regarding resources allocated, amount of authority, timelines, interim reports, action on problems, and contracts needed; (f) timeline for each division of the project or each objective; and (g) delegates' questions concerning the briefing.

Control is the monitoring of the delegate's progress and accomplishment of the tasks. Leaders institute different types of methods to control a project, such as involvement in all correspondence, written reports, oral reports, open-door policy for day-to-day updates, and formal progress meetings (Heller, 1998).

During the appraisal stage, the feedback mechanism operates, and information is shared between the administrator and delegate. The appraisal stage is also the time to reassess a delegate's abilities, assess performance, rectify problems encountered during the task, review the project, and identify practices and activities that could be improved (Heller, 1998).

Leadership Styles

Each public health nursing leader develops his or her leadership style. Leadership styles are not static. Public health nursing leaders must be adaptable and versatile enough to configure their leadership styles to situations as a means of achieving maximum effectiveness. Common leadership styles are autocratic, democratic, and laissez-faire. Autocratic leadership is directive, with no input from others into the decisions rendered. One individual renders the ultimate decision in autocratic leadership. Democratic leadership style is most inclusive, with participation of those individuals affected by or associated with the decision. The democratic leadership style provides stakeholders with equal input into the ultimate decision. In laissez-faire leadership, the leader deliberately and consciously is absent from providing direction or interference with the ultimate decision.

Other theorists have identified various leadership styles. Four leadership styles are described in path-goal leadership theory: directive, supportive, participative, and achievement oriented (Donnelly et al., 1997). Directive is similar to autocratic. Directive leadership directs subordinates with no input from the subordinates. Supportive leadership is friendly and interested in the subordinates as people. Participative is similar to democratic leadership. Participative leaders ask for and use suggestions provided by subordinates. Achievement-oriented leaders define challenging goals for subordinates but also demonstrate confidence in the subordinates' ability to achieve the goals. Vroom-Yetton theory identifies similar leadership styles, grouped into three major areas: autocratic (A), consultative (C), and group (G). Five leadership styles exist within these three major areas:

- A-I: Leader solves the problem using available information.
- A-II: Leader obtains information from followers, then makes the decision.
- C-I: Leader makes the decision after sharing the problem with followers individually rather than as a group.
- C-II: Leader makes the decision after sharing the problem with followers as a group.
- G-II: Leader shares problem with followers, group generates possible solutions together, group reaches consensus on the decision, with the leader serving as a group facilitator (Donnelly et al., 1997).

The Future of Public Health Nursing: Leading Change

Public health continues to be challenged with change. Forces driving global change are increased technology, international integration of economic and human resources, maturation of developing countries, and changes in multiple social structures (the fall of communism and increased immigration and migration). Globalization of the economy, along with international public health efforts, present increased opportunities and challenges for public health. The future of public health nursing is dependent on public health nurses' ability to effectively lead community members and other public health professionals through multiple times of continual change. Kotter (1996) has identified eight errors in effective leadership for change: (a) too much complacency, (b) failing to create a guiding coalition, (c) underestimating the power of a vision, (d) undercommunicating the vision, (e) permitting obstacles to block the vision, (f) failing to create short-term wins, (g) declaring victory too early, and (h) neglecting to anchor changes into the corporate culture (organizational sustainability). These eight mistakes guide the eight-stage process of effectively leading change.

Kotter's (1996) eight-stage process of effective change focuses on the use of both managerial and (primarily) leadership skills in the appropriate situations. The eight-stage process consists of

1. Establishing a sense of urgency—identify and discuss crises, potential crises or opportunities; competitive market analysis

2. Creating a guiding coalition—empowering a group through teamwork to lead the change

3. Developing a vision and strategy—creating a vision and strategic planning to achieve the vision

4. Communicating the change vision—constantly communicate the vision; relate all communication to the vision; role-model for the coalition

5. Empowering broad-based action—eliminate barriers; change systems or infrastructure that do not support the vision; encourage risk taking and nontraditional, creative ideas

6. Generating short-term wins—plan short-term goals; recognize the achievement of short-term goals (celebrate successes)

7. Consolidating gains and producing more change—change systems that don't fit the vision; hire, promote, and mentor nurses who are implementing the change vision

8. Anchoring the change in the culture—articulate success between new activities and behaviors to the organization's success; sustain change into the organizational culture

Implementation of this eight-stage process provides public health nurses with a framework to guide them during the change process.

Other Leaders

This chapter has focused on the public health nurse as a leader. Within communities, there are many types of leaders that exist in addition to the public health nurse and other public health professionals. Two additional leaders need recognition in public health practice: the servant leader and the community leader. Public health nurses, depending on their leadership philosophy, can also be considered servant or community leaders.

Servant leaders are individuals who become leaders out of their desire to serve the public more effectively. Servant leaders consider themselves as equals among others, use power honestly, understand the daily details of leadership, listen to and care for the constituency, facilitate the community's achievement of its goals, challenge their constituents to grow, and inspire others to serve their community. Developing as a servant leader involves listening to others, involving others, promoting teamwork rather than individual decision making, and enhancing problem solving (Greenleaf, 1976). Community leaders are community members who assume leadership within the community to achieve the community's goals. A community leader may also be recognized as a servant leader. Community leader is a general term used to identify key individuals with formal or informal leadership in a community.

Summary

Key issues in public heath–community health leadership are as follows.

- Characteristics of a good leader are the ability to control subordinates in a bureaucratic manner, certain personal characteristics or attributes, ability to maintain communication, ability to adapt behavior to the situation to foster the growth and development of others and still move forward, charisma, ability to envision the future and inspire and excite others, and political astuteness.
- Coaching, mentoring, and training are considered essential to develop the leadership ability of other community health nurses.
- Leadership is defined as a process in which a person or group aligns a diverse population of individuals with a vision as a means of enthusiastically pursuing mutually defined goals and objectives of the community.
- The influence that leaders exert over others is considered power.
- Principle-centered power is defined as the kind of power that inspires loyalty and devotion and that transcends time and place.
- Coercive power relies on control of other individuals and uses fear.
- Utility power is based on principles of negotiation.
- The type of power public health nurses use is matched to their values, experience, administrative position, and the professional situation requiring the use of power.
- Three levels of power sharing are (a) constituents or stakeholders providing ideas to the leader, (b) constituents or stakeholders participating in the decision-making process through exercises such as brainstorming, and (c) an equal sharing of power in decision making between the leader and the constituents or stakeholders.

- Administration is considered an umbrella term for management and leadership.
- Management is a process used by public health nurses to conduct, supervise, or coordinate the activities of multiple individuals to achieve defined goals and objectives.
- Mentorship is an intense relationship that promotes the personal, professional, and scholarly development of a novice nurse.
- Mentoring is the process that evolves from the formal and informal mentorship relationship and promotes the protégé's development.
- Delegation is the allocation of jobs and responsibilities to other individuals or teams.
- The process of delegation encompasses five stages: analysis, appointment, briefing, control, and appraisal.
- Common leadership styles are autocratic, democratic, and laissez-faire.
- Eight errors in effective leadership for change are too much complacency, failing to create a guiding coalition, underestimating the power of a vision, undercommunicating the vision, permitting obstacles to block the vision, failing to create short-term wins, declaring victory too early, and neglecting to anchor changes into the corporate culture.
- The eight-stage process of effective change involves establishing a sense of urgency, creating a guiding coalition, developing a vision and strategy, communicating the change vision, empowering broad-based action, generating short-term wins, consolidating gains and producing more change, and anchoring the change into the culture.
- Servant leaders are individuals who become leaders out of their desire to serve the public more effectively.
- Community leaders are community members who assume leadership within the community to achieve the community's goals.

References

Boedigheimer, S., & Gebbie, K. (2001). Currently employed public health administrators: Are they prepared? *Journal of Public Health Management Practice, 7*(1), 30-36.

Donnelly, J., Gibson, J., & Ivancevich, J. (1997). *Fundamentals of management* (10th ed.). Boston, MA: Richard D. Irwin.

Glanville, C., & Porche, D. (2000). Graduate nursing faculty: Ensuring cultural and racial diversity through faculty development. *Journal of Multicultural Nursing & Health Care, 6*(1), 6-13.

Goldman, K. & Schmalz, K. (2001). Follow the leader: Mentoring. *Health Promotion Practice, 2*(3), 195-197.

Greenleaf, R. (1976). *Servant leadership: A journey into the nature of legitimate power and greatness.* New York: Paulist.

Heller, R. (1998). *How to delegate.* London: Dorling Kindersley.

Kotter, J. (1996). *Leading change.* Boston, MA: Harvard Business School Press.

Lee, B. (1997). *The power principle: Influence with honor.* New York: Simon & Schuster.

Madison, J. (1994). The value of mentoring in nursing leadership: A descriptive study. *Nursing Forum, 29*(4), 16-23.

Magee, M. (2000). *Positive leadership.* New York: Spencer.

Maxwell, J. (2001). The right to lead: A study in character and courage. Nashville, TN: J. Countryman.

Mays, C. (1997). *Anatomy of a leader.* Aurora, IL: Successories.

Morton, J. (1999). A model of leadership for community nurses? *Journal of Community Nursing, 13*(5). Retrieved June 25, 2003, from http://www.jcn.co.uk

Roebuck, C. (1998). *Effective delegation: The essential guide to thinking and working smarter.* London: Marshall.

Romig, D. (2001). *Side by side leadership: Achieving outstanding results together.* Atlanta, GA: Bard.

Smith, L., McAllister, L., & Crawford, C. (2001). Mentoring benefits and issues for public health nurses. *Public Health Nursing, 18*(2), 101-107.

18

Communication, Collaboration, Negotiation, and Conflict

Collaboration, negotiation, and conflict have one common element: communication. Communication is the process used to get information from one individual to another to effectively create a collective understanding. This chapter focuses on describing the communication process, nonverbal communication, communication barriers, and communication flow; describing transcultural communication, communication plans, media communication, and risk communication; presenting conflict and conflict resolution; and defining and describing collaboration and collaboration models and processes.

Introduction

Public health nursing leaders and administrators engage in interactions with multiple public health disciplines, various community-based organizations, and public health agencies. This leadership and administration is accomplished through individual-to-individual, individual-to-group, and individual-to-community interactions, regardless of whether the interaction is between public health nurses or a public health nurse and community member. To effectively serve as a leader and manager of public health professionals and implement public health interventions, public health nurses must be competent in written and oral communication skills. Public health nurses use communication skills and techniques as community-level interventions that target particular populations.

Poor communication may be one cause of conflict between individuals and agencies. Management of conflict requires that public health nurses be skilled in conflict management and negotiation. In addition, public health nurses can use their negotiation skills to secure additional public health resources.

Negotiation of public health services or resources between and among public health agencies may lead to the development of collaborative relationships. Collaboration is an effective means of maximizing access to resources and reducing duplication of services. Collaborative public health models are dependent on public health nurses who can effectively communicate and negotiate the collaboration processes needed to provide public health services. This chapter will focus on communication, conflict management, negotiation skills, and collaboration.

The Communication Process

Communication is defined as the transfer of information and the understanding of this information from one individual to another. Communication is the process through which individuals share thoughts, ideas, facts, beliefs, values, and traditions. The communication process is influenced by many factors, such as language, ethnicity, culture, environment, personal background, and experience. These factors influence both the encoding of messages by the sender and the decoding of messages by the receiver. Communication is a process that requires the engagement of at least two individuals, the message sender and the message receiver.

The communication process is outlined in Figure 18.1. A thought or message originates in the sender's mind. The sender then encodes the message into a form or medium that the receiver can understand, such as words, symbols, pictures, charts, gestures or some other form, to transmit the message. The sender must consider the purpose of the message during this encoding process. The sender transmits the encoded message in the chosen medium to the receiver. The receiver then decodes the message. The receiver attempts to understand exactly what the sender meant when the message was sent. The communication process is completed when the receiver provides feedback to the sender. The communication process has been effective if the receiver responds in a manner that informs the sender that the intended message was interpreted correctly.

Nonverbal Communication

Nonverbal communication is the exchange of information through behaviors without the use of words. Nonverbal communication normally occurs during verbal communication, both consciously and unconsciously. During the communication process, the sender and receiver are both engaging in behaviors that are transferring messages to each other. The sender should ensure that his or her nonverbal communication is consistent with the verbal message. Any incongruence may lead the receiver to interpret the message in a manner that was not intended by the sender. Messages are communicated nonverbally through body type, shape, and size; clothing and personal appearance; body movements and gestures; facial expressions and eye behavior; personal space; touching behavior; voice characteristics and quality; smells and taste; and other environmental aspects.

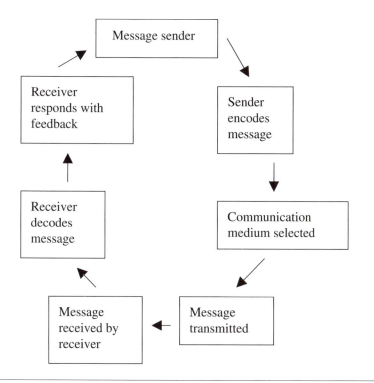

Figure 18.1 The Communication Process

Communication Barriers

The communication of a message is a complex transaction between two parties. Many potential barriers can interrupt this communication process. These barriers can be process, physical, semantic, or psychosocial in nature. Process barriers consist of noise, poor listening skills, perceptual differences, conflicting verbal and nonverbal messages, and reluctance to communicate. Physical barriers can consist of poor positioning, the presence of physical structures, or the selection of an inappropriate medium through which to communicate. Semantic barriers exist if there is not a common language, word usage, or idiomatic phrasing. Psychosocial barriers consist of differences in the sender's and receiver's personal backgrounds, values, beliefs, needs, biases, and expectations.

Communication Flow

Individuals exchange information in distinct communication patterns. These communication patterns outline the flow of communication. Communication flow can be classified as either vertical or horizontal. Public health nurses should effectively assess and use both vertical and horizontal communication flow, as appropriate. The public health nurse must be alert to the means through which communication flows in a community.

Vertical communication can flow either upward or downward. Upward communication is the exchange of information from individuals in lower levels to individuals in higher levels. Downward communication is the exchange of information from individuals in higher levels to individuals in lower levels. Horizontal communication is also known as lateral communication. Horizontal communication is the exchange of information among peers, colleagues, or community members who are at the same level. In addition, communication flows through the grapevine, which can be either vertical or horizontal. The grapevine is the informal circulation of information among members of the community. The informal flow of information is vital to understanding the flow of communication within a community. It is the public health nurse's challenge to know the communication flow patterns in a community and effectively use these to implement community-level population-based change.

Transcultural Communication

Public health nurses are engaged in communities that consist of a cornucopia of cultures. To effectively interact with representative members of the community, public health nurses need to be competent in transcultural communication. Transcultural communication is the successful exchange of ideas, feelings, and information between people from different cultures (Luckmann, 1999). Effective transcultural communication requires that the public health nurse be familiar with (a) starting conversations, (b) how to be understood (i.e., is an interpreter needed), (c) appropriate responses to gestures or questions, (d) sensitivity to reactions, (e) how to listen to concerns, and (f) illness- and health-related beliefs (Luckmann, 1999). Competence in transcultural communication starts with public health nurses assessing their own cultural background, becoming familiar with their own values, recognizing their own culture's influence in communication, and appreciating that many cultures interact in the community. Transcultural communication competence is further developed through studying various cultures. The public health nurse should always recognize the community member first as an individual with unique cultural communication needs, then as a member of a cultural group.

Barriers to transcultural communication inhibit the exchange of ideas and information between members of differing cultural groups. Common barriers to transcultural communication are (a) lack of cultural knowledge; (b) fear and distrust; (c) racism—individual, cultural, or institutional; (d) ethnocentrism; (e) stereotyping; (f) language—foreign language, dialect differences, regionalisms, slang, idioms, or street talk; and (g) conflicting perceptions.

Table 18.1 Transcultural Communication Techniques

- Approach slowly when first meeting
- Greet respectfully
- Establish a quiet environment
- Establish a comfortable distance—assess reaction to personal space
- Provide the opportunity to ask questions
- Mirror their communication style and posture
- Restate or paraphrase
- Seek validation of understanding
- Use reflection
- Use silence as appropriate
- Be alert to nonverbal communication—quality and tone of voice, posture, gestures, facial expressions, touch, eye contact
- Cautious use of touch
- Follow other individuals' use of eye contact as a guide

SOURCE: Luckmann (1999).

Communication is critical to establishing a relationship. Public health nurses must first convey empathy, show respect, build trust, establish rapport, listen actively, and provide feedback to communicate transculturally (Luckmann, 1999). Table 18.1 outlines communication techniques that can facilitate transcultural communication.

To assist with transcultural communication, public health nurses use the assistance of interpreters. An interpreter translates orally for individuals conversing in different languages. Interpreters are recommended unless the nurse is thoroughly fluent and effective in the language. It is generally recommended that family members not be used as translators or interpreters, especially with young children. Use of family members may raise issues of confidentiality and validity of the assessment information. There are three general styles of interpretation: voice box, excluder, and collaborator. In the voice-box style, communication is translated word for word. In the excluder style, the interpreter takes over the interaction, communicating with the other individual and then explaining to the public health nurse what was said. The collaborator is a combination of the voice-box and excluder styles. The collaborator style has the nurse and interpreter working together and interacting with the client (Hatton & Webb, 1993).

Communication Plan

Public health organizations should consider developing a communication plan to provide the public with sensitive or critical messages. A communication plan facilitates the communication process and assists in achieving the desired communication goal. The communication plan is a means through which the message is organized and critically thought through prior to its delivery. This is especially critical when speaking with groups in the community. The communication plan is developed through the answers and measures designed in response to the following critical questions:

- What are your communication goals?
- Who is your target audience? What is their preferred communication medium? Which medium will have the greatest public penetration?
- What is your public health organization's communication history? What has worked best in the past? What has worked worst in the past? What lessons have been learned?
- What resources and means does your public health organization have to communicate the message?
- What are potential barriers to your public health organizations communication? What alternative do you have? How can you manage these potential barriers?

Media Communication

Communication through the media is a community-level intervention used to target a large population at one time. The media is recognized as a channel through which information is transmitted from a news source—the radio, television, or print—to the general community population. The media can be used to announce new public health programs, create an awareness about public health issues, inform the community about community events, and transmit health education messages. The media can also be used in public health policy agenda setting (refer to chapter 24).

Media communication should be approached with a media communication plan. The media communication plan should identify the communication team members, identify the goals and objectives of the media communication, select the target audience, select the appropriate media format (radio, television, or print), draft the media message, pilot the media message, revise the media message, implement the media message, and evaluate the effectiveness of the media message (Wallack, Dorfman, Jerniagan, & Themba, 1993). The media message may be in the form of a "media bite": a 10- to 15-second quote or shorter phrase that provides the essential message and secures the audience's attention.

Public health nurses participate in media communication by participating in the development of the media communication plan. Additionally, public health nurses use small and large print media to provide health education information to individuals and groups in the community. Public health nurses also engage in the development of public service announcements, press conferences, and the writing of press releases.

Public Service Announcements

Public service announcements (PSAs) are short messages produced for radio or television stations that communicate a public health message to the community. The Federal Communications Commission (FCC) requires broadcast media to serve "in the public's interest," and most stations use PSAs as a method of meeting this requirement. PSAs are useful to increase awareness or communicate announcements of public health events. The writing of PSAs requires a clear purpose and goal.

PSAs are developed for a specific target audience. The media outlet selected should be consistent with the target audience and the message delivered. The message should be vivid, simple, and provide the audience with something that they remember—a "hook." Some guidelines for writing PSAs are (a) choose a focal point for the message, (b) brainstorm with colleagues and members of the target audience, (c) ensure that facts and information are valid and reliable, (d) identify a part of the message (a hook) that catches the audience's attention, (e) pilot and evaluate the message, and (f) revise as necessary.

Press Conference

Public health professionals, including public health nurses, usually must have permission from their public relations department prior to engaging in a press conference. A press conference is a carefully planned communication technique used to generate news and formally communicate announcements and information that is timely, significant, and relevant to the community in a public forum. In certain situations, the press conference may be superior to other media formats. A press conference permits the release of more information, allows interaction between the public health nurse and community members, and provides publicity.

Press conferences should be carefully planned, as a special media event. The steps to planning a press conference are (a) clarify the issue and essential messages into a few key points, (b) identify the audience intended to hear the message (which may not consist of the same individuals invited to the press conference), (c) select the date and time, (d) select a location that is related to or symbolic of the public health issue or message, (e) identify the contact individuals or organizational representatives, (f) notify the media, (g) develop small print media to be distributed, (h) conduct the press conference, and (i) evaluate the effect of the press conference (Taplin, 1993).

Press Release

A press release is considered small print media communication. A press release is a brief narrative summary that provides the public with a timed announcement. Press releases are designed to inform the public. Press releases can be used to announce an event or new program, provide factual information, or highlight special public health issues. Press releases are faxed, e-mailed, or mailed to the target audience.

Press releases have a typical format. The following are guidelines for the development and formatting of a press release: (a) label it as a press release in bold print; (b) place the date and location of origin of the press release in a clearly visible spot (press releases may be distributed with an embargo date to coordinate the timely dissemination of the information); (c) develop a short, interesting title; (d) make the first paragraph a summary statement that encourages the reading of the press release; (e) the narrative body of the text should be easy to read and double spaced; (f) the press release should be written in active tense; (g) quotes from experts or community members should be included; (h) contact information should be provided; and (i) the press release should identify associated organizations.

Risk Communication

Public health nurses and other officials engage in exchange of information during tense times in the community. Risk communication is the presentation of information to a population in a community regarding that population's level of risk in relation to a potentially harmful agent. During risk communication, the public health nurse attempts to exchange information with community stakeholders regarding the nature, magnitude, significance, and control of a community risk. This communication is generally of a highly scientific nature, with technical information that must be provided to an often non–scientifically informed or nontechnical population of community members who are anxious and concerned about their risk. Risk communication is the effective exchange of information to community members in a low-trust but high-concern context.

The EPA, which engages in risk communication with community members regarding actual or potential environmental exposures, has provided seven cardinal rules of risk communication (see Table 18.2).

The elements that make up risk communication are the message, messenger, audience, and context. The message is one of uncertainty or risk. The medium and format of the message must be given careful consideration. The messenger must be a trusted individual in the community. The culture, language, and educational level of the audience must be considered in planning the risk communication intervention. The context of the situation must be assessed during the planning of the risk communication message, to the point of delivering the information. The assessment, at a minimum, must include an examination of the amount of the community's anger or outrage (known as the outrage factor), the employment situation in the community, the socioeconomic status of the community, and any history or

Table 18.2   The Environmental Protection Agency's Seven Cardinal Rules of Risk
                  Communication

1.   Accept and involve the public as a partner

2.   Develop a communication plan and evaluate your efforts

3.   Listen to the public's specific concerns

4.   Be honest and open

5.   Partner with other credible community resources in communicating the risk

6.   Meet the needs of the media

7.   Speak clearly and with compassion

Table 18.3   Pitfalls to Avoid in Risk Communication

- Technical jargon
- Inappropriate humor in relation to safety and health
- Repeating negative allegations
- Using negative words or phrases
- Communicating with only words
- Temper
- Complex communication
- Abstract communication
- Nonverbal messages that are not consistent with verbal
- Attacking a person (focus only on issues)
- Grandiose promises
- Speculation on what will be done
- Blaming others
- Assuming something is "off the record"
- Being unprepared or off schedule
- Not knowing knowable information
- Lengthy presentations

previous relationship of public health professionals with the community
(trust factor). Some common pitfalls to avoid in risk communication are
presented in Table 18.3.

The risk communicator should make statements of personal concern, the
organization's intent, and the purpose and plan of the meeting. The presenter should acknowledge the existence of hostility in the community and practice self-management so he or she will not react to the level of hostility. The
presentation should be prepared and the message should be communicated
with empathy and care. Questions posed by community members should be
repeated, answered clearly, and the community member should then be
asked the extent to which their question has been answered. If questions get
off the specific topic, it is the presenter's responsibility to answer the unfo-
cused question in such a way that it returns back to the topic of discussion.

Conflict

Conflict is a part of everyday life. Conflict occurs at all levels in a community: individual, family, aggregate, organizational, institutional, and community. Conflict is frequently cited as being natural, inevitable, normal, and necessary for change (Robbins & Coulter, 2001).

Mayer (2000) describes conflict as occurring along three dimensions: cognitive, emotional, and behavioral. The cognitive dimension exists when one party perceives that his or her belief about or understanding of his or her own needs, interests, wants, or values is incompatible with someone else's. The emotional dimension consists of fear, sadness, bitterness, anger, or hopelessness resulting from a disagreement between two or more parties regarding a situation or interaction. The behavioral dimension consists of actions that express feelings or perceptions or that attempt to meet needs in some way that interferes with others' ability to meet their needs (Mayer, 2000).

The antecedent causes of conflict are multifactorial (Mayer, 2000). A lack of communication or incorrect communication could lead to wrongful perception of another's motives or actions. Emotions are fueled by interactions, situational circumstances, and previous experiences. Incongruence between emotional feelings can cause conflict to develop. Escalation of emotions can fuel a conflict that is in progress or create the perseverance to resolve the conflict. A powerful influence on conflict is the past history that has occurred between the involved parties. The historical context provides underlying momentum for conflict. The external structural framework between two parties influences the type of interactions that occur. The external structural framework consists of available resources, decision-making procedures, time constraints, communication patterns, and physical setting and facilities. Differences in values can lead to the development of conflict or escalation of conflict (Mayer, 2000).

Another common source of community conflict is the actual or perceived inequity or unfairness that occurs within defined populations or throughout the community. There are five types of justice that may contribute to the development or escalation of community conflict if they are not present: distributive justice, procedural justice, sense of justice, retributive and reparative justice, and scope of justice (Deutsch & Coleman, 2000). Distributive justice exists when scarce resources are equally allocated. Procedural justice is concerned with fair treatment in relation to decisions made and implementation of decisions among all parties. Sense of justice is the perception of equal or fair treatment. Retributive and reparative justice consists of an equitable response to the violation of moral norms and ways with which to equitably repair the moral community that has been violated. The scope of justice is concerned with who is and who is not included in the moral community. Scope of justice describes the boundaries of populations considered entitled to equitable treatment in the specific situation (Deutsch & Coleman, 2000).

Conflict is approached based on various attitudes or needs. Mayer (2000) describes five types of conflict: conflict based in power, rights, personal interests, principles, or manipulation. These can be sources of conflict but may also be used as methods of resolving conflict. Power-based conflict occurs when two parties are competing for the same power base or one is exercising power over the other. Rights-based conflict asserts an individual's privileges or rights in accordance with law, policy, regulation, or procedures. Interest-based conflict comes from the belief that one's needs or concerns are not being addressed as desired. Principle-based conflict uses the appeal of values, reasonableness, justice, or moral assertions as the cause of conflict or means of resolving conflict. Manipulation-based conflict can be constructive or destructive, as can the approaches previously discussed. Manipulation-based conflict encourages others to meet their needs or desires without directly confronting the issue or making needs directly known to others (Mayer, 2000).

Conflict Resolution

Prevention is the best alternative to conflict resolution. Individuals may avoid conflict through several approaches: aggressive avoidance, passive avoidance, passive-aggressive avoidance, avoidance through hopelessness, avoidance through surrogates, avoidance through denial, avoidance through premature problem solving, and avoidance by folding. Aggressive avoidance is the use of aggressive behavior to ward off conflict. Passive avoidance is the avoidance, removal, or lack of action in response to a conflict. Passive-aggressive avoidance is the use aggressive behavior by provoking others to engage in the conflict but remaining directly uninvolved in the conflict. Avoidance through hopelessness views the situation as beyond repair or denies that anyone has the ability to change the situation. Avoidance through surrogates lets others engage in the conflict to fight the battle. Avoidance through denial is not recognizing that conflict exists. Avoidance through premature problem solving resolves the immediate conflict but may not alter the underlying issues causing the conflict. This kind of "problem solving" may be superficial or misdirected. Avoidance by folding resolves the conflict by one party giving in to the other party to stop the conflict (Mayer, 2000).

Conflict resolution parallels the dimensions of conflict; the resolution may be cognitive, emotional, or behavioral. Cognitive conflict resolution uses the creation of cognitive dissonance and reframing. In cognitive dissonance, the mediator proposes a new cognitive framework that is amenable to both parties. Reframing attempts to alter perceptions about the nature of the conflict, the issues, or choices to facilitate resolution. In emotional conflict resolution, the disputing parties express their feelings and acknowledge each other's feelings. Emotional conflict resolution attempts to have the two parties work toward forgiveness and apology. Behavioral conflict resolution involves discontinuing the conflicting behavior and instituting or substituting the existing conflicting behavior with another acceptable behavior. Formal agreements, contracts, peace treaties, and consent decrees can be used in behavioral conflict resolution (Mayer, 2000).

The Negotiation Process

The negotiation process can be used to resolve conflict or to create a win-win situation in the allocation of scarce resources (Mayer, 2000). Negotiation can be distributive or integrative. Distributive negotiation focuses on each party getting as much as possible of what they want for themselves or their community. Distributive negotiators attempt to have the other party agree to an allocation of resources favorable to the negotiators' party. Integrative negotiation differs in that it focuses on maximizing the resources available to both parties and meeting both parties' needs in some manner (Mayer, 2000). Integrative negotiation may require the expansion of resources available.

Negotiators reach closure through several measures. Negotiators can reach closure through the convergence of distributive and integrative negotiation. This occurs by permitting each party to take as much as they want (distributive). When there is nothing more to take, then what was available is increased (integrative) so that both parties get what is wanted.

Negotiators can reach agreement through fractionalization. Fractionalization consists of breaking the conflict down into smaller, manageable parts. This makes it possible to work on smaller pieces of the conflict at a time and provides opportunities for tradeoffs. Negotiation can occur through agreements in principle. Agreements in principle means that both parties agree to the broad issues, which are then refined and specified until an operational agreement is reached. Reframing the issues can facilitate negotiation. In addition, maturation of the conflict facilitates negotiation. The needs, wants, and desires of each party may change or alter with time (Mayer, 2000).

Collaboration Defined

The ability to communicate is an essential element in forming collaborative relationships. Collaboration occurs at the individual, group, organizational, or institutional level. With limited resources available to deliver health-care services to the public, community-based and public health agencies are forming partnerships to use their resources efficiently. Collaboration can expand or enhance existing services.

Collaboration has multiple definitions. Collaboration is described as a process of mutual respect for differences in opinion and perspective (Hills et al., 1994), a process of negotiation and compromise integral to decision making (Henry, Schmitz, Reif, & Rudie, 1992), and an interpersonal process in which each member contributes to a common goal (Henneman, 1995). Sullivan (1998) defined collaboration as "a dynamic transforming process of creating a power sharing partnership for pervasive application in health care practice, education, research and organizational settings for the purposeful attention to needs and problems in order to achieve likely successful outcomes" (p. 6). For the purposes of this book, collaboration will be defined as a dynamic process of forming partnerships that share power and resources through mutual respect and negotiation to achieve mutual goals.

Collaboration is one method of building and sustaining relationships in the community. Collaboration facilitates the partnering of organizations and community members to solve common problems of the community. Multisector collaboration involves the aggregation of different resources from multiple sectors in the community—business, educational institutions, government, and nonprofit organizations—to meet community needs.

Collaboration Models

Community members and organizations can form multiple types of working relationships. Working relationships are generally initiated to share information or resources. Collaboration assists each party to expand or enhance existing capabilities.

The Systems Model of Collaboration

This collaboration model is based on open systems theory. Collaboration is considered an open system in which the attributes of each party are connected within a pattern of interrelations and actions that influence each other. An understanding of the collaborative process using this model can be best understood by studying the whole collaborative system. Collaboration is considered to consist of four major attributes or subsystems: processes, partnership, practice, and outcomes. These collaborative attributes are based on communication, respect and trust, shared vision and goals, and shared decision making. Using this model, the partners come together through dynamic processes to form a partnership of public health practice to achieve desired outcomes. Each component of this systems model is considered to influence another component (Sullivan, 1998). Some processes that facilitate collaboration will now be explored.

The Collaboration Process and Facilitation

The core processes of community collaboration are organizing the effort, convening the community, creating a shared vision, assessing current realities and

Table 18.4   Core Community Collaboration Processes

Organizing the Effort
- Write memorandum of collaboration
- Acknowledge contributions of all stakeholders
- Agree on processes, procedures, and roles
- Develop leadership capacity

Convening the Community
- Include relevant stakeholders
- Generate acceptance by all stakeholders
- Ensure credibility
- Create interest

Creating a Shared Vision
- Develop a shared vision through consensus
- Differentiate vision from individual values of each party
- Encourage continual refinement of vision

Assessing Current Realities and Trends
- Conduct assessments
- Measure assets
- Identify resources
- Link assessment to vision, action, and outcomes
- Gather relevant data and useful information

Action Planning
- Facilitate ownership of plan by all stakeholders
- Define actions for each objective
- Plan for training and resources needed
- Write collaborative action plan

Doing the Job
- Implement activities in collaborative action plan
- Link actions to vision

Monitoring and Adjusting
- Mutually agree on benchmarks and outcomes
- Develop monitoring procedures
- Use multiple methods of data collection
- Continuously document and share evaluation findings
- Use findings to alter processes during collaborative endeavor

SOURCE: Johnson et al. (1996).

trends, action planning, doing the job, and monitoring and adjusting (Johnson, Grossman, & Cassidy, 1996). Organizing the effort supports the formation of a partnership and the operationalization of multisectoral collaboration through the establishment of agreements, policies and procedures, and the formation of a coordinating committee. To facilitate the establishment of a collaborative endeavor between multiple individuals or organizations, a memorandum of collaboration is recommended. A memorandum of collaboration is a binding agreement between two or more parties that agree to the roles and responsibilities spelled out in the memorandum. The memorandum of collaboration is dated and signed by all parties, with each party receiving a copy.

The process of convening the community mobilizes the community into a collaborative effort. Creating a shared vision engages each party to envision what they want for their community. Assessing current realities and trends is the process of gathering accurate assessment data about each collaborative party and the community. Action planning develops an action plan that outlines the goals, objectives, strategies, timelines, and parties responsible for implementing the collaborative initiative. Doing the job is the implementation of the action plan. Monitoring and evaluation measures the process and outcomes of the collaborative partnership as a means of promoting continuous quality improvement. The steps for each of these collaborative processes are detailed in Table 18.4.

Summary

Key issues in communication, collaboration, negotiation, and conflict are as follows.

- Communication is defined as the transfer of information and the understanding of this information from one individual to another.
- Nonverbal communication is the exchange of information through behaviors without the use of words.
- Communication barriers can be process, physical, semantic, or psychosocial in nature.
- Communication patterns outline the flow of communication.
- Vertical communication can flow either upward or downward.
- Horizontal communication is the exchange of information among peers, colleagues, or community members who are at the same level.
- The grapevine is the informal circulation of information among members of the community.
- Transcultural communication is the successful exchange of ideas, feelings, and information between people from different cultures.
- Common barriers to transcultural communication are lack of cultural knowledge, fear and distrust, racism, ethnocentrism, stereotyping, different language or dialects, and conflicting perceptions.
- Public health nurses must first convey empathy, show respect, build trust, establish rapport, listen actively, and provide feedback to communicate transculturally.
- A communication plan is a means through which a message is organized and critically thought through prior to its delivery.

- The media is recognized as a channel through which information is transmitted from a news source.
- A media bite is a 10- to 15-second quote or shorter phrase that provides the essential message and secures the audience's attention.
- PSAs are short messages produced for radio or television stations that communicate a public health message to the community.
- A press conference is a carefully planned communication technique used to generate news and formally communicate announcements and information that is timely, significant, and relevant to the community in a public forum.
- A press release is a brief narrative summary that provides the public with a timed announcement.
- Risk communication is the presentation of information to a population in a community regarding that population's level of risk to a potentially harmful agent.
- Conflict is defined as perceived differences between two or more parties that are incompatible and that result in interference or opposition.
- Common causes of conflict are communication, emotions, history, structure, and values.
- Five types of conflict are conflict based in power, rights, personal interests, principles, or manipulation.
- Cognitive conflict resolution uses the creation of cognitive dissonance and reframing.
- Emotional conflict resolution occurs when the disputing parties express their feelings and acknowledge each other's feelings.
- Negotiation is the process that occurs when two parties try to meet their own and differing needs by reaching an agreement that is acceptable to both parties.
- Collaboration is defined as a dynamic process of forming partnerships that share power and resources through mutual respect and negotiation to achieve mutual goals.
- The core processes of community collaboration are organizing the effort, convening the community, creating a shared vision, assessing current realities and trends, action planning, doing the job, and monitoring and adjusting.
- A memorandum of collaboration is a binding agreement between two or more parties that agree to the roles and responsibilities in the memorandum.

References

Deutsch, M., & Coleman, P. (2000). *The handbook of conflict resolution: Theory and practice.* San Francisco: Jossey-Bass.

Hatton, D., & Webb, T. (1993). Information transmission in bilingual, bicultural contexts: A field study of community health nurses and interpreters. *Journal of Community Health Nursing, 10*(3), 137-147.

Henneman, E. (1995). Nurse-physician collaboration: A poststructural view. *Journal of Nursing Administration, 22*, 359-363.

Henry, V., Schmitz, K., Reif, L., & Rudie, P. (1992). Collaboration: Integrating practice and research into public health nursing. *Public Health Nursing, 9*, 218-222.

Hills, M., Lindsey, E., Chisamore, M., Bassett-Smith, J., Abbott, K., & Fournier-Chalmers, J. (1994). University-college collaboration: Rethinking curriculum development in nursing education. *Journal of Nursing Education, 33*, 220-225.

Johnson, K., Grossman, W., & Cassidy, A. (1996). *Collaborating to improve community health: workbook and guide to best practices in creating healthier communities and populations.* San Francisco: Jossey-Bass.

Luckmann, J. (1999). *Transcultural communication in nursing.* Boston, MA: Delmar.

Mayer, B. (2000). *The dynamics of conflict resolution: A practitioner's guide.* San Francisco: Jossey-Bass.

Robbins, S., & Coulter, M. (2001). *Management* (7th ed.). Upper Saddle River, NJ: Pearson Education.

Sullivan, T. (1998). *Collaboration: A health care imperative.* St. Louis, MO: McGraw-Hill.

Taplin, S. (1993). *Holding press conferences: Why, when, and how.* Palo Alto, CA: Stanford University.

Wallack, L., Dorfman, L., Jerniagan, D., & Themba, M. (1993). *Media advocacy and public health: Power for prevention.* Newbury Park: Sage.

Public Health–Community Health Decisional and Causal Analysis

Public health nurses are challenged with multiple problems at various levels: individual, programmatic, organizational, political, and community. Effective methods of analyzing the causative elements of a problem are required for effective decision making. This chapter focuses on presenting causal analysis models and methods for problem analysis.

Introduction

Behavioral, public health, environmental, and community assessments identify community assets and health problems in addition to identifying population-based health needs in a community. These assessments provide data that can be used in further analysis of community or public health problems encountered by public health nurses. Causal analysis models and methods are used in public health decision-making processes. Causal analysis models and methods will be presented as tools needed for public health nursing managers to use in identifying solutions to actual or potential community- and population-based problems. Various types of health-care and industrial organizations use these models in problem solving.

Causal Analysis Models and Methods

In addition to quality improvement measures and program monitoring and evaluation, public health nurses employ a variety of causal analyses to solve population-based community health problems or organizational problems. A causal analysis consists of techniques used to describe or analyze factors or conditions that contribute to the existence of an identified problem (Witkin & Altschuld, 1995). Several techniques that public health nurses can add to their problem-solving skills are root-cause analysis, the "fishbone" or cause-and-effect diagram, cause-and-consequence analysis, faulty tree analysis, and force-field analysis.

Root-Cause Analysis: The Five Whys

Root-cause analysis uses the "five-whys" technique, asking the question "Why?" five times. The repeated asking of "Why?" is expected to identify the root or deep cause of the problem being explored. This technique is simple, identifies potential root causes, and can determine relationships between different root causes of a problem. The five-why root-cause analysis can be conducted individually or using a group.

The analysis begins with writing down the specific need or problem, as a means of formalizing the essential problem under analysis. The next step consists of asking why the problem occurs. The answer to this question is written down below the problem. If the written answer does not provide the root cause, the next question posed is "Why does _____ contribute to the problem?" This process is continued for a series of about five times, thus the name "five-whys" technique. This technique provides the public health nurse with a series of successive questions that ask why each answer is potentially contributing to the need or problem identified previously.

The following is an example of the five-whys root-cause analysis technique. The initial problem is that the immunization rate in the community continues to remain at a low level.

Question 1:   Why does the immunization rate remain at a low level?

Answer: Mothers are not bringing their children for their childhood immunizations.

Question 2:   Why are mothers not bringing their children to receive their immunizations?

Answer: Mothers do not understand the immunization schedule, reasons for immunization, or where to get immunizations.

Question 3:   Why do mothers not understand the immunization schedule, reasons for immunization, or where to seek immunizations?

Answer: Mothers are not educated about immunizations after delivery.

Question 4:   Why are mothers not educated about immunizations?

Answer: Immunization education is not consistently provided.

Question 5:   Why is immunization education not consistently provided?

Answer: It is not part of the patient education standards after a delivery.

In this example, public health nurses can provide literature and work with acute care facilities to ensure the integration of such information into patient education materials.

Fishbone or Cause-and-Effect Diagram

The "fishbone" or cause-and-effect diagram is also known as the Ishikawa diagram. This diagram is used in causal analysis of various types of problems identified, including community health and organizational problems. The fishbone diagram provides a systematic method with which to analyze an effect and the causes that create or contribute to it. The fishbone diagram is a heuristic tool that can be used to study a problem or issue to determine the root cause, to study all possible reasons for problems, to identify areas of further data collection, and to study why a process is not performing as desired.

The fishbone diagram can be used in three types of cause-and-effect analyses: cause enumeration, dispersion analysis, and process analysis. Cause enumeration is frequently used in quality improvement and evaluation to identify all possible types of causes and their influence on the identified problem. Dispersion analysis consists of thoroughly analyzing each major cause by investigating subcauses and their impact on the effect in question. Process analysis seeks to identify causes in the sequence of operations that may have led to a certain effect (Reshef, 2003).

The procedure for developing a fishbone diagram is simple. A group is convened to develop the diagram. The "fishbone" is drawn with a head, a backbone and at least four rib structures, as shown in Figure 19.1. The community need or problem is placed in the head of the fishbone (Figure 19.2). The community need or problem (effect) is analyzed using any of the following major categories (potential causes) or a combination thereof:

- Four Ms: methods, machines, materials, and manpower
- Four Ps: place, procedure, people, and policies
- Four Ss: surroundings, suppliers, systems, and skills (Reshef, 2003; Witkin & Altschuld, 1995)

Each of the major categories is placed on one of the rib structures along the fishbone backbone structure. An idea-generating technique such as nominal technique or brainstorming is used to identify factors within each category structure that may have caused the community need or problem. This process is continued until no other potential causes are identified. The group facilitator typically reviews each potential cause identified under each category. Through group consensus, restructuring of the fishbone diagram is completed by adding or deleting from the fishbone. At the conclusion, there is general discussion regarding the fishbone diagram in its entirety. This process concludes the identification of the major likely causes of the community need or problem (effect) (Witkin & Altschuld, 1995).

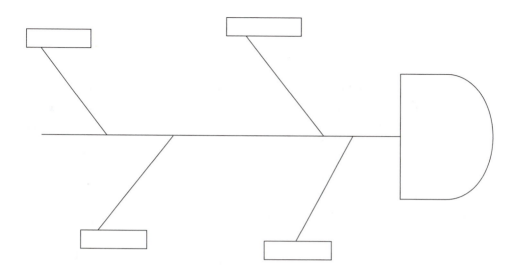

Figure 19.1   Basic Fishbone Structure

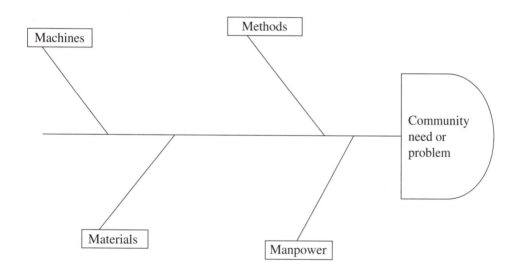

Figure 19.2   Fishbone Diagram Using the Four Ms

Public health nurses can use data from a fishbone causal analysis in multiple situations: community assessments, program planning, and organizational management. Specifically, the data can be used to comprehensively explore an expressed need and its contributing factors, narrow the focus of an assessment, and identify areas where it is necessary to focus evaluation and quality improvement efforts (Witkin & Altschuld, 1995).

Cause-and-Consequence Analysis

Cause-and-consequence analysis promotes the identification of both the causes and effects of present problems and potential effects in the near future. Cause-and-consequence analysis is also considered a risk assessment technique. This technique works best with a small group of key informants from the community. The end result of this technique is priority ranking of the potential problems based on the severity of causes and the potential consequences of not eliminating the causes (whether this will result in the identified problems; Witkin & Altschuld, 1995).

Five to eight key informants work individually to generate ideas that fit into one of five columns. The five columns in the cause-and-consequence analysis table include the following information:

- Column 1 lists the problems, needs, or adverse situations identified in the community.
- Column 2 lists all possible causes of each problem, need, or adverse situation.
- Column 3 lists all potential consequences that may result if the causes are not eliminated and the problem continues to exist.
- Column 4 rates the level of difficulty in correcting the problem as low, medium, or high.
- Column 5 rates the critical nature of the problem, need, or adverse situation if it is not resolved, with 1 being least critical and 5 being most critical (Witkin & Altschuld, 1995).

Each of the key informants rates each of the problems individually in columns 4 and 5. The scores for all the group members are tallied to reach a total rating score for the difficulty and critical nature of each problem. Problems that are rated as highly critical with low or moderate difficulty are generally the best problems to solve with short-term planning. Long-term planning is needed for problems rated both highly critical and difficult (Witkin & Altschuld, 1995).

Faulty Tree Analysis

Faulty tree analysis (FTA) is a system-centered approach to causal analysis. FTA is considered a form of risk assessment. This multicausal type of analysis outlines the contribution of each causal consequence to other causal consequences. Each event on the FTA tree is a potential failure or a contributor to an undesired event. The purpose of FTA is the avoidance of failures and the enhancement of success (Witkin & Altschuld, 1995).

Failure events are placed in boxes and connected to other failure events by logic gates. The steps of an FTA are

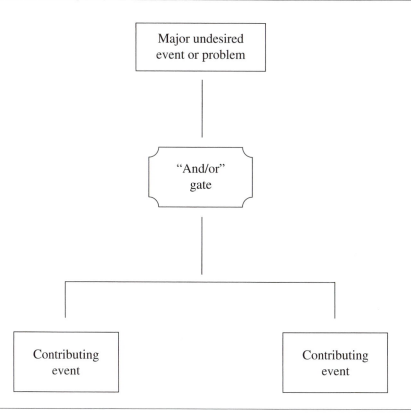

Figure 19.3 Faulty Tree Analysis Structure

- Perform a success analysis
- Select one or more undesired events
- Gather concerns and supporting data regarding the undesired event and place them as events on the tree
- Synthesize the events by constructing a faulty tree (Witkin & Altschuld, 1995)

The success analysis defines "what should be." This can be accomplished through the development of a mission statement, establishing goals and objectives, or defining criteria for a desired state of affairs. Defining the desired or success analysis assists community members in identifying the undesired event that exists within the system. This undesired event is the cause or contributing factor that is impeding what should be.

The faulty tree is constructed by placing the major undesired event or problem at the top of the tree. Logic gates connect the relationships between the major undesired event or problem and the other contributing events. The logic gates depict the relationships that exist among events. Figure 19.3 provides a structure of a faulty tree analysis. Logic gates are either *and* or *or* in nature. The *and* gate is used when two or more events must coexist to

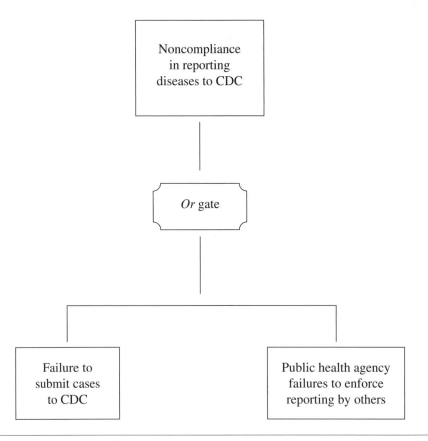

Figure 19.4 Sample Faulty Tree Analysis

produce the major undesired event. The *or* gate is used when any one of the two events must exist to produce the major undesired event. An example is presented in Figure 19.4.

Force-Field Analysis

The implementation of organizational or community-level change is the result of problem identification and resolution. Force-field analysis is a technique used frequently in organizational change to explore the causal implications of proposed changes. Force-field analysis provides a technique with which to identify the forces that may effect an organizational change. The theory supporting force-field analysis assumes that a state of equilibrium exists within any system. If a change is recommended within the organization, it will disturb the existing state of equilibrium. Force-field analysis provides the public health nurse with a strategy to use in analyzing the forces that will drive or restrain the recommended change. The driving forces are those that are identified as pushing and supporting the organizational change. The restraining forces are those blocking the organizational change. Using force-field analysis, the public health nurse can analyze the causal forces that may support or restrain a change (Witkin & Altschuld, 1995).

Summary

Key issues in public health–community health decisional and causal analysis are as follows.

- A causal analysis is a technique that describes or analyzes factors or conditions that contribute to the existence of an identified problem.
- A root-cause analysis uses the five-whys technique, in which the question "Why?" is asked five times.
- Fishbone diagrams are used to examine a problem or issue to determine the root cause, to study all possible reasons for problems, to identify areas of further data collection, and to study why a process is not performing as desired.
- Cause-and-consequence analysis promotes the identification of the causes and effects of present problems and of potential effects in the near future.
- Faulty tree analysis is a system-centered approach to causal analysis that outlines the contribution of each causal consequence to other causal consequences.
- Force-field analysis is a technique used frequently in organizational change to explore the causal implications of proposed changes.

References

Reshef, Y. (2003). *Fishbone diagram*. Retrieved June 23, 2003, from http://courses. bus.ualberta.ca/orga432-reshef/fishbone.html

Witkin, B., & Altschuld, J. (1995). *Planning and conducting needs assessments: A practical guide*. Thousand Oaks, CA: Sage.

20 Fiscal and Human Resource Management

The budgeting process is a management function of public health nurses. Its purpose is to allocate and control the fiscal resources of a public health organization. Human resources (HR) is also a management function, concerned with securing, retaining, and developing the human resources of a public health organization. This chapter focuses on funding sources; provides fiscal definitions; discusses budgeting, budgeting types, and approaches; presents information on nonprofit and tax-exempt status, and concludes by providing information on human resource management, such as performance appraisals and public health job classifications.

Introduction

Public health organizations, both government oriented and community based, are responsible for ensuring the public's health. Government-based public health organizations have formal responsibilities appropriated through public health policy and laws. In contrast, community-based organizations are generally nonprofit organizations with a socially driven mission to ensure the public's health.

The delivery of health-care services to the public occurs within a complex and dynamic health-care system. Public health organizations are only one kind of organization that exists within this system to provide efficient, effective, and quality health care that is population based. The delivery of these health-care services is dependent on a competent workforce. From an organizational perspective, health-care services are delivered through public health leadership and management activities. Fiscal and human resources management are two critical elements in the coordination of public health services. This chapter focuses on information necessary for public health nurses in the management of population-based public health organizations.

Funding Sources

Public health organizations are funded through a mixture of federal, state, and grant-related sources. The specific types of funding sources are dependent on the structure of the public health system within the particular state. Generally, funds are disbursed from federal organizations through the implementation of federal policies and laws. Federal policies and laws also direct some fiscal oversight responsibilities for the allocation of these funds. In most states, there is one central government body that oversees the funding of public health services: the state health department (Leviss, 2001). Under this structure, the state health department assists with and provides management and oversight of fiscal resource allocation for public health services.

Nonprofit public health organizations are frequently funded through grants or contracts. Fiscal management in these organizations is governed through the contract or resources requested through the grant. Nonprofit public health organizations with grant or contract services are fiscally responsible to the granting organization and to local, state, and national laws, as applicable.

Fiscal Definitions

Fiscal management consists of multiple terms that are generally not germane to public health nursing. These terms are often unfamiliar to public health nurses yet are necessary for public health nursing leaders and managers to understand (Table 20.1). Fiscal management is a subset of management that focuses on financial information used in public health decision-making processes. Fiscal management encompasses the areas of accounting and finance. Accounting is the system for documenting a public health organization's fiscal status. Accounting consists of two types: managerial and financial. Managerial accounting relates to the general financial information that managers use to improve the organization's functioning. Financial accounting provides retrospective information in the form of records that summarize and report fiscal activities (Finkler, 2001; Lee & Johnson, 1998). Accounting is explored further here.

Accounting

Accounting consists of the process that documents, classifies, analyzes, and interprets the financial records of a community-based or public health organization. Accounting practices permit organizations to keep track of their financial status and analyze the results of each financial transaction.

Table 20.1   Fiscal Definitions

Accrual basis	Accounting system that matches revenues and expenses in the same fiscal year
Allocation	The process of taking cost from one area to another
Bottom-up budget	A budget formed by managers that informs top management
Calendar year	A 1-year period that extends from January 1 to December 31
Capital assets	Resources that extend beyond the year in which they are acquired
Creditors	An individual or organization to whom the organization owes money
Cost center	The unit, department, or division to which a cost is assigned
Deficit	The excess of spending over income (revenue)
Direct costs	Costs incurred with the organizational unit
Fiscal year	A 1-year period that begins at any point designated by the organization
Fixed costs	Costs that do not change in total as the volume changes
Full-time equivalent (FTE)	A unit of staffing measurement related to the amount of time worked in 1 year—typically, 2080 hours per year or 40 hours per week
Indirect costs	Costs that are assigned to an organizational unit but that are derived from elsewhere in the organization
Off-budget	Items that are not included during the budgeting process
On-budget	Items included during the budgeting process
Overhead	Indirect costs
Revenue	Financial resources received in exchange for goods or services (income)
Surplus	The excess of income (revenue) over spending
Top-down budget	A budget prepared by top management and provided to managers
Uncollectibles	The estimated amount that is expected not to be collected for goods or services
Variable costs	Costs that vary in direct proportion to volume changes

SOURCE: Finkler (2001).

Accounting procedures are expedited with comprehensive and accurate bookkeeping procedures. Bookkeeping consists of the accurate entering of information into an organization's financial records. Accounting processes consist of conducting financial transactions, analyzing transactions, recording transactions in journals, posting the journal transaction to the general ledger, and analyzing the general ledger account (Finkler, 2001).

Accounting systems consist of the accounting records that are analyzed during an audit (checkbooks, ledgers, journals, and spreadsheets). A chart of accounts lists each item that the accounting system tracks. A general ledger organizes information by accounts. The general ledger maintains a year-to-date balance for each account in the accounting system. Journals record all the accounting transactions before they are entered into the general ledger. Journals organize information chronologically and by type of financial transaction. An audit is a comprehensive review of the accounting system to assess the accuracy and completeness of all these financial records (Finkler, 2001).

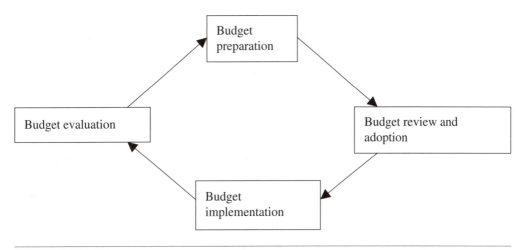

Figure 20.1   Budget Cycle

Finance focuses on the securing of funds to provide public health services. Finance also includes financial markets that provide other means of generating funds to operate the public health organization.

Budgeting

A budget is a plan that allocates the organization's financial resources in relation to the mission, goals, and objectives of the public health organization. The budget details the amount of money the organization is expected to receive in relation to the amount of money expected to be spent in various budget categories. The typical categories of a budget are personnel, equipment, capital expenditures, supplies, operating expenses, travel, consultations, and miscellaneous (Finkler, 2001). This plan is developed through a process known as budgeting. Budgeting is the process that plans and controls the budget in relation to the manner in which resources were allocated.

The budget process includes multiple activities that occur in a cyclic pattern. This cyclic pattern is referred to as the budget cycle. The budget cycle includes the following activities: budget preparation, budget review and adoption, budget implementation, and budget evaluation (Finkler, 2001). Figure 20.1 diagrams this cycle.

Budget preparation is the first step in the budget cycle. Budget preparation consists of assigning measures in terms of dollars or units for the resources needed to achieve the mission, goals, and objectives. The budget is prepared in response to budget guidelines that define what procedures should be used to forecast expenditures and designate expenditures to the appropriate budgetary categories. Most budget guidelines require the justification of forecasted expenditures. Budget guidelines for public health organizations are developed by the organization in accordance with state laws and organizational policies and procedures. Some budget guidelines require a budget justification for each line item; others require budget categories for new expenditures or expenditures that exceed a predetermined amount.

The next step in budgeting is budget review and adoption. Budgets are reviewed at multiple administrative levels, such as that of the immediate administrator, the business manager, and the budget officer. Budgets are reviewed for calculation errors, appropriate budget category designation, and for approval of requested expenditures. During budget review, budgets are frequently negotiated between the public health manager submitting the budget and the administrative superior. Once the budget from each respective department or division within the public health organization is reviewed, the entire organizational budget is prepared and reviewed. At this time, the budget is typically presented to the final approving body. The presentation should focus on justifying the relationship of the budgetary request to the mission, goals, and objectives of the public health organization. After the final approving body adjusts and approves the final budget, a vote is cast to appropriate the funds as presented in the budget (Finkler, 2001).

Once the budget is approved and appropriated, it can be executed and implemented. Budget execution and implementation permits the initiation or continuation of public health programs and projects as budgeted. The last activity in the budgeting cycle is budget evaluation. Budget evaluation consists of analyzing the accomplishment of public health program goals and objectives in relation to expenditures. Budget evaluations are best accomplished in sequence with strategic plans; however, budget evaluations should be conducted at least midyear and at the completion of the budget year. Accountability for fiscal management is achieved through budget evaluations. Budget evaluation is one strategy to ensure that fiscal resources are used efficiently and effectively (Finkler, 2001).

Budget Types

Public health organization budgeting yields different types of budgets, depending on the focus and funding sources of the public health organization and the public health program's objectives and scope. The type of budget developed may also be dependent on the format and specifications of the parent public health organization or funding agency. A master budget summarizes all expenditure categories forecast for the next budget year. The master budget serves as the master plan for allocating expenditures during the year. Within the master budget, there is generally an operating and financial budget. Some public health organizations develop these budgets as separate budgets rather than as a component of a master budget.

Table 20.2 Typical Budget Expenditures

	Budgeted Amount	Encumbered Amount	Actual Expenses	Previous Year
Personnel				
Base salary				
Overtime wages				
Merit increases				
Bonuses				
On-call pay				
Fringe benefits				
Consultant services				
Honorarium				
Travel expenses				
Meals				
Hotel				
Contract services				
Equipment and furniture				
Operating expenses				
Supplies (consumable products)				
Travel				
Space rental				
Miscellaneous				

Operating Budget

The operating budget is a plan of public health expenditures and revenues generated during a specific period of time, usually a year. The operating budget is categorized into revenues and other fiscal support and expenditures. The difference between the revenues and expenditures is presented in another category, labeled surplus or deficit. Table 20.2 outlines some typical expenditure categories. The operating budget provides the public health manager with fiscal information regarding the ongoing generation of revenues in relation to organizational expenditures. The provided information generally contains an analysis of the fiscal resources required to operate the organization and provide the necessary programmatic services.

Financial Budget

The financial budget is composed of two components: the cash budget and the capital budget. The cash budget consists of expected cash revenue generated from the delivery of services or selling of goods. The capital budget consists of the acquisition or purchase of resources that will last past the present budget year. Items often budgeted for in the capital budget are building purchases, building renovations, and some types of equipment purchases. The capital budget is planned for the acquisition of long-term assets.

Special-Purpose Budget

A special-purpose budget is developed for a specific project, program, or activity that was not budgeted for in the master budget. This type of budget has no money already planned for it or set aside. A special-purpose budget is not always forecast during the budgeting process. The fiscal resources allotted to this budget may have external revenue sources, special funding from a grant, or the master budget may be reallocated to cover the special-purpose budget expenses.

Budgeting Approaches

Public health organizations take multiple approaches to their budgeting process. The type of approach used depends on the type of public health organization, source of public health funds, profit or nonprofit status, and the ability to carry fiscal resources from one budget year to the next. Several budgeting approaches will be discussed.

Traditional Budgeting

The traditional budgeting approach is also known as the fixed or incremental budgeting approach. In this approach, fiscal resources are allocated at the organizational unit level for specific amounts. These funding levels are maintained throughout the budget period. The distribution of fiscal resources to programs or activities is determined at the unit level. The budget that is developed in this approach uses the previous year's budget to forecast the next year. The previous year's budget is adjusted for the next year using a predetermined incremental factor of increase or decrease. This predetermined incremental factor can be consistent over time or vary depending on the appropriation of funds, such as the state appropriation of health service funding to the state office of public health combined with any federal or grant funding.

Variable Budgeting

Variable budgeting is also known as flexible budgeting. The basic assumption of variable budgeting is that the expenditures (especially personnel and supplies) will vary in relation to the volume of goods and services. Flexible budgets focus on the output measure. Flexible budgeting requires the ability to forecast which budget categories are likely to vary and which ones are likely to remain constant. This budgeting approach uses a more flexible budgeting process that is dependent on revenue generation or increased funding through grants or contracts.

Functional Budgeting

Functional budgeting forecasts expenditures and revenues in relation to the main functions of the public health program, such as counseling and diagnostic testing, and the typical budget categories. This permits the budget analyst to determine the expenditures for each program function in relation to the budget category. For example, for counseling services delivery, a functional budget would determine the amount of personnel cost, supplies, operating, and other expenses incurred to deliver counseling.

Program Budgeting

Program budgets are developed to plan the expected revenues and expenses for a specific public health program. Fiscal resources in a program budget are earmarked for the delivery of program-specific goods and services and the achievement of specific program objectives. A program budget may be federally allocated through a block grant; therefore there may be restrictions on the manner in which the funds are allocated, and the funds are typically restricted to that program's expenses. A program budget could be a one-time program (making it similar to the special-purpose budget) or a recurring program.

Performance Budgeting

Performance-based budgeting attempts to focus on the outcomes produced by the public health program. Performance budgets provide line-item expenditures for those activities necessary to produce a desired program outcome. Performance budgets require the following processes: (a) program objectives are clearly defined, (b) an operating budget is established, (c) the percentage of operating resources allotted for each objective is determined, (d) performance measures are established for each activity, (e) an expected outcome level is developed for each activity, and (f) program performance is determined based on the amount of resources consumed compared to the expected outcome level and compared to the amount of resources consumed to produce a certain activity.

Zero-Base Budgeting

Zero-base budgeting is designed to eliminate any budget excess. Zero-base budgeting requires a careful examination of each line item each year. Items that are determined not to add value or which are not needed to produce the goods or services are to be eliminated from the budget. Each year the organizational unit begins with a zero-base budget, and all expenditures must be justified. No expenditure is permitted without a sound budget justification related to the program's mission, goals, and objectives.

Nonprofit and Tax-Exempt Status

Community-based and public health organizations are primarily nonprofit organizations, with tax-exempt status. *Nonprofit* and *tax-exempt status* do not mean the same thing. The majority of organizations that are nonprofit are also tax-exempt. The petition processes for nonprofit and tax-exempt status are different and are completed at different times. Nonprofit status is conferred on an organization by the state, whereas tax-exempt status is provided by the federal government. Nonprofit status is a prerequisite to apply for tax-exempt status.

A nonprofit organization is any organization in which the owner or the controlling board does not earn a profit. Nonprofit status does not mean that the organization cannot earn a profit in a fiscal year. A nonprofit organization can earn a profit, but the profit must be invested back into the organization. Essentially, with a nonprofit organization, there is no profit sharing with the owner or controlling board. The three types of nonprofit organizations are a corporation, an unincorporated organization, or a trust.

Several types of federal tax-exempt status may be granted by the federal government. The most common is the 501(c)(3), which is also known as the charitable tax exemption status. This status permits the organization to be exempt from federal corporate and income taxes for most revenue. These organizations can solicit tax-deductible contributions from interested stakeholders and philanthropists. A new organization that is applying for federal tax-exempt status will be provided with a letter of determination from the Internal Revenue Service. Some organizations will receive automatic recognition as having 501(c)(3) status. Subordinate organizations that are evaluated by a parent organization, churches, church organizations or associations, and organizations that are not private foundations that gross receipts not greater than $5,000 will receive automatic 501(c)(3) status.

In addition to federal tax-exempt status, an organization can apply for state tax exemption. The laws governing state tax exemption vary by state; therefore, each state's laws should be reviewed prior to applying. State tax exemption status could provide the organization with exemptions from sales tax, income tax, and property tax.

Human Resources

The greatest public health resources are the people who make up the public health workforce. These resources are known as public health's human resources. Human resources are our most precious commodity, essential to the delivery of public health services. Public health nurses who are savvy in human resource management can maximize the full potential of the public health workforce. An essential function of human resource management is personnel management. Personnel management consists of recruitment, selection, promotion, retention, position classification, compensation including benefits, personnel record keeping and documentation, counseling, corrective and disciplinary actions, training, competency requirements, staffing, and performance appraisals (Thielen, 2001). This chapter will be limited to an examination of professional development, performance management and appraisals, and job classifications and analysis.

Professional Development

Professional development can increase employee satisfaction. In addition, professional development assists in ensuring that public health nurses have the necessary knowledge and skills to perform their assigned duties. Professional development consists of employee orientation, training, academic education, and developmental plans.

Public health organizations must conduct an employee orientation that presents the new public health nurse with information regarding job responsibilities, legal requirements, and organizational policies and procedures. Public health nurses must be provided with opportunities for training through continuing education programs. These continuing education programs should reflect the expected public health competencies and job description for the public health nurse. In addition, public health continuing education should include attending local, state, and national public health conferences as a means of keeping current in emerging public health issues.

Academic education formally prepares public health nurses for public health practice. The completion of an academic program of study results in the awarding of a degree that entitles the public health nurse to all the honors, rights, and privileges associated with the respective degree. Academic credentials are one definitive method of documenting that a specific level of public health competency has been achieved. Glanville and Porche (2000) created a faculty development model that can also be used by public health professionals to achieve professional development. This model consists of three phases: an individual enhancement plan, a professional development plan, and resource allocation that results in a competent public health professional.

Phase one consists of public health nurses developing individual enhancement plans. Individual enhancement plans include personal and professional goals and objectives in alignment with the nurse's current position or a position to which the nurse would like to be promoted. The public health nurse also identifies the resources that may be needed to achieve personal and professional goals and objectives. In the second phase, the public health nurse and the administrator meet to review the individual enhancement plan and write a professional development plan. The professional development plan uses the negotiated and agreed-on goals and objectives from the public health nurse's individual enhancement plan. Resources identified as necessary are reviewed. During this time, the administrator reviews the mission, goals, and objectives of the public health organization or unit with the public health nurse. Collaboratively, the public health nurse and administrator write a professional development plan that meets the individual's personal and professional goals and that are consistent with the needs, mission, goals, and objectives of the public health organization or unit. Phase three consists of the public health nurse assuming responsibility for engaging in activities that achieve the objectives outlined in the professional development plan and the administrator allocating resources to assist the public health nurse in achieving the objectives. Additionally, in phase three, the administrator may engage in mentoring the public health nurse (Glanville & Porche, 2000). Mentoring programs are another strong method of conducting professional development. Chapter 17 discusses mentoring.

Performance Management and Appraisals

Performance management and appraisals are the responsibility of the public health nurse's administrator. Performance management is a managerial function that ensures that the employee is functioning in accordance with duties and responsibilities outlined in the job description. The performance appraisal is the written document that results from performance management activities. Performance appraisals are used to determine salaries, promotions, transfers, layoffs, demotions, and terminations (Thielen, 2001). Performance appraisals should use a personnel instrument that validly and accurately measures the individual's performance according to various levels in relation to all the duties and responsibilities designated for the job position.

The performance appraisal is a good time to develop the professional development plan. Performance data should be reviewed during a meeting between the public health nurse and administrator. This meeting should maintain a positive tone focusing on personal and professional improvement. This will facilitate open and ongoing communication after the performance appraisal.

Public Health Job Classifications

Public health professionals who work in a governmental organization are generally classified according to a civil service system. In 1912, the federal government passed the Civil Service Commission legislation (Thielen, 2001). This was a measure to eliminate political favoritism in personnel management of government employees. The job description, not the employee, is classified in relation to the duties performed. Factors considered in the classification of a position are job requirements, difficulty of work, level of responsibility, independence in decision making, number of employees supervised, budgetary management, relationship with other decision makers and administrators, complexity of work, working environment, and level of accountability (Thielen, 2001). Educational requirements can be established for the public health position as a minimal requirement. Compensation is derived in accordance with the job classification level in the civil service system. Additional compensation is not provided for educational preparation above what was designated as a minimal requirement.

Summary

Key issues in fiscal and human resource management are as follows.

- Community-based organizations are generally nonprofit organizations, with a socially driven mission to ensure the public's health.
- Public health organizations are funded through a mixture of federal, state, and grant-related sources.
- Nonprofit public health organizations are frequently funded through grants or contracts.
- Fiscal management is a subset of management that focuses on financial information used in public health decision-making processes.
- Accounting is the system for documenting a public health organization's fiscal status.
- An audit is a comprehensive review of the accounting system to assess the accuracy and completeness of all financial records.
- Finance focuses on the securing of funds to provide public health services.
- A budget is a plan that allocates a public health organization's financial resources in relation to the mission, goals, and objectives of the organization.
- The typical categories of a budget are personnel, equipment, capital expenditures, supplies, operating expenses, travel, consultations, and miscellaneous.
- Budgeting is the process that plans and controls the budget in relation to the manner in which resources were allocated.

- The budget cycle consists of budget preparation, budget review and adoption, budget implementation, and budget evaluation.
- A master budget summarizes all expenditure categories forecast for the next budget year.
- The operating budget is a plan of public health expenditures and revenues generated during a specific period of time, usually a year, that is categorized into revenues and other fiscal support and expenditures.
- The financial budget is composed of the cash budget and the capital budget.
- A special-purpose budget is developed for a specific project, program, or activity that was not budgeted for in the master budget.
- The traditional budgeting approach is also known as the fixed or incremental budgeting approach.
- Variable budgeting is also known as flexible budgeting; expenditures vary in relation to the volume of goods and services.
- Functional budgeting forecasts expenditures and revenues in relation to the main functions of the public health program.
- Program budgets are developed to plan the expected revenues and expenses for a specific public health program.
- Performance-based budgeting attempts to focus on the outcomes produced by the public health program and provides line-item expenditures for those activities necessary to produce a desired program outcome.
- Zero-base budgeting begins each year with a zero-base budget. All expenditures must be justified yearly.
- A nonprofit organization is any organization in which the owner or the controlling board does not earn a profit.
- Federal tax-exempt status is granted by the federal government.
- State tax-exempt status can provide an organization with exemptions from sales tax, income tax, and property tax.
- An essential function of human resource management is personnel management.
- Personnel management consists of recruitment, selection, promotion, retention, position classification, compensation including benefits, personnel record keeping and documentation, counseling, corrective and disciplinary actions, training, competency requirements, staffing, and performance appraisals.
- Professional development assists with ensuring that public health nurses have the necessary knowledge and skills to perform their assigned duties and consists of employee orientation, training, academic education, and developmental plans.
- The faculty development model can also be used to achieve professional development of public health professionals. It consists of three phases: an individual enhancement plan, a professional development plan, and resource allocation that results in a competent public health professional.

- Performance management is a managerial function that ensures that the employee is functioning in accordance with duties and responsibilities outlined in the job description.
- Civil Service Commission legislation was passed as a measure to eliminate political favoritism in personnel management of government employees.
- Factors considered in the classification of a position are job requirements, difficulty of work, level of responsibility, independence in decision making, number of employees supervised, budgetary management, relationship with other decision makers and administrators, complexity of work, working environment, and level of accountability.

References

Finkler, S. (2001). *Financial management: For public, health, and not-for-profit organizations.* Upper Saddle River, NJ: Prentice Hall.

Glanville, C., & Porche, D. (2000). Graduate nursing faculty: Ensuring cultural and racial diversity through faculty development. *Journal of Multicultural Nursing & Health,* 6(1), 6-13.

Lee, R., & Johnson, R. (1998). *Public budgeting systems* (6th ed.). Gaithersburg, MD: Aspen.

Leviss, P. (2001). Financing the public's health. In L. Novick & G. Mays (Eds.), *Public health administration: Principles for population-based management* (pp. 413-430). Gaithersburg, MD: Aspen.

Thielen, L. (2001). Human resource management. In L. Novick & G. Mays (Eds.), *Public health administration: Principles for population-based management* (pp. 397-412). Gaithersburg, MD: Aspen.

21

Public Health Informatics

The rapid development of technology has expanded the ability to rapidly communicate public health information and data through various systems. Public health informatics is a developing area that will continue to expand, resulting in better communication networks to protect the public from horrific events such as bioterrorism attacks. This chapter focuses on providing definitions, presenting the public health informatics agenda and describing various databases and information system categories, and discussing developing issues of privacy in relation to informatics.

Introduction

Public health organizations require integrated information systems to effectively and efficiently use and communicate a plethora of health-related data among various organizations. These information systems facilitate the daily decision-making processes of public health nurses in areas such as epidemiology, health-related assessments (behavioral, community, and environmental), staffing effectiveness, program planning, program monitoring and evaluation, public health legislation, and policy development. Information systems facilitate the analysis and synthesis of large amounts of health-related data about defined public health populations to assist in population-based decision making.

The increased need for and dependence on information systems is a result of the increased amounts of data available, advances in information technology, and an increased awareness of the benefits of information systems to support public health decision making (Parente, 2001). The major goals of health information systems for public health organizations are the integration of multiple public health data sources, the creation of a network of public health information systems that will promote seamless interaction and information flow, and the use and integration of health-care delivery information systems with public health information systems (Parente,

2001). The integration of multiple information systems can provide great benefits through information sharing and facilitation of public health program planning, but it also raises concerns regarding privacy and security of information. This chapter provides a general introduction to the use of health information systems in the public health arena. Public health nurses will be involved in and expected to be knowledgeable about these systems, are likely to participate in their development, and will certainly use them.

Definitions

The terminology used in public health informatics is continuing to evolve as the sophistication of information systems evolves. The terminology used to describe the area of health informatics does not have consistent definitions across the various health-related disciplines. Public health practitioners are adopting some of the existing terminology but are also developing terminology that specifically describes the use of informatics in public health. Some general definitions are provided in this chapter.

Data are the raw facts and figures collected. These facts and figures are processed and analyzed in a formal and intelligent manner so that they may be used by public health professionals as what is known as *information*. This information is used for public health decision making (Austin & Boxerman, 1995). Knowledge is gained through the use of the information and is used to explain the context of the public health problem (Parente, 2001).

Informatics is a general term that encompasses the methods, systems, and technologies used to provide information. The American Medical Informatics Association defined public health informatics as the systematic application of information and computer sciences and technology to public health practice, research, and learning (Yasnoff et al., 2001). The information and computer technology hardware and software that permits the use of this information is known as the *information system*.

The National Public Health Informatics Agenda

A national public health informatics agenda was articulated though 74 recommendations in 19 categories during the 2001 Spring American Medical Informatics Association Congress (Yasnoff et al., 2001). The recommendations in the 19 categories are grouped together in the following framework: funding and governance; architecture and infrastructure; standards and vocabulary; research, evaluation, and best practices; privacy, confidentiality, and security; and training and workforce. Table 21.1 summarizes the 74 recommendations that articulate the national public health informatics agenda.

Table 21.1   Public Health Informatics Recommendations: Brief Summary

Funding and Governance

1. Fund information management as part of the core public health budget

2. Fund the vision of information, not information technology

3. Create diverse funding sources

4. Allocate adequate funding throughout the information system life cycle—planning, start-up, implementation, and maintenance

5. Provide dedicated funding for public health information systems

6. Provide leadership as needed

7. Create planning and management structures that include stakeholders

8. Ensure that public health and information technology representation is broad

9. Develop a merged superset of public health and informatics planning and evaluation models

10. Establish a business case for continued investment in information systems

11. Establish a business case for public health information architecture

Architecture and Infrastructure

12. Provide dedicated Internet access, workstations, and training

13. Provide software tools and access to data

14. Develop an implementation plan for the information architecture

15. Develop a public health data repository with person-based, integrated data

16. Establish a process to develop a model data repository

17. Establish procedures for monitoring compliance with audit and evaluation criteria of data systems

18. Implement access control measures and computational disclosure in data systems

19. Consider establishing a unique personal identifier for data system integration

20. Provide effective communication and workflow management capability between health-care and public health agencies

21. Minimize the impact of public health data collection on health-care providers

Standards and Vocabulary

22. Increase awareness of and participation in current standards development

23. Develop and maintain a comprehensive Web-accessible list of standards

24. Identify gaps in standards

25. Promote consistent use of standards across governmental agencies

26. Increase use of CDC public health conceptual data model

27. Develop additional standard messages for public health reporting

(Continued)

Table 21.1 (Continued)

28. Establish a mechanism for expanding standardized codes

29. Develop a model state regulation to promote disease reporting

30. Develop specific implementation guidelines for creating and transmitting electronic laboratory messages

31. Harmonize key guideline formats

32. Create database versions of ICD-CM codes

Research, Evaluation, and Best Practices

33. Agree on process for developing and disseminating best practices

34. Establish standards for performance at all levels

35. Establish a repository of best practices

36. Establish a program to fund demonstration project of best practices

37. Link evaluation to Healthy People 2010

38. Standardize outcome measures

39. Evaluate data quality, economics, transferability, and individual measures

40. Evaluate existing programs first

41. Develop a research agenda for public health informatics

42. Use existing informatics knowledge, techniques, and methods in public health informatics research

43. Involve multidisciplinary teams

44. Integrate informatics into all public health research proposals

45. Provide additional research funds for public health informatics

46. Establish and fund a lead research agency for privacy, confidentiality, and security

Privacy, Confidentiality and Security

47. Create a national forum on privacy policy

48. Establish a community advisory board for privacy policy

49. Consider creation of public health ethics committee

50. Include front-line public health workers in policy development

51. Develop model public health privacy legislation

52. Develop regulations and policies that are dynamic

53. Develop policies for cross-jurisdictional data exchange

54. Require public health data systems to have a state purpose, privacy board, and confidentiality agreements

55. Develop model security policies

(Continued)

Table 21.1   (Continued)

56. Adopt the provisions of the Health Insurance Portability and Accountability Act

57. Review security preparedness for potential attacks

58. Consider indirect funding options for security

Training and Workforce

59. Establish academic programs in public health informatics

60. Develop a national competency-based program in public health informatics

61. Enhance CDC public health informatics fellowship program

62. Establish instructional design guidelines for public health informatics curriculum

63. Establish curriculum guidelines for public health informatics

64. Develop a comprehensive and consistent curriculum about data security, privacy, and confidentiality

65. Consider establishing an ethical, legal, and social issues program in public health informatics

66. Involve appropriate public health groups when developing academic programs

67. Develop a career track in public health informatics

68. Expand opportunities for public health and informatics professionals

69. Strengthen prevention and public health special interest groups

70. Use the National Network of Libraries of Medicine to arrange meetings for public health informatics outreach

71. Define public health informatics

72. Support the CDC's effort to develop core competencies in public health informatics

73. Examine informatics competencies in other health-related fields

74. Adopt the American Association of Medical Colleges medical school informatics objectives for public health informatics

The public health agenda for public health informatics is further articulated through the Centers for Disease Control and Prevention's Information Network for Public Health Officials (INPHO) framework for public health information and practice. This framework was developed based on the public health needs to connect fragmented systems, link public health professionals at various levels, empower communities with information, and lead and respond to the information technology boom. INPHO works from the three concepts of linkage, information access, and data exchange as a means of strengthening the public health information infrastructure. The vision of INPHO is to create an integrated telecommunications network that links the public health community and provides for the exchange of data and information in a secure and private manner (Baker, Freide, Moulton, & Ross, 1995; Parente, 2001).

The CDC INPHO concepts can be used to develop a public health informatics system that is comprehensive and secure. This infrastructure must have the capability to meet the internal needs of the public health agency as well as connect the agency to other public health agencies or health-care agencies within the community and at other levels, such as state or national.

Databases and Information System Categories

Information systems are designed based on the data sources. Databases are characterized as wide, deep, or multidimensional. A wide database has many variables. A deep database contains many observations. A multidimensional database has variables that can be linked across different periods of time and databases (Parente, 2001). There are various types of data to be included in databases to develop an information system. Data sources are described as containing transaction, registry, survey, or relational data.

Transaction data is the most prevalent form of data. Transaction data consist of the date of the medical services, procedures performed, and diagnosis (Parente, 2001). Registry data are organized at an individual personal level. Registry data are collected through health information questionnaires. Other types of registry data are lists of health-care providers, lists of members in professional organizations, and state or national lists of individuals with a particular illness or condition. Survey data are generated when registry data are not sufficient, and a national health survey is conducted. Relational data identify key variables that can be linked to other databases (Parente, 2001). The data linkages that permit health-care professionals to access public health information are formed through the creation of information systems.

Information systems are generally categorized into four types: clinical, administrative, strategic decision-support, and electronic networking (Austin & Boxerman, 1995). Clinical information systems are designed to support patient or population-based care. Clinical information systems consist of computerized patient record systems; automated medical instrumentation; computer-aided diagnosis and treatment; systems that contain behavioral, environmental, public health organization, or community assessment data; and other information systems that support research and education. Administrative information systems support the nonpatient care activities needed to manage and administer the public health agency. Administrative information systems consist of financial information systems, payroll, inventory control, workforce data, and purchasing systems. Strategic decision-support systems assist the administrative team with public health strategic planning, managerial control, and quality control and program evaluation. Electronic networking information systems permit the exchange of information with other agencies through electronic means. Electronic networking information systems consist of electronic submission of billing and claims processing, online purchasing, and electronic communications (Austin & Boxerman, 1995).

Information systems, regardless of their categorization, must be capable of eight basic functions. These basic functions can also provide the general framework from which to evaluate the utility of information systems. Essential information system functions are data acquisition, data verification, data storage, data classification, data update, data computation, data retrieval, and data presentation (Tan, 1995). To provide a perspective on the use and capability of public health information systems, information about local health networks, the national electronic disease surveillance system, and geographic information systems is presented here.

Local Health Networks

Communication technology permits public health nurses to communicate rapidly and reliably during routine provision of services, especially in times of emergencies. Public health and community-based agencies are using these advanced communication systems to establish local health networks. Local health networks are an integrated communication system that links key public health planners and responders into one secure and private communication system using computer technology and telephone technology. These local health networks enhance routine public health functions such as surveillance and reporting of diseases. In addition, these systems enhance the speed and coordination of communication among various public health and community-based agencies during times of national emergencies (Doniger, Labowitz, Mershon, & Gotham, 2001).

The development of local health networks links public health professionals such as public health nurses with other entities and professionals, such as administrative agencies (e.g., the mayor's or governor's office), the police, the fire department, emergency medical teams, and other acute care health agencies, using public health informatics systems. The CDC desires not only the creation of local health networks but national health networks that link together all key planners and responders to protect the health of the public (Doniger et al., 2001). These local health networks can also be used to promote training and planning of public health services in nonemergency situations.

The National Electronic Disease Surveillance System

The CDC used informatics principles to develop the National Electronic Disease Surveillance System (NEDSS). NEDSS is a broad-based initiative focused on the use of data and information systems to advance the development of efficient, integrated, and interoperable surveillance systems at the local and state levels. This system is designed to permit the automatic capture and analysis of surveillance data, permitting greater integration of information between public health and other health-care agencies. Surveillance data from this integrated system will permit critical assessment of the population's health status, detect disease outbreaks, assist with program planning, and provide data for evaluative purposes (NEDSS Working Group, 2001).

The NEDSS includes eight critical elements to ensure a seamless information system: (a) Web-browser–based data entry and management, (b) electronic message processing, (c) integrated data repository, (d) active data translation and exchange, (e) programming practices, (f) data recording and visualization ability, (g) shareable directory of public health personnel, and (h) consistent security standards to protect sensitive public health records (NEDSS Working Group, 2001). NEDSS can serve as an integrated approach to public health surveillance that other agencies can use to develop information systems at the local, state, and national level.

Geographic Information Systems

Geographic information systems (GISs) permit the integration, storage, retrieval, analysis, and communication of data with respect to a spatial or geographic component (Melnick, 2001). GISs allow the epidemiological analysis of data according to time, person, and place (geographic location). GISs provide a graphic display of an area, with an overlay of diseases or disease risk factors related to the specific geographic locations on the map. This provides the public health nurse with the ability to visualize and analyze "hot spots" of disease within a community in relation to the geographic location of the population. Multiple variable overlays can be used to simultaneously visualize the spatial association of multiple variables within a geographical area in the community.

Privacy Issues

Information systems share confidential information, thus creating issues of privacy. The public's concern regarding the privacy of individuals' health information is a major public health policy issue at this time. Much of the data in public health information systems consist of personal identification information, health history, and risk behavior information that could be used in a manner harmful to individuals. Additionally, population-based data could be used to stigmatize specific communities.

In 1996, Congress passed the Health Insurance Portability and Accountability Act (HIPAA) to protect the privacy of medical information (Lumpkin, 2001). HIPAA's final rule was effective as of August 17, 2001, with a compliance mandate of October 16, 2002. Currently, further revisions to this legislation by the secretary of the Department of Health and Human Services are proposed and under review.

The Center for Medicare and Medicaid Services is the agency responsible for the implementation of various unrelated provisions of HIPAA. HIPAA Title I protects health insurance coverage for workers and their families during job change or loss. HIPAA Title II requires the establishment of national standards for the protection of electronic information (Center for Medicare and Medicaid Services, 2002).

Summary

Key issues in public health informatics are as follows.

- Public health organizations require integrated information systems to effectively and efficiently use and communicate a plethora of health-related data among various organizations.
- Information systems facilitate the analysis and synthesis of large amounts of health-related data about defined public health populations to assist in population-based decision making.
- Major goals of health information systems for public health organizations are the integration of multiple public health data sources, the creation of networks for public health information systems to promote seamless interaction and flow of information, and the use and integration of health-care delivery information systems with public health information systems.
- Data are the raw facts and figures collected.
- Data are processed and analyzed in a formal and intelligent manner so that they may be used by public health professionals as information.
- Informatics is a general term that encompasses the methods, systems, and technologies used to provide information.
- Public health informatics is the systematic application of information and computer sciences and technology to public health practice, research, and learning.
- A national public health informatics agenda was articulated though 74 recommendations in 19 categories during the 2001 Spring American Medical Informatics Association Congress.
- The CDC's INPHO framework is based on the three concepts of linkage, information access, and data exchange as a means of strengthening the public health information infrastructure.
- Data sources are described as containing transaction, registry, survey, or relational data.
- Databases are characterized as wide, deep, or multidimensional.
- Information systems are generally categorized as clinical, administrative, strategic decision-support, or electronic networking.
- Essential information system functions are data acquisition, data verification, data storage, data classification, data update, data computation, data retrieval, and data presentation.

- The local health network is an integrated communication system that links key public health planners and responders into one secure and private communication system, using computer technology and telephone technology.
- NEDSS is a broad-based initiative focused on the use of data and information systems to advance the development of efficient, integrated, and interoperable surveillance systems at the local and state levels, permitting the automatic capture and analysis of surveillance data and allowing greater integration of information between public health and other health-care agencies.
- GISs permit the integration, storage, retrieval, analysis, and communication of data with respect to a spatial or geographic component.
- Congress passed HIPAA to protect the privacy of medical information.

References

Austin, C., & Boxerman, S. (1995). *Information systems for health services administration* (5th ed.). Chicago, IL: Health Administration Press.

Baker, E., Freide, A., Moulton, A. & Ross, D. (1995). CDC's information network for public health officials (INPHO): A framework for integrated public health information and practice. *Journal of Public Health Management and Practice, 1*(1), 43-47.

Center for Medicare and Medicaid Services. (2002). *The Health Insurance Portability and Accountability Act of 1996 (HIPAA)*. Retrieved June 24, 2003, from http://www.cms.hhs.gov/hipaa/

Doniger, A., Labowitz, D., Mershon, S., & Gotham, I. (2001). Design and implementation of a local health alert network. *Journal of Public Health Management and Practice, 7*(5), 64-74.

Lumpkin, J. (2001). Air, water, places and data: Public health in the information age. *Journal of Public Health Management and Practice, 7*(6), 22-30.

Melnick, A. (2001). Geographic information systems in public health. In L. Novick & G. Mays (Eds.), *Public health administration: Principles for population-based management* (pp. 248-265). Gaithersburg, MD: Aspen.

National Electronic Disease Surveillance System Working Group. (2001). National electronic disease surveillance system (NEDSS): A standards-based approach to connect public health and clinical medicine. *Journal of Public Health Management Practice, 7*(6), 43-50.

Parente, S. (2001). Using information systems for public health administration. In L. Novick & G. Mays (Eds.), *Public health administration: Principles for population-based management* (pp. 221-247). Gaithersburg, MD: Aspen.

Tan, J. (1995). *Health management information systems: Theories, methods and applications.* Gaithersburg, MD: Aspen.

Yasnoff, W., Overhage, J., Humphreys, B., LaVenture, M., Goodman, K., Gatewood, L., et al. (2001). A national agenda for public health informatics. *Journal of Public Health Management & Practice, 7*(6), 1-21.

Part VI

Public Health Policy, Law, and Ethics

22

Public Health Policy and Politics

Public health policy and political processes are strategies that public health nurses can use to implement population-based community and societal level change. Policy development, implementation, analysis, and evaluation are considered population-based interventions useful in affecting the nation's health. This chapter focuses on defining public health policy and politics, describing the types and forms of policy and policy decision-making processes, and discussing the nursing role of policy, politics, and the intersection of these with scholarship.

Introduction

Public health nurses at all levels of practice must become politically knowledgeable and increase their participation in public health policy decision making. Greipp (2002) states that the number of people involved in the policy process or in a debate relative to a policy, plus their intensity and commitment to the values and beliefs related to the policy, equals a significant impact on policy outcomes. Mason, Leavitt, and Chaffee (2002) identified four spheres in which nurses can influence policy: government, workplace, organizations, and community. Therefore, public health nurses have a clear role, based on their numbers in the profession and the intensity of their commitment, to affect health-care policy decision making and policy outcomes. Nurses, especially public health nurses, need to capitalize on their collective potential to influence public health policy that affects the health, welfare, and safety of large populations.

Public Health Policy Defined

An understanding of public health policy requires comprehension of the definitions of health and policy, respectively. Health is a concept that is accepted as important to individuals and communities. Whether health is a right or privilege is frequently debated in the public health arena. Health is defined by some as the absence of disease and others as maximal states of positive concepts that exist to produce what is known as "health." A generally accepted definition of health is WHO's definition. WHO defines health as "the state of complete physical, mental, and social well-being, and not merely the absence of disease or infirmity" (World Health Organization, 1998).

Policy may be defined as the principles that govern an action directed toward a given outcome (Titmus, 1974). Health policy, in general terms, is any policy that affects the health of individuals or communities. Health policy is a general term that includes public health policy. WHO (1988) defined healthy public policy as "any course of action adopted and pursued (by a government, business, or other organization) that can be anticipated to improve (or has improved) health and reduce inequities in health" (p. 4).

The definitions of public policy are numerous, with no common agreement. However, there are some similarities. Dye (2002) defines public policy as whatever governments choose to do or not to do to regulate behavior, organize bureaucracies, distribute benefits, or extract taxes. Peters (1999) defines public policy as the sum of government activities, whether the government is acting directly or through agents, as it has an influence on the life of citizens. Birkland (2001) defines public policy as "a statement by government of what it intends to do or not to do, such as a law, regulation, ruling, decision, or order, or a combination of these" (p. 132). Longest (2002) defines public policy as "authoritative decisions made in the legislative, executive, or judicial branches of government that are intended to direct or influence the actions, behaviors, or decisions of others" (p. 11). Most of these definitions have common themes of governmental activity and the influence or regulation of something or some entity.

Public health policy intersects the definitions of health, policy, and public policy into one comprehensive definition. Therefore, for the purposes of this book, public health policy is defined as the administrative decisions made by the legislative, executive, or judicial branches of government that define courses of action affecting the health of a population through influencing actions, behaviors, or resources.

Types and Forms of Policy

Public health policy is a type of public policy. Public policy is basically any policy formed by a governmental body or entity. In addition, there are four other types of policy: social, health, institutional, and organizational (Mason et al., 2002). Social policy is policy that is formulated to affect the welfare of the general public. Health policy is a policy that is formulated to affect the health of individual community members. Institutional policies are policies developed by or to affect an institution. Institutional policies frequently govern the institution's workplace, such as those policies regarding the goals and operational procedures of the institution. Organizational policies are administrative decisions or statements developed by an organization such as the American Nurses Association. Organizational policies could be in the form of resolutions, procedures, or position statements.

The various types of policies developed—public, social, health, institutional, or organizational—can assume many forms. Policies can assume the form of laws, rules or regulations, operational decisions, or judicial decisions. Laws are enacted at all levels of government. The formulation of public health law and the scope of public health law will be presented in chapters 26 and 27. Laws are considered freestanding legislative enactments aimed at achieving some specific predetermined objective. The executive branch of the government formulates rules or regulations. Laws enacted at the federal or state level are implemented through the formation of rules or regulations by agencies in the executive branch. In addition to the formation of rules and regulations, agencies in the executive branch develop operational decisions to further implement the laws. Operational decisions can be in the form of procedures or protocols. Judicial decisions, made through the judicial branch, are also a type of policy. Administrative decisions made in the judicial branch of government establish precedence, which is a form of policy, and which sometimes invalidates other forms of policy developed, such as the constitutionality of some laws.

Public Health Policy Decision Making

Multiple forces affect the public health policy decision-making process. Greipp (2002) developed a model based on general systems theory to describe the forces that affect policy decision making. Greipp identifies three major forces that affect policy decision making: consumers, providers, and regulatory bodies. In addition, she identified motivating and inhibiting factors that affect the decision-making process.

Consumers are considered clients, families, and communities. Consumer forces are represented by those who have a perceived need for health-care services and products. Providers are caregivers and scientists or researchers. Providers include health-care providers and family caregivers. The last driving force in health policy decision making is regulatory bodies. Regulatory bodies include governments, legal systems, third-party payers, political action committees, other special interest groups, and ethics and institutional review board committees. These three driving forces intersect and influence each other during health policy decision making, with the greatest influence being that of the force or forces whose perspective on the issue has been adopted (Greipp, 2002).

Motivators and inhibitors are the intervening variables that can influence the perspective of consumers, providers, or regulatory bodies. Motivators are the positive variables that serve to influence the decision making in the direction of what is best for the common good. Inhibitors are negative variables that serve to influence the perspective in the direction of self-interest rather than public interest (Greipp, 2002).

Politics Defined

In nursing, politics is frequently considered to have a negative connotation. The mention of politics seems to create negative feelings, such as anger, disgust, and a sense of injustice. However, all nurses engage in some form of politics or political maneuvers at one time or another. Politics is the process of influencing someone or something to allocate resources as you desire. The political process includes the use of power. In addition to policy, Mason et al. (2002) consider that nurses engage in politics in four spheres of action: government, workplace, organizations, and community.

The Role of Nurses in Policy and Politics

Nurses must become more politically involved in public health policy formulation, modification, analysis, and evaluation. These are core public health functions that must be included in public health nursing job descriptions and used as evaluative measures in the performance appraisal process. Cohen et al. (1996) developed a conceptual model to describe nursing's political development processes. These authors identified four stages that encompass the political development of the nursing profession.

Stage one began in the 1970s and 1980s. Known as the "buy-in" stage, this stage was reactive, characterized by the increase of nursing's political sensitivity. Stage two, termed the self-interest stage, occurred from the 1980s to 1990s. Stage two is characterized by the development of nursing's political voice. Nursing began to be recognized as a special interest group, and the American Nurses Association Political Action Committee was formed. Stage three, the political sophistication stage, emerged during the 1990s. In this stage, nurses began to be recognized as policymakers and health-care leaders who had a valuable perspective and expertise in health policy. Stage four, our current stage, is characterized as the leadership stage. Nursing is actively involved in leading health-care policy through the establishment of policy agendas (Cohen et al., 1996). Additionally, nursing is assuming leadership as a key interest group or stakeholder through organized political participation.

Political participation is defined by Schlozman, Burns, and Verba (1994) as any formal or informal activity that is mainstream or unconventional and that occurs as a result of individual or collective action to either directly or indirectly influence what the government does. Organized political participation is the engagement in activities of groups or associations whose goals are to politically affect something.

Verba, Schlozman, and Brady (1995) developed a civic voluntarism model to describe the factors that influence nurses' decisions to engage in organized political participation. They identified three key factors that influence nurses' participation: resources, engagement, and networks of recruitment. Nurses must have the *resources* or wherewithal to engage in the political process. The resources that influence nurses' participation are free time, available money, and civic skills. The second influencing factor is the nurses' motivation to *engage* in political activity. Political interest, political information, personal efficacy, and partisanship influence the nurse's decision to engage in organized political activities. The last influencing factor is opportunity, or the *network* of recruitment. Simply, this consists of requests or cues to action that stimulate the nurse to become involved in an organization's political activities.

According to Verba et al.'s (1995) civic voluntarism model, engagement is a necessary factor to influence political participation but is not sufficient in itself. The greatest emphasis is placed on the nurse having the wherewithal or resources with which to engage in political activity. Public health nurses can use this model to understand why a nurse is hesitant to participate or to facilitate the organization of public health nurses into political activity.

Policy and Scholarship

Nurses should maximize all of their resources to influence public health policy. Nursing scholars who engage in the dissemination of nursing science through publication have an opportunity to relate their theoretical discourse or research findings to policy. Nurse scholars can use publication as a forum from which to state their own unique position or link their research to the policy-making process or content of political debates (Wakefield, 2001). This is an excellent maneuver to influence public health policy decision making based on evidence. Table 22.1 outlines guidelines to use in linking scholarly nursing publications to public health policy.

Summary

Key issues in public health policy and politics are as follows.

- Four spheres in which nurses can influence policy are government, workplace, organizations, and community.
- WHO defines health as the state of complete physical, mental, and social well-being, not merely the absence of disease or infirmity.

Table 22.1   Guidelines for Linking Publications to Policy

- Explicitly link manuscript topic to public health policies
- Frame the research findings or theoretical information in the current public health policy debate
- Manuscript should address populations of interest to policy makers
- Language of manuscript should be understandable to policy makers and general public
- Manuscript should include policy-relevant content in the literature review and discussion sections
- Manuscript should have information that can be used in all phases or should focus on one particular phase of the policy-making process
- Manuscript content should be useful to political action committees, advocates, or special interest groups
- Media and general public should be able to glean useful content from manuscript

SOURCE: Wakefield (2001).

- Policy may be defined as the principles that govern an action directed toward a given outcome.
- Health policy, in general terms, is any policy that affects the health of individuals or communities.
- Public health policy is defined as the administrative decisions made by the legislative, executive, or judicial branches of government that define courses of action affecting the health of a population through the influencing of actions, behaviors, or resources.
- Public policy is, basically, any policy formed by a governmental body or entity.
- Social policy is policy that is formulated to affect the welfare of the general public.
- Health policy is policy that is formulated to affect the health of individual community members.
- Institutional policies are policies developed by or to affect an institution.
- Organizational policies are administrative decisions or statements developed by an organization.
- Policies can assume the form of laws, rules, or regulations; operational decisions; or judicial decisions.
- Politics is the process of influencing someone or something to allocate resources as you desire.
- Political participation is any formal or informal activity, mainstream or unconventional, that occurs as a result of individual or collective action to either directly or indirectly influence what the government does.
- Three key factors that influence nurses' participation are resources, engagement, and networks of recruitment.
- Nursing scholars who engage in the dissemination of nursing science through publication have an opportunity to relate their theoretical discourse or research findings to policy.

References

Birkland, T. (2001). *An introduction to the policy process: Theories, concepts, and models of public policy making.* Armonk, NY: M. E. Sharpe.

Cohen, S., Mason, D., Kovner, C., Leavitt, J., Pulcini, J., & Sochalski, J. (1996). Stages of nursing's political development: Where we've been and where we ought to go. *Nursing Outlook, 44,* 259-261.

Dye, T. (2002). *Understanding public policy.* Upper Saddle River, New Jersey: Prentice Hall.

Greipp, M. (2002). Forces driving health care policy decisions. *Policy, Politics and Nursing, 3*(1), 35-42.

Longest, B. (2002). *Health policymaking in the United States* (3rd ed.). Washington, DC: Association of University Programs in Health Administration.

Mason, D., Leavitt, J., & Chaffee, M. (2002). *Policy and politics in nursing and health care* (4th ed.). St. Louis, MO: Saunders.

Peters, G. (1999). *American public policy: promise and performance.* Chappaqua, NY: Chatham House/Seven Rivers.

Schlozman, K., Burns, N., & Verba, S. (1994). Gender and the pathways to participation: The role of resources. *Journal of Politics, 65*(4), 963-990.

Titmus, R. (1974). *Social policy: An introduction.* New York: Pantheon.

Verba, S., Schlozman, K., & Brady, H. (1995). *Voice and equality: Civic voluntarism in American politics.* Cambridge, MA: Harvard University Press.

Wakefield, M. (2001). Linking health policy to nursing and health care scholarship: Points to consider. *Nursing Outlook, 49*(4), 204-205.

World Health Organization. (1988). *Second International Conference on Health Promotion, Adelaide, South Australia, 5-9 April 1998: Adelaide recommendations on healthy public policy (WHO/HPR/HEP/95.2).* Retrieved July 3, 2003, from http://www.who.int/hpr/NPH/docs/AdelaideRecommendations.pdf

World Health Organization. (1998). *Health for all: Origins and mandate.* Retrieved June 27, 2003, at http://www.who.int/archives/who50/en/health4all.htm

23

The Development of Public Health Policy

A core function of public health practice is policy development. The policy development process is dynamic and has a profound impact on multiple public health systems and populations. This chapter focuses on presenting the context in which policy development occurs and describing the sources of public health policy, the roles of policy makers, and multiple policy development models.

Introduction

Public health policy development is a core function of public health practice and is listed as one of the 10 essential public health services. Therefore, all public health professionals should engage in the public health policy development process. Specifically, public health nurses should engage in developing policies and plans that support population-based and community health efforts. Public health nurses should engage in the development of public health legislation and other types of policy to guide the practice of public health nursing. This chapter focuses on the influential factors of policy development. Chapter 24 will focus on the policy development process of formulating and modifying policy.

The Context of Policy Development

The context in which public health policy is developed is a weave of interdependent discourse among scientific, social, and political public health interests. Public health policy is developed within a sphere of political processes. Stakeholders engaged in public health policy development negotiate with policy makers for scarce resources and balance the public's need against multiple competing interests. The context of public health policy development consists of the public's need, special interest groups, political party agendas, social and economic pressures, personal desires, and governmental influence. The type of policy developed and the level at which policy is developed depends on the extent to which national, state, and local governments exercise separate and autonomous authority over their elected officials, taxation, and policy development. This is frequently referred to as American federalism. In addition to American federalism, the public's perspectives influence the context in which policy is developed.

Federalism

Dye (2002) describes federalism as a political system that has units of government that exist at the national, state, and local levels, all of which have governmental authority and protection. According to the United States Constitution, only national and state governments are protected; local governments are delegated certain powers but are considered subdivisions of state governments. Federalism is considered to provide for the existence of both federal and state governments. Federalism assures protection against tyranny, policy diversity, manages conflict between levels of government, disperses power, increases participation in policy making, improves efficiency, ensures policy responsiveness, and encourages policy innovation (Dye, 2002). The practice of and emphasis on federalism set the tone and political context surrounding the policy-making process.

Throughout history, the United States has moved through various types of federalism—state centered, dual, cooperative, centralized, "new," coercive, and representational (Dye, 2002). The amount of federalism present depends on the majority political parties represented at each level of government, stakeholders' power structure, and the public's desires. State-centered federalism (1787-1865) considered the states as the most important unit of government in the American federal system. Dual federalism (1865-1913) maintained that governmental powers are divided between the federal and state government. Cooperative federalism (1913-1964) shifted the governmental focus to the federal level with the creation of federal income tax. This type of federalism shifted the financial resources of the nation to the federal government, which allocated resources. Centralized federalism (1965-1980) centralized federal-state relations. The states' roles were to be responsive to federal policy initiatives and conform to federal regulations. The bureaucracies of federal, state, and local governments were indistinguishable and centralized. The "new federalism" (1980-1985) was a strategic shift in the flow of power, back to the state and local governmental levels and away from the federal government. Coercive federalism (1985-?) was a maneuver by the federal government to indirectly influence activities at the state and local governmental levels. Coercive federalism allocates resources based on the state or local government's compliance with "special strings" attached to funding streams. This coerces the states to comply and abide by federal mandates, or the state or local government will not qualify for federal resources. Representational federalism is an idea of no constitutional division of powers between the federal and state governments. Representational federalism considers that the amount of federalism that exists is dependent on the states' role in electing the United States president and members of Congress. Therefore, state protections are dependent on state-elected congressional members' ability to protect their state's power and promote the allocation of resources to their respective states through political processes at the national level (Dye, 2002).

The type of federalism currently in use affects federal actions, especially federal preemptions and mandates. Federal preemptions occur with the supremacy of federal laws over state or local laws and are permitted through the national supremacy clause of the United States Constitution. This permits Congress to decide when and whether state laws will be preempted by federal laws. There are various levels of preemption. Total preemption occurs when the federal government assumes all powers over state laws. Partial preemption permits state laws concerning similar topics to be valid as long as the law in question does not conflict with the federal law on the same topic. Standard partial preemption permits state laws or regulatory agencies to regulate activities in a field regulated by the federal government as long as the state regulatory standards are at least as stringent as those of the federal government. For example, many states have developed occupational health standards under standard partial preemptions that meet, at a minimum, Occupational Safety and Health Administration (OSHA) standards (Dye, 2002).

Mandates are direct orders or regulations to state or local governments that require them to conduct specific activities or to comply with specific federal laws. Examples of federal compliance mandates are the Age Discrimination Act of 1986, Safe Drinking Water Act of 1986, and Americans with Disabilities Act of 1990. Unfunded mandates are mandates from the federal government that require states and local governments to comply with cost requirements but do not allocate federal funds to offset the expense of implementing such policies (Dye, 2002).

Public Health Policy Perspectives

The public's perspective regarding health policies can influence the context in which public health policy is developed. Two primary perspectives influencing public health policy are pluralistic and elitist. The pluralist perspective embraces the idea of multiple special interest groups affecting public health policy development as a way of representing everyone's interest. Pluralists contend that special interest groups that are representative of the public should play a critical role in public health policy development. From this perspective, the various interest groups are seen as counterbalancing each others' perspectives in the policy development process, leading to the best policy in the best interests of the public. The pluralist perspective fits with the group theory of politics (Truman, 1993). Truman summarizes the essential tenets of the group theory of politics as (a) interest groups are essential linkages between the people and government; (b) interest groups compete with each other, creating a counterbalance of interest; (c) no interest group is likely to become too dominant; and (d) interest group competition is fair (Longest, 2002; Truman, 1993).

In contrast, the elitist perspective considers interest groups to be ineffective and powerless (Longest, 2002). This perspective sees the "real" political power of the United States as being in the hands of a very small proportion of the public population, consisting generally of those individuals who control key national institutions or organizations. The amount of power these people have is greatly influenced by their wealth. The elitist perspective is considered to be primarily concerned with self-interest. This group seen as controlling the power is frequently referred to as the "power elite." The power elite has a financial basis from which to directly or indirectly influence public health policy development. The central tenets of the power elite theory are (a) real political power rests with a small proportion of the population, (b) members of the power elite have similar values and interests, (c) incremental change is preferred, and (d) elites protect their power bases (Longest, 2002; Dye, 2002)

Sources of Public Health Policy

Public health policy at the federal, state, or local level is made through actions of the three governmental branches: executive, legislative, and judicial. Within these three branches of government, the three main suppliers of public health policy are executives or bureaucrats, legislators, and judiciary officers.

Presidents, governors, mayors, and city council officials, as executive officials, influence or develop policy proposals for legislators to enact. The executive officials have a great base of public responsibility for the development of policy. These officials are held accountable by their public constituency, as are legislators. Bureaucrats or civil servants who are members of regulatory agencies are responsible for the development of rules and regulations that operationalize the implementation of public health policy. These bureaucrats also collect, analyze, and transmit information that can influence the development of public health policy (Longest, 2002).

Executive officials and legislators are elected by the public and are responsible to the public. Legislators at all levels of government are essential players in the formation of public health policy. Legislators are responsible for weighing the pros and cons of each aspect of a policy based on the public's best interest. Legislators are the primary drafters of public health policy at the federal or state level as laws; however, bureaucrats in regulatory agencies also draft another level of public health policy to make federal or state laws into operational rules and regulations that implement the federal or state law (Longest, 2002).

Judicial officials supply policies through the interpretation of ambiguous law, interpretation of state and federal constitutions, and the establishment of judicial procedures (Longest, 2002). The judicial branch holds the power to declare laws as constitutional or unconstitutional, which sets precedent for future public health policy development. Judicial officials also interpret the intent and meaning of public health policy, which directly influences the manner in which the policy is implemented.

The Role of the Nurse as Public Health Policy Maker

Public health nurses assume multiple roles throughout the public health policy-making process. The public health nurse-researcher generates or validates the scientific base that provides the foundation of evidence to support the public health policy. Public health nurses can join or organize special interest groups, which engage in all stages of public health policy formulation and modification (refer to chapter 24). Lobbying is the process of influencing public health policy making through political processes (Longest, 2002). Public health nurses can conduct lobbying activities but usually not in their role as employees of a governmental agency. However, public health nurses can serve as informants to lobbyists. Electioneering is the process of using available resources to aid political candidates in securing an elected office. Public health nurses can engage in electioneering activities as private citizens, but as with lobbying, they must not engage in these activities as employees of a governmental agency. As electioneers, their role is to mobilize community votes for political candidates.

Legislative advocacy is a process of working with policy makers and policy-making bodies to gain support or influence public health policy. The process of legislative advocacy consists of (a) marshaling allies, (b) coordinating an organizational advocacy structure that supports communication and decision making among allies, (c) developing coalitions, (d) collecting all available data regarding the public health policy issue, (e) defining and piloting the message, (f) revising the message and developing a communication network, (g) cultivating the media, and (h) diffusing the message into the public and political structures that influence the public health policy issue.

Public health nurses can provide testimony regarding public health policy issues. The testimony can be as an expert public health professional or a personal story. Expert testimony substantiates a position supported by the representative authority of public health information based in scientific evidence. In contrast, personal testimony provides a personal dimension on the "real-life" impact a public health policy may have on individual public citizens. Personal testimony provides a first-hand account of the impact of public health policy.

Conceptual Models of
Public Health Policy Process

Conceptual models of public health policy processes specify the evolutional steps through which a policy moves, beginning with the point at which a public health issue or problem emerges to the point at which a public health program is created to deal with the problem. There are multiple models that characterize the process of public health policy development. These conceptual models are used to understand, influence, analyze, and evaluate the public health policy process. A brief discussion of some common policy development models is presented here.

Kingdon's Policy Stream Model

Kingdon (1995) describes the policy development process as occurring in three streams: problem, policy, and political. Kingdon envisions these streams as floating around and waiting for the "window of opportunity" to open through the fusing together of two streams. This window of opportunity offers an environment that is considered prime for policy development.

The problem stream consists of the challenge of getting policy makers to focus on one problem. The goals and ideas of policy subsystems, such as legislative staff, researchers, congressional committee members, and interest groups, are all part of this stream. In the policy stream, Kingdon (1995) envisions ideas floating around the policy circles in search of public health problems or a person who is ready to assume the policy development challenge. The political stream characterizes the political environment that influences the policy agenda. Once two of these streams align, the window of opportunity opens for policy development (Mason, Leavitt, & Chaffee, 2002). This model can also be used to analyze public health policy: It identifies some of the key elements that should be assessed during a policy analysis.

The Stage-Sequential Model

The stage-sequential model is a systems model that considers the policy development process as occurring in sequential stages. This model consists of four stages: policy agenda setting, policy formulation, program implementation, and policy evaluation (Mason et al., 2002).

Stage one is policy agenda setting. The identification of a problem warranting a policy initiates this stage. The problem is then framed into a policy issue. This stage attempts to place the identified policy issue on the public health policy agenda. Placement on the public policy agenda can assume one of three levels of consideration: discussion, action, or decision. The discussion agenda simply places the public policy issue within the policy makers' scope of attention. The action agenda signifies that the public policy issue is moving through to the policy formulation phase. The decision agenda is the last phase of legitimization by policy makers during legislative or regulatory processes.

Policy formulation is stage two. Policy formulation consists of collecting information on the issue, analyzing the information, disseminating the information, and drafting legislation. All interested stakeholders should provide input during the policy formulation phase.

Program implementation is stage three. During program implementation, the executive agency or regulatory body charged with implementing the program begins to draft guidelines, rules, or regulations from which to implement the legislation. Proposed drafts of the guidelines, rules, or regulations are published for a period of public comment in documents such as the *State Register*, *Federal Register*, or the official publication of the regulatory agency.

Program evaluation is the last stage of the stage-sequential model. This stage attempts to answer the question, "Did the policy effectively achieve what it was formulated to do?" The policy evaluators determine the extent to which the program has accomplished its goals and objectives, comparing the result to the legislative mandate. In addition to this outcome evaluation, the processes of implementing the policy are also evaluated (Mason et al., 2002).

The Richmond-Kotelchuck Model

The Richmond-Kotelchuck model of health policy was developed to influence public health prevention. This model posits that there are three necessary elements for prevention: knowledge base, political will, and social strategy. All three of these elements must be present in some amount for preventive policy to occur (Atwood, Colditz, & Kawachi, 1997).

The first component of the Richmond-Kotelchuck model is the knowledge base. The knowledge base is the scientific and administrative database used as the foundation of informed policy decisions (Richmond & Kotelchuck, 1991). This first component is considered to be where public health researchers should concentrate their efforts so that they may use scientific knowledge to influence public health policy.

The second component that influences policy is political will. Political will is defined by Richmond and Kotelchuck (1991) as society's desire and commitment to develop and fund new programs and support or modify existing programs in alignment with the knowledge base and social strategies. Political will is highly dependent on the ability to influence politicians, legislators, stakeholders, and special interest groups in alignment with policy issues. The knowledge base and political will are considered interdependent. Scientific knowledge influences political will, and vice versa.

Social strategy is the last component of the Richmond-Kotelchuck model. Social strategy is defined as the plan that uses the scientific knowledge base

Table 23.1   The Processes and Activities of the Local Public Health Policy Model

Prepare to Act
- Know the community's history
- Identify the issue's strengths and weaknesses
- Select the appropriate process

Clarify Role and Approach
- Determine source of authority for action
- Establish decision-making process
- Identify realistic expectations

Community Involvement
- Appoint a diverse task force
- Create an open process of collecting information
- Collect pertinent information
- Review all options
- Evaluate information and cultivate a commitment from the community
- Establish a timeline
- Assign responsibilities and authority

Communicate Policy and Rationale
- Draft policy
- Summarize rationale for policy
- Communicate policy and rationale through multiple communication channels
- Conduct public hearings
- Collect public input
- Respond to public input regarding policy and revise policy as necessary

Adopt, Implement, and Evaluate Policy
- Adopt policy
- Implement policy
- Provide resources to implement policy
- Monitor compliance with policy
- Evaluate policy
- Identify areas for policy modification

SOURCE: Upshaw and Okun (2002).

and political will to develop public health policy that improves or initiates the program desired (Atwood et al., 1997).

The Local Public Health Policy Model

Upshaw and Okun (2002) describe a public health policy model that was used on a local level to influence livestock operations that were affecting the public's health. This model consists of processes that can assist in formulating local public health policy. The model's five major processes are preparing to act; clarifying role and approach; community involvement; communicating rule and rationale; and adopting, implementing, and evaluating the rule. Table 23.1 outlines the recommended activities for each process in this model.

Summary

Key issues in public health policy development are as follows.

- Public health policy development is a core function and essential service of public health practice.
- The context in which public health policy is developed is a weave of interdependent discourse among scientific, social, and political public health interests.
- Federalism is a political system that has units of government that exist at the national, state, and local levels and have governmental authority and protection.
- National and state governments are protected; local governments are delegated powers by the state.
- Total preemption occurs when the federal government assumes all powers over state laws.
- Partial preemption permits state laws to be valid as long as they do not conflict with federal laws on the same topic.
- Standard partial preemption permits state laws or regulatory agencies to regulate activities in a field regulated by the federal government as long as the state regulatory standards are at least as stringent as those of the federal government.
- Mandates are direct orders or regulations to state or local governments that require them to conduct specific activities or comply with specific federal laws.
- Unfunded mandates are mandates from the federal government that require states and local governments to comply with cost requirements but do not allocate federal funds to offset the expense of implementing the policies.
- The primary perspectives influencing public health policy are either pluralistic or elitist.
- Public health policy at the federal, state, or local level is made through the actions of the three governmental branches: executive, legislative, and judicial.
- Lobbying is the process of influencing public health policy making through political processes.
- Electioneering is the process of using available resources to aid political candidates to secure an elected office.
- Legislative advocacy is a process of working with policy makers and policy-making bodies to gain support or influence public health policy.
- "Window of opportunity" denotes an environment that is considered prime for policy development.
- The stage-sequential model is a systems model that considers the policy development process as occurring in sequential stages.

- The Richmond-Kotelchuck model of health policy assumes that public health policy is influenced through the elements of knowledge base, political will, and social strategy.
- The local public health policy model consists of five processes: preparing to act; clarifying role and approach; community involvement; communicating rule and rationale; and adopting, implementing, and evaluating the rule.

References

Atwood, K., Colditz, G., & Kawachi, I. (1997). From public health science to prevention policy: Placing science in its social and political contexts. *American Journal of Public Health, 87*(10), 1603-1605.

Dye, T. (2002). *Understanding public policy.* Upper Saddle River, NJ: Prentice Hall.

Kingdon, J. (1995). *Agendas, alternatives, and public policies.* North Scituate, MA: Duxbury.

Longest, B. (2002). *Health policymaking in the United States* (3rd ed.). Washington, DC: Association of University Programs in Health Administration.

Mason, D., Leavitt, J., & Chaffee, M. (2002). *Policy and politics in nursing and health care* (4th ed.). St. Louis, MO: Saunders.

Richmond, J., & Kotelchuck, M. (1991). Coordination and development of strategies and policy for public health promotion in the United States. In W. Holland & R. Detels (Eds.), *Oxford textbook of public health.* Oxford, England: Oxford Medical.

Truman, D. (1993). *The governmental process.* Berkeley, CA: University of California Institute of Governmental Studies.

Upshaw, V., & Okun, M. (2002). A model approach for developing effective local public health policies: A North Carolina county responds to large-scale hog production. *Journal of Public Health Management Practice, 8*(5), 44-54.

24

Public Health Policy Formulation, Implementation, and Modification

A continuation of the policy development process is the actual formulation, implementation, and modification of public health policy. This process occurs in a context of high political diplomacy and negotiation. This chapter focuses on presenting agenda setting and the processes of policy formulation, implementation, and modification.

Introduction

The public health policy development process is a dynamic and continuous process that occurs within a political context of constant negotiation. This process consists of a series of activities or subprocesses that occur within the political arena. Dye (2002) identifies the processes of public health policy development as problem identification, agenda setting, policy formulation, policy implementation, and policy evaluation. Chapter 25 focuses on the processes of public health policy analysis and evaluation, with some discussion of differentiating public health problems from public health issues.

Two approaches to public health policy making are the rational and incremental approaches (Mason, Leavitt, & Chaffee, 2002). These two approaches provide some explanations into the sequence of activities that occurs during the political process of policy making.

The rational approach is considered to reflect "real-world" goals. In this approach, policy makers define the problem; identify and rank social values within the policy goals; examine policy alternatives in relation to positive and negative consequences of the policy, along with costs and benefits; compare and contrast the options; and select the policy that achieves the problem resolution, fits with social values, and reflects the best alternative policy (Mason et al., 2002).

In contrast to the rational approach, the incremental approach makes small changes over time. Most public health policy is made using the incremental approach. This approach begins with the existing status quo and alters it through the formulation of a policy that changes incrementally in relation to a desire expressed by some political subsystem (Mason et al., 2002). This process permits greater involvement and permeation over time of various political factions within the political arena. Both approaches to policy formulation are dependent on the policy issue being adequately placed onto the public health policy agenda.

Public Health Policy Agenda Setting

The first activity of the public health policy process, which many believe is the most critical, is agenda setting (Longest, 2002). Use of the word "agenda" indicates that there is a prioritization of issues or some listing of which issues are most relevant and pertinent. In the policy formulation process, policy makers must be aware of the multiple and competing agendas that may be influencing public opinion. Generally, there are at least four agendas in relation to policy issues: the media's agenda, the public's agenda, the politician's agenda, and the government's agenda (Prouty, 2000).

Agenda setting is the activity of determining what public health problems are deserving of public health policy solutions. Placement of a public health issue on the policy agenda is a pivotal point in promoting the development of a public health policy. Kingdon's policy development model identified the interaction of three streams: problem, policy, and political circumstances (refer to chapter 23). The convergence of these three streams increases the chance of a public health issue making it onto the public health policy agenda (Smith, 1997). In addition, the convergence of these three streams—problems, policy, and political circumstances—into an alignment creates a window of opportunity for policy development. A policy entrepreneur is an individual who secures this opportunity in the favorable political climate, ensuring that the policy is brought to the forefront of the public policy agenda (Smith, 1997).

The media plays a critical function in agenda setting. The media's power lies in the hands of editors, producers, anchors, reporters, columnists and prestigious sources of press (Dye, 2002). The media exerts a considerable amount of influence in agenda setting. The media influences the public health agenda through newsmaking, determining what is "news" and who or what is "newsworthy" (Dye, 2002). According to Prouty (2000), the media is "not telling us what to think but telling us what to think about."

The media exerts an influence on the public health policy agenda through two activities, priming and framing. Priming is the psychological process the media uses to increase the salience of an issue through the activation of previously acquired information. Priming uses cognitive psychology. In priming, an idea or concept is planted in an individual's mind and related to other ideas or concepts through semantic pathways. This process uses these pathways as a filter, an interpretive frame, or a premise for the processing or judging of future information. The media uses priming to influence information storage and retrieval in the mind (Domke, Shah, & Wackman, 1998). Priming gets us ready for the message that the media intends to deliver later.

Framing is the activity of focusing attention on particular aspects of an issue and obscuring the focus on other aspects (Prouty, 2000). It is frequently referred to as the "maps" drawn by the media for the public to influence the manner in which information is assimilated on the public health issue. These maps, or frames, essentially provide the boundaries within which we think about the issue. There are two primary forms of frames: episodic and thematic (Dubber, 2000). Episodic frames focus on the people in trouble or the current point of conflict in relation to the public health issue. In comparison, thematic frames focus on the context within which the public health issue is unfolding. Thematic framing places the public health issue within a broader social, political, and economic context for the public. Both priming and framing influence and guide our thinking in relation to the public health policy agenda. These activities can actively be used by public health nurses when working in concert with the media to influence the public health agenda.

In addition to the media, interpersonal social or political networks exert considerable influence on agenda-setting activities. This is known as interpersonal agenda setting. Interpersonal agenda setting is the use of social networks (or social interest groups) to mediate the relationships between any or all of the involved parties: policy makers, governmental representatives, media, and public (Dubber, 2000).

Other forces driving public health policy agenda setting are the problem's magnitude, research, political forces, public opinion, and the government's executive officer. Problems that typically are placed on the agenda for policy formulation are those that are broadly identified by policy makers as important or urgent in regard to the public's health or safety. Other factors influencing the perceived magnitude of the problem is public salience and the amount of conflict surrounding the problem. A public health problem is considered salient if there is real or potential public interest. Conflictive problems are those that generate intense disagreements among interest groups or other stakeholders who may place the interest of these groups in opposition to the public's interest (Longest, 2002). Public health problems known to have widespread implications are frequently placed on the agenda. A problem's level of perceived importance for placement on the agenda changes as the social and political contextual circumstances of the given time change.

Research data that are presented in terms that create a perceived threat or risk typically generate considerable public interest for the given issue. Public health research determines the extent and nature of the problem, clarifies the associative factors, and provides evaluative data regarding possible solutions. Research data that assist in clarifying the public health problem for placement on the agenda can also serve as baseline comparative data to evaluate policy effectiveness in the future (Longest, 2002).

Political forces that favor a public health problem influence its placement on the agenda. Public health issues that are directly related to a political party's platform may be more readily placed on their agenda. Public health problems that generate a lot of public health attention can be used politically to influence the allocation of multiple types and sources of resources in the favor of the political group.

Public opinions are shared through direct correspondence with elected officials, special interest polls, and communication with the press. Public opinion serves an iterative process. It can place items on the public health policy agenda but can also serve to shape public opinion once a problem is placed on the policy agenda.

The governmental executive officer (e.g., president, governor, mayor) commands the public's attention and communicates frequently with the public through the media. Through their directive leadership, government executive officers communicate their position on public health problems and their expected direction for solutions. Through their communication, governmental executive officers raise issues that are directly or indirectly critical to influencing the policy agenda. These issues are frequently raised during "State of the State" or "State of the Union" addresses (Longest, 2002). They frame our thinking and pave the way for placement of the issues on the public's agenda for improvements or changes.

The Public Health Policy Formulation Process

Public health agenda setting, discussed earlier, is recognized as an integral part of the public health policy formulation process. Public health policy formulation consists of legislation development. Legislation development generally occurs at the governmental level. The outcome of public health policy formulation is the development of new public health laws or amendments to existing laws. This text broadly defines policy; therefore the generation of rules and regulations is considered an essential part of the public health policy formulation process. Policy formulation occurs in multiple settings and contexts—government bureaucracies, special interest group offices, association or specialty organization offices, legislative committee rooms, meetings of special commissions, think-tank groups, and at the hands of legislative staff (Dye, 2002; refer to chapter 26 to review the process of developing a law). Some aspects of policy formulation are presented here: proposal drafting, introduction of legislation, and legislative oversight.

Public Health Policy Proposal Drafting

The ideas for public health policy originate in multiple areas. The executive branch of government is generally expected to initiate public health policy proposals, although Congress is the arbiter of the policy (Dye, 2002). "Executive communication" from the executive branch of government strongly influences or initiates public health policy initiation. However, members of the legislative branch of government can also initiate public health policy proposals. In addition, citizens, organizations, and special interest groups can petition the government, through the First Amendment, to formulate policy. The proposed public health policy may be given in the form of public health ideas, solutions, or actually in a drafted proposal (Longest, 2002).

A very influential and frequently overlooked group that affects or directly drafts proposed public health policy is that composed of legislative staff members or governmental executive officers—the president, governor, or mayor. Once an issue is brought to the attention of legislators or governmental executive officers, they may delegate the proposal drafting to a member of their legislative staff team. In addition, legislative staffers control access to the legislators. By controlling access to the legislators, these staffers can directly influence public health policy agenda setting and who has input into policy formulation. Legislative staff have an essential role in selecting the small number of issues addressed in public health policy proposals (Weissert & Weissert, 2000). Legislators and executive officers change office, but legislative staff remain in office. Legislative staff may orient the new legislator to the current or critical issues, therefore shaping the public health agenda. The influence level of the legislative staff is dependent on the level of trust between the legislator and staff members (Weissert & Weissert, 2000). Sometimes the person who has been consistently in the policy formulation process and who has both historical and current political perspective on the public health policy agenda or problem may be the legislative staff member who remains in office after the legislator is gone.

Legislative staff affect public health policy proposal development through multiple responsibilities. Legislative staff research issues, schedule legislative meetings and hearings, line up experts and interest groups for testimony, remain abreast of competing or similar proposals, stay current on executive communication through contact with the executive office, and write the draft proposal (Dye, 2002).

Drafting a bill is a team effort. Any member of the legislature or executive branch can draft a bill. The legislative council's office in either the Senate or House of Representatives can provide assistance with drafting the appropriate language of a bill (Longest, 2002). Drafting a bill involves multiple meetings with special interest groups, association or organization members, or the constituency. Once a legislator agrees to officially sponsor a bill, that legislator is responsible for the language of the bill.

Introduction of the Policy
Proposal Into the Legislative Process

A public health policy proposal can be drafted through multiple avenues. Members of the public can draft public health policy proposals. However, only members of the legislative branch can actually introduce proposed public health legislation, regardless of who originated the proposal (Longest, 2002). A public health policy proposal that originated through the executive branch is submitted to a committee chairperson for introduction into the legislative process. For example, the state or federal budget submitted to the legislature each year is considered one source of regular executive communication that occurs between the executive and legislative branches. Even this proposed appropriation bill that originates in the executive branch is submitted to the legislative branch through the appropriate legislative committee for consideration, approval, and enactment into law. The approved bill returns to the executive branch for the president or state official to sign into law.

Legislative Oversight of Public Health Policy Proposal

Bills introduced into the legislature for consideration are numbered sequentially by date of introduction and referred to the appropriate standing committee. Each committee of the legislature has jurisdiction over certain areas of legislation. Bills that pertain to that respective area are referred to that standing committee. Bills with a broad focus may be referred to more than one standing committee for consideration; bills regarding the same public health problem with two different foci may be assigned to two different committees, depending on the overall intent of the proposed bill. Each committee has a professional staff person that assists with administrative functions. In addition, expert consultants can be appointed to assist with the standing committee's work on the proposal.

Public health nurses should be familiar with the focus of each standing committee that routinely manages public health proposals. As a general rule of thumb at the federal level, health-related bills are referred to the House Committee on Energy and Commerce and to the Senate Committee on Health, Education, Labor, and Pensions. Any bill that involves taxation and revenues must be referred to the House Committee on Ways and Means and the Senate Committee on Finance (Longest, 2002). Each of these standing committees has subcommittees to which the health proposal may be directed for consideration. Some examples of subcommittees of standing committees are

- Committee on Finance subcommittee on health care
- Committee on Health, Education, Labor and Pension subcommittees on aging, on children and families, and on public health
- Senate Committee on Appropriations subcommittees on labor, health and human services, and education and on veterans, housing, and urban development
- Committee on Ways and Means subcommittee on health
- Committee on Energy and Commerce subcommittees on health and on environment and hazardous materials

- House Committee on Appropriations subcommittees on labor, health and human services, and education; on veteran affairs, housing and urban development, and independent agencies; and on agriculture, rural development, and the Food and Drug Administration (Longest, 2002)

These standing subcommittees can hold hearings on proposed bills, or the proposal can be handled directly by the standing committee. If proposals are referred to the subcommittee, the subcommittee provides the standing committee with a draft of the proposed bill and a recommendation for consideration.

Public Health Policy Implementation

Once a bill is legislatively passed, the governmental executive officer must sign the proposed bill into law. With the signing of the bill into law, the policy-making process moves from policy formulation to policy implementation. This transition from formulation to implementation is accompanied by a transition of the process from the legislative branch to the executive branch of government. Policy implementation is generally a function of the executive branch. The executive departments and agencies of the executive branch are established and maintained to carry out the intent of public health laws, and, sometimes in cooperation with legislative committees, these departments and agencies have oversight responsibility for the public health laws (Longest, 2002). Policy implementation consists of two cyclical processes: rule making and operation.

Rule Making

Rule making is defined as the establishment of the formal rules and regulations necessary to fully operationalize the public health law (Longest, 2002). The language of the public health law is typically not explicit. Therefore, the implementing agency must determine the intent and develop rules and regulations consistent with this intent. The promulgation process of rules and regulations requires publication of the proposed rules for a period of time that allows public comment. The process of promulgating rules and regulations is as follows:

- A "notice of proposed rulemaking" is published in the *State Register* or *Federal Register*. This notice is actually a draft of the proposed rules and regulations.
- A comment period is permitted, during which reactions and recommendations are obtained from interested parties and the public.

- Proposed rules and regulations are revised as necessary.
- The wording of the final rule is published in the *State Register* or *Federal Register*.
- The rules is operationalized (Longest, 2002).

Rule making is sometimes referred to as the policy legitimization process. Legitimization is considered the final process in policy making. Policy legitimization occurs as a result of the open, public stage of the policy-making process of publishing rules and regulations for public feedback (Dye, 2002).

Operation

Once the rules and regulations have been promulgated, operationalization of the rules begins the operation process. Operation in this context means the actual activities involved in carrying out the law, such as conducting inspections, imposing fines, and issuing permits (Longest, 2002). The operationalization of the public health law is dependent on well-written laws that contain clearly articulated goals and objectives either in the law, rules, or regulations.

Legislative Oversight of Public Health Laws

The same legislative committees and subcommittees that maintain legislative oversight of the public health proposal assume legislative oversight of the law after it is passed and implemented. These committees review reports and other evaluations conducted on the public laws as a means of assuring legislative oversight of the public health law. The most powerful source of public health law oversight is the continued appropriation of funds for each of the respective public health programs initiated as a result of public health laws.

The Legislative Reorganization Act of 1946 mandates oversight of public health laws by the legislative branch (Longest, 2002). This oversight is intended to achieve the following:

- Ensure adherence to the intent of the public health law
- Improve the efficiency, effectiveness, and economy of the government's operations
- Assess the ability of the implementing agency to manage and achieve the implementation
- Ensure that policies are implemented in the public's best interest

Public Health Policy Modification

Public health policies are never perfect. Mistakes of omission and commission inevitably occur during the policy-making process. Policies are modified as an attempt to limit the negative aspects of the law and meet the legislative intent and the public's need. Policy modification differs from policy formulation in that policy formulation is the initial establishment of an original public health law (Longest, 2002); policy modification is the result of analysis or evaluative information that is discovered after policy formulation and requires a change in the policy. This information goes back to earlier stages such as agenda setting, legislation development, or rule-making stages to stimulate changes in the legislation, rules, or operations as originally formulated. The modification can occur as an alteration to the original law (an amendment), a modification in the development of rules and regulations of the program, or a change in the way the program is operationalized.

Summary

Key issues in public health policy formulation, implementation, and modification are as follows.

- Two approaches to public health policy making are rational and incremental.
- Agenda setting is the most critical element of the public health policy-making process.
- Priming is the psychological process used by the media to increase the salience of an issue through activation of previously acquired information.
- Framing is the activity of focusing attention on particular aspects of an issue and obscuring the focus on other aspects.
- Interpersonal agenda setting is the use of social networks to mediate the relationships between any or all of the involved parties.
- Forces driving public health policy agenda setting are the problem's magnitude, research, political forces, public opinion, and the government's executive officer.
- Public health policy formulation consists of legislation development.
- The executive branch of government is generally expected to initiate public health policy proposals, but Congress is the arbiter of the policy.
- Any member of the legislature or executive branch can draft a bill.
- Only members of the legislative branch can actually introduce proposed public health legislation.
- Bills that pertain to a specific area are referred to the appropriate standing committee.
- At the federal level, health-related bills are referred to the House Committee on Energy and Commerce and to the Senate Committee on Health, Education, Labor, and Pensions.
- With the signing of a bill into law, the policy-making process moves from policy formulation to policy implementation.

- Policy implementation is generally a function of the executive branch.
- Policy implementation consists of two cyclical processes: rule making and operation.
- Rule making is defined as the establishment of the formal rules and regulations necessary to fully operationalize the intent of the public health law.
- Operation means the actual activities involved in carrying out the law, such as conducting inspections, imposing fines, and issuing permits.
- The most powerful source of public health law oversight is the continued appropriation of funds.
- Policies are modified as an attempt to limit the negative aspects of the law and meet the legislative intent and the public's need.
- Policy modification is a result of analysis or evaluative information that is discovered after policy formulation and requires a change in the policy.

References

Domke, D., Shah, D., & Wackman, D. (1998). Media priming effects: Accessibility, association, and activation. *International Journal of Public Opinion Research, 10,* 51-75.

Dubber, A. (2000). *Agenda-setting-theory.* Retrieved September 11, 2002, from http://home.aut.ac.nz/~adubber/html/agenda_essay.html

Dye, T. (2002). *Understanding public policy.* Upper Saddle River, NJ: Prentice Hall.

Longest, B. (2002). *Health policymaking in the United States* (3rd ed.). Washington, DC: Association of University Programs in Health Administration.

Mason, D., Leavitt, J., & Chaffee, M. (2002). *Policy and politics in nursing and health care* (4th ed.). St. Louis, MO: Saunders.

Prouty, J. L. (2000). *Agenda setting function of Maxwell McCombs & Donald Shaw.* Retrieved June 25, 2003, from http://oak.cats.ohiou.edu/~jp340497/agsapp.htm

Smith, A. (1997). *Agenda setting by John W. Kingdon.* Retrieved June 25, 2003, from http://www.tamucc.edu/~whatley/PADM5302/theo13b.htm

Weissert, C., & Weissert, G. (2000). State legislative staff influence in health policy making. *Journal of Health Politics, Policy and Law, 25*(6), 1121-1148.

25 Public Health Policy Analysis and Evaluation

Public health policies that have been formulated and implemented must be continually analyzed and evaluated for currency with the political climate and social issues and must also be evaluated for effectiveness. Public health policy analysis and evaluation continually provide valuable data that can assist with policy modifications. This chapter focuses on differentiating public health problem analysis and issue analysis and presenting public health policy analysis and evaluation processes.

Introduction

Public health policy formulation and modification is not the end of the policy-making process. Public health policies are continually analyzed during all phases of the policy-making process, including agenda setting, policy formulation, policy drafting, rule making, policy implementation, and policy modification. Policy analysis is critical to the correct identification of a public health issue. Policy analysis influences the initial formulation of public health policy and future modifications to public health policy (Dye, 2002; Longest, 2002).

Some public health policy experts refer to public health policy analysis and evaluation as synonymous. For the purposes of this book, public health policy analysis and public health policy evaluation will be differentiated: Public health policy evaluation measures the extent to which a public health policy has achieved its intent, goals, and objectives; public health policy analysis critically appraises the context in which the public health issue or policy exists. Public health policy analysis is initiated with an interpretive analysis of the policy. Public health policy analysis may generate information regarding the amount of congruence between the present public health policy and the present political and social context. If there is significant incongruity, the analysis may initiate the need to conduct a thorough public health policy evaluation. These two processes can be iterative in nature.

Public Health Problem or Issue Analysis

The first step in conducting an analysis of a public health policy is to clearly analyze the public health problem or issue framing the need for a public health policy. Public health problem or issue analysis is a systematic approach to describing and explaining the interrelationships of multiple antecedents or background variables affecting a public health problem or issue (Mason, Leavitt, & Chaffee, 2002). Public health problem or issue analysis is used to structure the public health problem or issue and identify relevant underlying problems or issues.

A critical step in problem or issue analysis is distinguishing whether the public health area of concern is a real problem or merely an issue of concern. The ability to differentiate among problem situations, policy problems, and policy issues is critical to the understanding of the most appropriate policy solutions. Problem or issue formulation is heavily dependent on stakeholders' perceptions of the public health concern. A public health policy failure can result from the inability to adequately state or characterize the public health problem or issue. Public health areas of concern may be considered issues at one point but can later evolve into what are determined to be public health problems. There are multiple issues that frame public health problems. Therefore, the first step typically is to analyze the public health area of concern as an issue, then determine whether it is an issue or a problem. If it is determined to be a problem, then a public health problem analysis is conducted.

Public Health Issue Analysis

A public health issue is generally an area of public health concern. However, it is not defined as the etiologic root cause of the public health condition but as an associated factor. Analysis of a public health issue consists of a 10-step process. During the analysis, debate and inquiry into the public health issue is encouraged to achieve insightfulness, inquisitiveness, and refusal to accept simple answers for complex queries. The following steps outline the public health issue analysis process:

1. *Public health issue identification.* Identification of the issue clarifies the underlying public health issues. Causes, potential effects, and interested parties are identified. The manner in which the issue received attention on the public health agenda is analyzed.

2. *Background.* The context of the issue is analyzed through an assessment of social, economic, ethical, political, and legal factors that are forcing the issue on the public health agenda.

3. *Stakeholders.* All direct and indirect stakeholders are identified.

4. *Position analysis*. Stakeholders' and governmental officials' (in the executive, legislative, and judicial branches of government as necessary) positions on the issue are analyzed.

5. *Political analysis*. The political climate is analyzed.

6. *Issue statement*. A narrative statement of the identified issue is written. A tentative issue statement can be written after the public health issue is identified. The issue statement may be altered throughout the issue analysis process.

7. *Issue interaction analysis*. The interrelationship of this public health issue with other public health issues or problems is analyzed.

8. *Policy identification*. Potential public health policy options and alternatives are analyzed.

9. *Outcome identification*. Desired outcomes are identified.

10. *Policy recommendation*. The optimal policy solution for the public health issue is recommended.

The final determination of whether the public health area of concern is an issue or problem is largely decided by interested parties and policy makers within the context of the area of concern. The magnitude of the concern frequently differentiates issue from problem. A public health area of concern considered a legitimate public health problem that needs public health policy intervention is frequently subjected to a public health problem analysis. This process further structures the problem. There is some redundancy in the process of conducting an analysis of public health issues and problems, but this only leads to further clarification of the public health area of concern.

Public Health Problem Analysis

A public health problem is the identifiable cause of the public health concern that needs resolution. Public health problem identification consists of the following four steps: problem sensing, problem search, problem definition, and problem specification. Problem sensing is the recognition and felt existence of a public health problem. The problem sensing step analyzes the problem situation. The problem search step discovers the multiple representations of the problem, multiple stakeholders involved, and multiple worldviews of the problem. Problem definition formally characterizes the problem as a substantive problem. In the problem definition step, the problem is characterized in basic and general terms, and a conceptual framework of the problem is presented. The last step, problem specification, formalizes the public health problem through agenda setting, identifying constituents' needs, conducting public opinion polls, and assessing the opposition's position on and strength in relation to the problem.

Several methods are used to structure or define a public health problem. The following methods and their aims are presented to assist the public health nurse in structuring the public health problem:

- *Boundary analysis*. Identify the boundaries of the problem by asking, What are the various facets of the problem? Who are the interested stakeholders and groups? What are the multiple views regarding the problem?
- *Concept analysis*. Analyze the multiple concepts presented and discussed in the problem.
- *Hierarchy analysis*. Analyze the potential causes as possible, plausible, or actionable causes.
- *Synectics*. Analyze the similarities and differences of the problems.
- *Brainstorming*. Use this technique to generate goals, ideas, and policy strategies.
- *Multiple perspectives analysis*. Generate multiple insights into the problem and potential policy strategies.
- *Assumption analysis*. Identify and synthesize multiple assumptions underlying the public health problem and policy solutions.
- *Argumentation mapping*. Assess the accuracy of each assumption.

Public health problem structuring is critical to public health policy development. In summation, public health problem structuring identifies the problem from the eye of the beholder, discovers and analyzes hidden assumptions about the problem, diagnoses possible causes, maps policy solutions, synthesizes conflicting views, and assists in designing new policy outcomes. The critical nature of problem structuring ensures that the correct public health problem is identified and that it is correctly characterized and solved.

The Public Health Policy Analysis Process

Once a public health policy is formulated, public health policy analysis is conducted, by multiple groups and for different reasons. Analysis of a public health policy can facilitate a clearer understanding of the policy's intentions, expected outcomes, and interrelationships with other policies. Public health policy analysis must also be conducted by regulatory agencies as a measure of rule making to implement required programs. Analysis of public health policies is also conducted prior to recommending public health policy modifications.

Public health policy analysis is a systematic methodology that critically appraises the extent to which the public health policy is a viable and implementable solution to a public health problem and whether the policy will be acceptable to affected populations given the current social fabric of society

(Taub, 2002). There is a lack of clearly articulated processes with which to structure the public health policy analysis process. Therefore, the following process is recommended as one possible method of conducting public health policy analysis:

1. *Critical policy review.* The public health policy needs to be read repeatedly until there is clear understanding of the policy's intent and the various directives buried in the policy. The essential components of the policy should be outlined and correlated to public health issues or problems. The policy should be reviewed for inconsistencies or gaps. The critical policy review should include an analysis of any components of the policy that are unrelated amendments to the policy.

2. *Policy search.* Conduct a comprehensive policy search for other policies that focus on the same public health problem. Policies that are affected by or related to the public health policy may also need to be analyzed. The related impact of one policy on another or contradictions in two related policies should be assessed. Each of the related policies may need to undergo policy analysis.

3. *Historical analysis.* The time period in which the policy was developed should be reviewed in relation to social, economic, political, and environmental factors that influenced the policy. The values, beliefs, and political affiliations of the policy makers who drafted the policy at that time should be reviewed.

4. *Budgetary analysis.* Analyze the appropriation of funds to support the policy. Determine which components of the policy had the largest appropriation of resources. This provides some idea of legislative priorities in regard to the policy.

5. *Public health issue and problem analysis.* The public health issues surrounding the policy should be analyzed, and analysis should also be made of the public health problems identified in the policy as it currently exists.

6. *Stakeholder identification.* Actual or potential stakeholders and special interest groups should be identified. Their positions regarding the public health problem and policy under analysis should be assessed.

7. *SWOT analysis.* Identify the strengths, weaknesses, opportunities, and threats (SWOT analysis) to the public health policy. The SWOT analysis should focus on the current analysis of the public health problem and the viability and adequacy of the existing policy to solve the problem.

8. *Gap analysis.* The provisions of the current public health problem in relation to the current needs to solve the public health problem should be appraised. The gap between the policy and the needs should be identified as potential areas for policy modification or development.

9. *Summation.* An executive summation of each of these steps should be developed and presented to policy makers. The summation should include recommendations on policy modification and development.

10. *Prioritization.* Recommendations provided in the summation should be prioritized for policy development and implementation.

Public Health Policy Evaluation

Public health policy evaluation assesses the overall effectiveness of a policy to determine if the policy is achieving its objectives (Dye, 2002). Public health policy evaluation is a systematic, empirical assessment of the effects of ongoing policies and programs developed from the policies (Nachmias, 1979). This evaluative process focuses on measuring the impact of a policy and the implementation of that policy as intended by the policy makers.

Dye (2002) recommends evaluation of the policy's effects on real-world conditions. Real-world effects that should be assessed are (a) impact on the target problem, (b) impact on the targeted group, (c) impact on nontargeted groups (spillover effects), (d) impact on future and immediate conditions of the problem, (e) direct cost in terms of resources devoted, (f) indirect costs, and (g) net analysis of benefits to costs.

Various methods are used to evaluate the effectiveness of public health policy. Dye (2002) identified the most common methods of conducting a policy evaluation: (a) congressional or oversight committee hearings, (b) annual program reports to Congress or an oversight committee, (c) on-site visits, (d) tracking program benchmarks, (e) comparison of program to some professional standard, and (f) ongoing evaluation of constituent complaints. The reader is referred to chapters 13 and 14 to review program monitoring and evaluation and performance measurement and improvement measures that can also be used to assess the effectiveness of public health policies.

The General Accounting Office (GAO) is an arm of Congress established in 1921. The GAO maintains broad authority to audit federally funded programs' operations and finances. The GAO submits its findings to Congress and other oversight committees as appropriate, as an evaluative measure of programs developed and implemented as a result of public health policy (Dye, 2002; Longest, 2002).

Accountability to the public requires a comprehensive evaluation of the impact of public health policies on the public's health. The following process is recommended as a procedure to evaluate public health policies:

1. Conduct a public health policy analysis.

2. Identify the goals and objectives of the policy.

3. Identify public health data to measure the effectiveness of the public health policy.

4. Identify the articulated timelines in the public health policy.

5. Collect data on the chronological implementation of the policy.

6. Collect public health data indexes that measure the impact of the policy on the public's health.

7. Determine the extent to which the public health policy objectives have been met.

8. Identify intervening variables or circumstances that may have a negative impact on the maximum effectiveness of the public health policy.

9. Provide recommendations to improve the impact of the public health policy.

10. Disseminate findings to policy makers, stakeholders, and special interest groups.

Summary

Key issues in public health policy analysis and evaluation are as follows.

- Public health policy evaluation measures the extent to which the public health policy has achieved its intent, goals, and objectives.
- Public health policy analysis critically appraises the context in which the public health issue or policy exists.
- Public health problem or issue analysis is a systematic approach to describing and explaining the interrelationships of multiple antecedents or background variables affecting a public health problem or issue.
- A public health issue is an area of public health concern. It is not, however, defined as the etiologic root cause of the public health condition but is an associated factor.
- A public health problem is the identifiable cause of the public health concern that needs resolution.
- Public health policy evaluation assesses the overall effectiveness of a policy.

References

Dye, T. (2002). *Understanding public policy*. Upper Saddle River, NJ: Prentice Hall.

Longest, B. (2002). *Health policymaking in the United States* (3rd ed.). Washington, DC: Association of University Programs in Health Administration.

Mason, D., Leavitt, J., & Chaffee, M. (2002). *Policy and politics in nursing and health care* (4th ed.). St. Louis, MO: Saunders.

Nachmias, D. (1979). *Public policy evaluation*. New York: St. Martin's.

Taub, L. (2002). A policy analysis of access to health care inclusive of cost, quality, and scope of services. *Policy, Politics and Nursing Practice, 3*(2), 167-176.

26

Public Health Law and the Legal System

Public health law is a form of public health policy. The development and use of public health law is considered a population-based, community-level intervention that protects and maintains the public's health and safety. This chapter focuses on defining public health law, describing the United States legal system and law formulation, and presenting the role of the public health officer in public health law.

Introduction

Public health law integrates concepts from law, medicine, health care, and public health (Gostin, 2000). Public health law provides the legal basis for public health practice. In addition, the implementation of public health law is a function of public health practice. Implementation of public health law is an essential element to ensuring population-level health, especially through governmental entities. Through public health law, public health officers, including public health nurses, are empowered to act on behalf of the greater population to ensure "healthy" living conditions.

Public Health Law Defined

Definitions of public health law abound. The general term of "law" is frequently used to refer to the legal system, legal processes, the legal profession, and legal knowledge and learning. Public health law is frequently defined within the context of public health policy, since public health law is considered public policy. Longest (2002) defines public health law as laws related to health, which can be enacted at any level of government. The definition of public health law adopted for this book is based on Gostin's perspective. Gostin (2000) defines public health law as

The study of the legal powers and duties of the state to assure the conditions for people to be healthy (e.g., to identify, prevent, and ameliorate risks to health in the population) and the limitations on the power of the state to constrain the autonomy, privacy, liberty, proprietary, or other legally protected interests of individuals for the protection or promotion of community health. (p. 4)

His definition goes on to list five essential characteristics of public health law: (a) the government is responsible for public health activities, (b) a population-based focus is assumed, (c) public health addresses relationships between the state and the population, (d) population-based services are delivered grounded in science, and (e) public health officers have the power to coerce individuals and businesses into actions that protect the health of the population.

The United States Legal System

The United States Constitution forms the legal basis of the United States legal system. The three primary functions of the United States Constitution are to allocate power between the federal government and the states (federalism), divide power among the three branches of government (separation of power), and limit the amount of government power (protection of individual liberties).

Federalism

Federalism separates the legal scope of authority into two governmental tiers, federal and state. Federalism grants the federal government limited authority but allows the state governments plenary powers to protect the public. The chief powers for public health purposes are the powers to tax, to spend, and to regulate interstate commerce (Gostin, 2000). In addition to delegated powers, states maintain the powers that they had prior to the ratification of the United States Constitution. The "reserved powers" doctrine holds that states can exercise all powers inherent in government to protect the public (Gostin, 2000; Grad, 1990). Also in the domain of federalism is the supremacy clause, which declares that the Constitution and other laws of the United States shall be considered the supreme laws of the land and therefore preempt any state public health laws (Gostin, 2000).

Through federalism's separation of the government into federal and state, states are delegated police power. Police power provides the basis for public health nurses' legal authority to ensure the health, safety, and welfare of the population. In addition, states are granted *parens patriae* (patriarchal power) and taxation power.

Police Power

Police was the original term used to describe the powers that permitted the sovereign government the right to control its citizens. The purpose of this was to promote the general health, safety, comfort, morals, and prosperity of the public (Gostin, 2000). Gostin defines police power as

> the inherent authority of the state (and, through delegation, local government) to enact laws and promulgate regulations to protect, preserve, and promote the health, safety, morals, and general welfare of the people. To achieve these communal benefits, the state retains the power to restrict, within federal and state constitutional limits, private interest—personal interests in autonomy, privacy, association, and liberty as well as economic interest in freedom to contract and uses of property. (p. 48)

Police power has three underlying principles—to promote the greater public good, permit the restriction of private interest to promote public good, and permit pervasiveness of state powers.

Parens Patriae Power

Parens patriae means "parent of the country." Parens patriae power means that the states have an inherent power through sovereignty to safeguard the community's welfare. This form of power gives states the legal authority to protect the interest of minors and incompetent persons: States may make decisions on behalf of individuals who are incapable of making decisions for themselves. Parens patriae also allows states to assert their own general interest regarding communal health, safety, comfort, and welfare (Gostin, 2000).

Taxation Power

The power to tax citizens is a primary public health intervention. Taxation is a means of achieving public health goals and objectives. Public health taxation regulates individual private behaviors through economic penalties. Taxation is an indirect measure to reduce risky behaviors. For example, taxation of cigarettes is a measure to deter individuals from smoking by placing an increased economic penalty on smoking. At the same time, this public health intervention generates revenue for the state or federal government. The power to tax is frequently referred to as the power to govern people's individual behaviors (Gostin, 2000).

Separation of Power

Power is separated among the three governmental branches (executive, judicial, and legislative). Executive power is vested in the president of the

United States, judicial power is vested in the U.S. Supreme Court, and legislative power is vested in the U.S. Congress. Each respective state maintains a similar governmental structure that separates delegated state powers within the state among three governmental branches.

The executive branch executes the law through the enforcement of public health policy. The executive branch also proposes law to the legislature, issues and enforces regulations, and signs or vetoes bills. The judicial branch interprets the law and resolves disputes. The judicial branch is the final interpreter of constitutional and federal statutory law, preserves individual rights and constitutional structure, and develops a body of case law for precedence. The legislative branch creates law and creates public health policy that funds legislative mandates (Aiken, 2002; Gostin, 2000).

Protection of Individual Liberties

In addition to providing broad powers to the government, the United States Constitution also provides some limits to governmental power. The Constitution limits the government's power for the purpose of protecting individual liberties. An individual's personal rights are preserved in the Constitution, and this influences the scope of the legal authority of public health nurses.

Formulation of Public Health Law

Public health law must first be drafted as a bill. In addition to a bill, legislation can assume the form of joint resolutions, concurrent resolutions, or a simple resolution. These resolutions can be amendments to an existing bill or an alternative proposal to an existing bill. A bill can be drafted by anyone but can only be introduced into legislation by congressional members or state legislators. The official legislative process is considered initiated when a bill is numbered, either in the House of Representatives (HR#) or in the Senate (S#).

A bill can be introduced in either house or in both houses simultaneously. There can also be different versions of a bill introduced in each house. Figure 26.1 outlines how a bill becomes law. After the bill is introduced, the bill is referred to a standing committee. The committee reviews the bill and either kills the bill, approves it with or without changes, or drafts a new bill. A bill can be killed in committee if the committee fails to forward the bill out of committee or refuses to act on the bill. When this happens, the bill is said to have "died in committee."

At the committee level, the bill can be referred to a subcommittee rather than be considered by the whole committee. At this point, the committee or subcommittee can hold hearings on the bill or conduct studies on the bill.

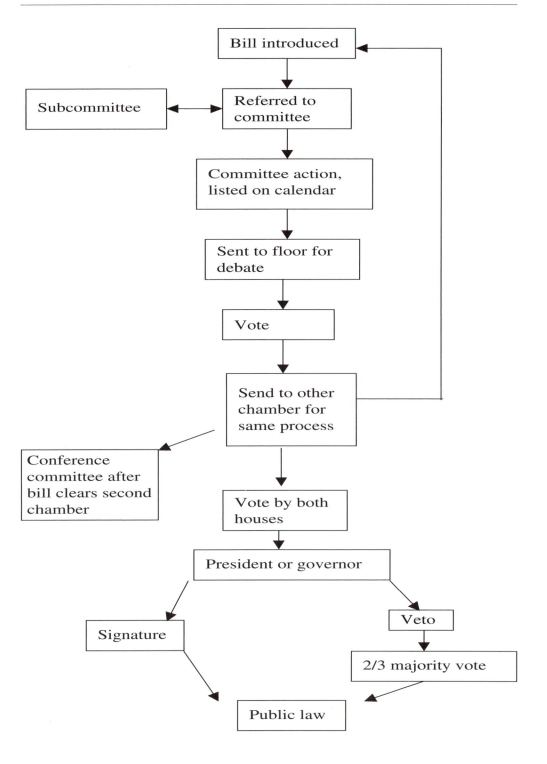

Figure 26.1 Bill to Law

A bill that is referred to a subcommittee generally is "marked up"; that is, changes and amendments are made to the whole bill. If a bill is referred to a subcommittee and the subcommittee does not refer the bill back to the whole committee, it can die in subcommittee.

Once the committee refers a bill for approval, it is placed on the committee's calendar, and a written report on the bill is drafted. The written report describes the intent, scope, impact, views of dissenting members, and position of the executive branch in regard to the bill. Once the bill is approved, the report is written, and the bill is placed on the calendar, it may be sent to the rules committee to be cleared for debate in the appropriate house. The rules committee determines the rules or procedures governing the debate on the bill. After the bill is debated by the entire house, if approved, it is referred to the other house ("chamber"), where it follows the same procedures.

In the second chamber, if only minor revisions are made to the bill, it will go back to the chamber of origin for a concurrence vote. If there are significant alterations to the bill, a conference committee with representation from both houses will be formed to reconcile any differences in the bill. If differences cannot be reconciled, the bill may die in conference committee. If agreement is reached, a conference report is prepared and both houses must approve the report. Once both houses approve the bill, it is signed by the speaker of the House and president of the Senate and forwarded to the president or governor for signature. Once it is signed, it becomes law. If no action is taken within a defined period of time and Congress or the state legislature is in session, it automatically becomes law. If the president or governor opposes the bill, he or she may veto it. If there is no action taken after Congress or the state legislature adjourns, the bill can be "pocket vetoed," and it dies. This means the bill action dies due to inaction on the bill by Congress or the legislature. This bill can be reentered in the next session. A presidential or gubernatorial veto can be overridden by a two thirds majority vote of Congress or the state legislature.

Role of the Public Health Officer in Public Health Law

The public health officer's role in public health law is multifaceted. The public health nurse is considered a public health officer as defined by the legal laws or statues of the respective states and in accordance with the position description and respective credentials of the public health nurse. The public health nurse is responsible for involvement in every phase of public health policy and law development, implementation, and evaluation. In addition to the role of public health law developer, implementer, and enforcer, the public health nurse assumes roles such as advocate, educator, researcher, and consultant. Some of the activities that public health nurses engage in are educating legislators and congressional leaders, agenda setting, and lobbying. Public health nurses may engage in lobbying activities such as face-to-face meetings, personal letters, mailgrams, telegrams, telephone calls, public testimony, petitions, reports, position papers, fact sheets, letters to the editor, news releases, public service announcements, speeches, coalition building, and litigation to ensure that public health laws protect the population's health.

The public health nurse is responsible, as defined by state laws, for ensuring the enactment of public health laws, regulations, ordinances, and statutes to protect the health of the population. This requires that public health nurses be aware of the scope of their legal abilities within their state. State statutes authorize the scope of practice of public health nurses to encompass the protection and enhancement of the public's health and safety. Public health nurses should know whether their mandated scope of practice consists of mandatory or discretionary functions. Mandatory functions are those that the public health agency must implement as required by legislative mandates. Discretionary functions are those that involve the exercise of judgment or discretion in connection with the decision to implement agency activities (Grad, 1990). Being knowledgeable regarding the scope of practice and mandatory and discretionary functions can alleviate some liability. In addition, public health nurses must be aware of the scope of the immunity provided to them in their role as public health official.

Legal Immunity

Common law provides sovereign immunity that is applied to federal and state government but not necessarily to any geopolitical subdivisions within the state. Sovereign immunity is complete immunity; it bars lawsuits against federal and state governmental agencies. The purpose of sovereign immunity is to (a) protect the operation of the government so it can operate to its full potential, (b) protect the government from the expense and time required for legal defenses, and (c) protect public funds (Grad, 1990). Sovereign immunity continues to exist but has variable levels of protection in each state, of which the public health nurse should be completely knowledgeable.

The three levels of government, judicial, executive, and legislative, are protected through governmental immunity. Governmental immunity protects the state from liability for torts (wrongful acts) committed by its officers, agents, or employees. In contrast to sovereign immunity, governmental immunity also applies to counties (or, in Louisiana, parishes) and cities. To designate the scope of governmental immunity, a distinction must be made regarding governmental and proprietary functions. Governmental functions are those activities implemented under the government's exercise of its power to promote the comfort, health, safety, and overall welfare of the public. Proprietary functions are those activities implemented to realize a profit or activities carried out by private citizens. The public health nurse must be knowledgeable regarding immunity legislation in his or her respective state.

Public health nurses, acting under the legal auspices of their public health office, may be required to testify at public hearings. During this time, the expert opinion of the nurse as a public health officer is critical. In addition, the actions taken that are legally permitted may be critiqued; therefore, the public health nurse must be sure to engage only in activities that are legally permitted. The public health nurse should also be competent in providing public testimony.

Public Testimony

Testifying may be required to provide the judicial branch of government with evidence in court. Public testimony may also be given to the press through press conferences. In both instances, information given by the nurse may be used as the basis for a decision regarding the health and safety of the public. In preparation for public testimony, the public health nurse should write down the testimony prior to the oral presentation. Oral statements should be short and accurate and should engage the audience in the issue and in political debate with relevant examples and stories. The public health nurse must first discuss the oral presentation with the respective employing agency. Your written testimony should include who you are, whom you represent, what you are testifying about, your position on the issue, and the facts that support your position. When you are giving your oral presentation, the most important points should be made first without reference to the written statement. The written testimony should focus on the issue under discussion. Copies of the testimony should be made available to members of the press; this can alleviate some errors in quotations (Aiken, 2002).

The public health nurse may be required to testify in public as an expert witness. This may be done through a deposition. A deposition is a statement that is taken under oath and considered "on the record." Depositions are required statements initiated through the issuance of a subpoena. The subpoena dictates the date, time, and location of the deposition. Public health nurses who are subpoenaed should notify the legal office in their agency immediately and provide them with a copy of the subpoena. Table 26.1 provides guidelines for the preparation of a deposition. A deposition is a stressful event that requires careful and conscious communication. Table 26.2 provides guidelines for the performance of the deposition (Aiken, 2002; Buppert, 1999).

Public health nurses may be required to provide expert testimony during a trial. The trial process is frequently an intimidating and novel experience for public health officers; therefore, public health nurses need to be aware

Table 26.1 Deposition Preparation

- Review the purpose of the deposition in the subpoena
- Compile and review all pertinent documents and evidence related to the deposition
- Plan your response to the opposing attorney
- Discuss and prepare for any weaknesses in your testimony
- Prepare a simple explanation for technical or complicated information you may need to communicate
- Plan for the use of any exhibits
- Role play with your attorney

SOURCE: Aiken (2002).

Table 26.2 Deposition Guidelines

- Speak clearly. All answers should be oral. Use minimal nonverbal communication.
- Do not make assumptions, exaggerate, or speculate.
- Make eye contact with the questioning attorney.
- Provide the court reporter and attorneys with a glossary of any governmental terms, acronyms, or technical terms.
- Always pause before answering a question. This provides your attorney with time to object and time for you to plan your response.
- Listen carefully. If you don't understand, ask to have the question explained or repeated.
- Answer only the question asked, and give a short, succinct answer. Provide no additional information.
- Avoid absolute answers such as "always."
- Control your emotions, especially fear and anger.
- Maintain your composure.
- Request a break if you are feeling tired or confused.
- Provide truthful answers. Do not make excuses.
- Do not discuss the deposition with anyone other than your attorney.
- Carefully read the written deposition after transcription. Note areas of correction to the transcriber and your attorney.

SOURCE: Aiken (2002).

of the trial process. There are five phases of a trial testimony: trial preparation, direct examination, cross-examination, re–direct examination, and re–cross-examination. Trial preparation may include the deposition discussed earlier. Trial preparation consists of reviewing pertinent documents and discussing in depth all aspects of the legal issues with your attorney. Direct examination occurs when the nurse is called to take the stand to provide testimony under oath. During the direct examination, the public health attorney will ask you questions regarding the case. The purpose of the direct examination is to ensure that your testimony is heard in a manner favorable to the public health agency. The opposing attorney conducts the cross-examination. During the cross-examination, the opposing attorney questions you regarding the information provided during direct examination in an attempt to cast doubt on your testimony. The opposing attorney will attempt to diminish your credibility by challenging your expertise,

Table 26.3   Trial Testimony Guidelines

- Prepare by reviewing all evidence and documents prior to the trial, including your deposition.
- Convey confidence, sincerity, and impartiality.
- Control your emotions.
- Speak clearly and address the judge or jury.
- Maintain eye contact.
- Provide short, succinct and precise answers. Answer only the question asked.
- Remain within the limits of your knowledge, expertise, credentials, and public health position.
- Explain any terms that may be unfamiliar to the judge or jury.
- When not on the stand, write notes to your attorney regarding important points.
- Dress conservatively and in a professional manner.
- Use demonstrative evidence to teach the jury.
- Do not discuss the case in public areas.
- Do not talk to any juror.

SOURCE: Aiken (2002).

challenging your memory or ability to recall information, highlighting inconsistencies, and demonstrating any bias in your testimony. Re–direct examination permits the public health attorney to ask any follow-up questions to clarify testimony given during the cross-examination. The re–cross-examination provides the opposing attorney with the opportunity to pose any remaining questions regarding the re–direct examination testimony. The public health nurse should be aware of each phase of the trial testimony to anticipate the attorney's line of questioning. Table 26.3 provides some guidelines for trial testimony.

Summary

Key issues in public health law and the legal system are as follows.

- Public health law integrates concepts from law, medicine, health care, and public health.
- Implementation of public health law is a function of public health practice.
- Public health law is defined as laws related to health that may be enacted at any level of government.
- The three primary functions of the United States Constitution are to allocate power between the federal government and the states (federalism), divide power among the three branches of government (separation of power), and limit the amount of government power (protection of individual liberties).
- Police power provides the basis for the public health nurse's legal authority.
- Power is separated among the three governmental branches: executive, judicial, and legislative.

- The public health nurse is considered a public health officer, as defined by the legal laws or statutes of the respective states.
- The public health nurse is responsible for involvement in every phase of public health policy and law development, implementation, and evaluation.
- Sovereign immunity is complete immunity that bars lawsuits against federal and state governmental agencies.

References

Aiken, T. (2002). *Legal, ethical, and political issues in nursing* (2nd ed.). Philadelphia, PA: F. A. Davis.

Buppert, C. (1999). *Nurse practitioner's business practice and legal guide.* Gaithersburg, MD: Aspen.

Gostin, L. (2000). *Public health law: Power, duty, restraint.* Los Angeles: University of California Press.

Grad, F. (1990). *The public health law manual* (2nd ed.). Washington, DC: American Public Health Association.

Longest, B. (2002). *Health policymaking in the United States* (3rd ed.). Washington, DC: Association of University Programs in Health Administration.

27

The Scope of Public Health Law

Public health nurses must practice within the scope of public health law as defined by their respective state. Public health law typically includes certain public health interventions of a legal nature. This chapter focuses on presenting the types of laws and legal interventions used in public health, describing malpractice and negligence, and examining public health laws.

Introduction

Public health law provides public health nurses with the legal basis for their practice and defines the scope of their practice. Public health nurses can use the legal authority granted by virtue of their public health officer position to intervene in unsafe public health conditions within a community. Therefore, public health law is and should be considered an appropriate community-level intervention for public health nurses.

The implementation of public health law as a community-level intervention may result in some restriction or infringement of individual rights. Therefore, it is imperative that public health nurses become familiar with public health law. This chapter will briefly familiarize the public health nursing professional with general law and public health law.

Types of Law

There are four main types of law in the United States: constitutional, legislative, judicial or common, and administrative law. Laws are established at the local, state, and federal levels. Lower level law should not conflict with higher level law and should be consistent with higher law. It is generally permissible for laws generated at the lower level to be more specific but consistent with the higher law of the land.

Constitutional law is considered the supreme law of the land. Constitutional law is derived from state and federal constitutions. The U.S. Constitution establishes the general government of the nation and grants certain powers to both federal and state governments. The U.S. Constitution is the highest law that exists, and no other law can overrule it. The state constitution is the highest law at the state level, and it can be invalidated by the federal constitution (Aiken, 2002).

Legislative law is generated through formal legislative processes at the national or state level. Passage of laws by Congress or the state legislature results in legislative law. These laws are frequently known as state statutes. Local governing bodies such as city councils can also promulgate laws. These laws are known as ordinances (Aiken, 2002).

Judicial or common law is also known as case law. Judicial law is generated through decisions rendered in the courts. Judicial law is based on principles such as justice, reason, and common sense. Every decision made in a courtroom by a judge contributes to the body of judicial law. Judicial law is either civil or criminal. Civil law protects individuals and enforces the rights, duties, and other legal relations that exist between private citizens in the community. Criminal law consists of concerns that threaten society: crimes committed against the state or unlawful behavior toward another individual (Aiken, 2002).

In addition, executive agencies of the government promulgate regulations. These regulations are administrative laws. Administrative laws are frequently created in response to legislation from the executive branch of government. Laws that are generated from regulatory agencies are considered or known as regulations. These agencies frequently enjoy the police power to enforce these regulations.

The remainder of this chapter focuses on public health law issues that are considered germane to public health nursing. The following public health legal issues are presented: individual rights, compulsory examination, quarantine and isolation, licensure and registration, inspection and searches, embargo and seizures, nuisances, and malpractice and negligence.

Individual Rights: Due Process

An individual's rights are protected through the Bill of Rights in the U.S. Constitution and bills of rights developed at state levels. The Bill of Rights in the Constitution consists of the first 10 amendments and a portion of the Fourteenth Amendment. Table 27.1 provides a brief summary of the Bill of Rights. The Fourteenth Amendment provides individuals with dual citizenship in the nation and their state of residence, entitling them to the rights outlined at the national and state level (Grad, 1990). In addition, the Fifth and Fourteenth Amendments prohibit the government from depriving individuals of "life, liberty, or property, without due process of law" (Gostin,

Table 27.1   Bill of Rights of the U.S. Constitution*

1. Congress shall make no law respecting an establishment of religion, or *prohibiting the free exercise* thereof; or *abridging the freedom of speech*, or of the press; or the *right of the people to peaceably assemble*, and to *petition the Government* for a redress of grievances.

2. A well regulated Militia, being necessary to the security of a free State, the right of the *people to keep and bear Arms*, shall not be infringed.

3. No Soldier shall, in time of peace, be quartered in any house, without the consent of the Owner, nor in time of war, but in a manner to be prescribed by law.

4. The *right of the people to be secure* in their persons, houses, papers, and effects, *against unreasonable searches and seizures*, shall not be violated, and no warrants shall issue, but upon probable cause, supported by Oath or affirmation, and particularly describing the place to be searched, and the persons or things to be seized.

5. No person shall be held to answer for a capital, or otherwise infamous crime, unless on a presentment or indictment of a Grand Jury, except in cases arising in the land or naval forces, or in the Militia, when in actual service in time of War or public danger; nor shall any person be subject for the same offence to be twice put in jeopardy of life or limb; nor shall be compelled in any criminal case to be a witness against himself, *nor be deprived of life, liberty, or property without due process of law, nor shall private property be taken for public use*, without just compensation.

6. In all criminal prosecutions, the accused shall enjoy the right to a speedy and public trial, by an impartial jury of the State and district wherein the crime shall have been committed, which district shall have been previously ascertained by law, and to be *informed of the nature and cause of the accusation*; to be confronted with the witness against him; to *have compulsory process for obtaining witnesses in his favor*, and to have the Assistance of Counsel for his defense.

7. In suits at common law, where the value in controversy shall exceed twenty dollars, the right of trial by a jury shall be preserved, and no fact tried by a jury, shall be otherwise reexamined in any Court of the United States, than according to the rules of the common law.

8. Excessive bail shall not be required, *nor excessive fines imposed*, nor cruel and unusual punishments inflicted.

9. The enumeration in the Constitution, of certain rights, shall *not be construed to deny or disparage others* retained by the people.

10. The *powers not delegated to the United States by the Constitution*, nor prohibited by it to the States, are *reserved to the States* respectively, or to the people

11. Section 1. *All persons born or naturalized* in the United States, and subject to the jurisdiction thereof, *are citizens of the United States* and of the State wherein they reside. No State shall make or enforce any law that abridges the privileges or immunities of citizens of the United States; *nor shall* any State deprive a *person of life, liberty, or property, without due process of law*, nor deny to any person within its jurisdiction the *equal protection* of the law.

---

* Important public health concepts are shown in italics.

2000, p. 72). This ensures that parts of an individual's life are not the government's business without due process.

The due process clause provides two separate obligations: a "substantive" element and a procedural element. The substantive element requires the government to provide sound reasons and justifications for invading an individual's personal freedoms. The procedural element requires the government to subject the individual to a fair process. A fair process must be ensured before an individual is deprived of life, liberty, or property. The fair process consists of a notice, a hearing, and access to an impartial decision maker (Gostin, 2000).

Compulsory Examination

Mandatory examinations and treatments require careful consideration and justification. The right to refuse treatment is embedded in ethical principles (see chapter 28) and the concept of informed consent. This right to refuse examination and treatment is grounded in common law. Public health statutes can override the common law and authorize mandatory examination and treatment.

States support the public health provision for compulsory examination and treatment based on three interests: health preservation, harm prevention, and preservation of effective therapies (Gostin, 2000). Public health officers have statutory authority for compulsory examination if there is sufficient belief that a communicable disease exists; a compulsory examination cannot be based on mere suspicion (Grad, 1990). Compulsory examination can also be mandated as a requirement for licensure, such as testing for sexually transmitted disease prior to the issuance of a marriage license. Periodic screenings of school children and compulsory immunization can be required (with exceptions for religious or medical reasons). Public health officials can require compulsory examinations, without concern for due process, if there is evidence of a threatened epidemic (Grad, 1990).

Quarantine and Isolation

Quarantine capabilities originate principally from local and state powers. The state power to quarantine is preempted by federal law pursuant to the federal government's power over commerce. The First International Quarantine Rules were adopted in 1852. The current promulgation of international quarantine laws originates from the World Health Organization (Gostin, 2000).

Public health nurses enacting quarantine orders must have a writ of habeas corpus that is proof of communicability (Grad, 1990). Quarantine orders must be enacted based on reasonable belief, not merely suspicion. Quarantine consists of complete restriction of a person or persons to an identified location (Grad, 1990). It basically consists of restricting the activities of a healthy person who has been exposed to a communicable disease during the period of communicability (Gostin, 2000).

Isolation is the separation of individuals who are known to be infected from the rest of the public during the period of communicability. The public health purpose of quarantine and isolation is to prevent or reduce the likelihood of a communicable disease being transmitted during the incubation period or period of infectiousness within a population (Gostin, 2000).

Licenses and Registration

Licensure power originates at the local or state government level. Licensure process is initiated through the passage of legislation that prohibits certain acts without a license (Grad, 1990). This legislation generally empowers an executive agency of the government to promulgate rules and regulations governing certain prohibited acts. The acceptance of a license by an individual or institution implies consent to submit to the conditions of continued regulatory control by the agency. Courts permit public health authorities to administer licenses, provided the public health organization has delegated administrative authority to issue such licenses (Gostin, 2000). A license is formal permission by the government to engage in specific acts not allowed to those without the license (Gostin, 2000).

Licensure establishes a system of continued monitoring and supervision for the purpose of protecting the public's health, safety, and welfare (Gostin, 2000; Grad, 1990). Licensure also provides an individual with property rights and triggers the right to procedural due process. Licenses can be denied, suspended, or revoked. These disciplinary actions require a clear notice to the affected party, a hearing, a right to counsel, a right to secure evidence by subpoena, and the right to confrontational cross-examination of an accuser (Grad, 1990). Licensure cannot be suspended or revoked without proper notice and hearing.

Public health uses licensure at the institutional and business levels, and at the individual level for protected occupations. Professional or occupational licensure occurs at the individual level to exclude certain individuals who do not meet the minimal standards established for engaging in certain activities (Grad, 1990).

Registration is a process of identification of and record keeping on certain individuals. Registration is simply a listing; no prior conditions or special circumstances are necessary. Licensure specifies requirements that must be satisfied prior to being licensed (Grad, 1990). For example, licensure as a registered nurse specifies that completion of a nursing program and successful passage of the National Council of Licensure Examination is required before the license can be granted.

Inspection and Searches

A *search* implies that the public health officer is looking for conditions that violate laws or for an instrument that may have been used in criminal activity. An *inspection* is a visitation or survey to determine if conditions that are deleterious to the public's health exist. Inspection does not include the aim of uncovering criminal evidence. An inspection is generally conducted on a routine basis and involves compliance with public health regulations or laws. A "random" inspection that is within the scope of the public health agency according to a schedule is permissible. The Fourth Amendment provides protection from unreasonable searches (Grad, 1990).

Administrative search warrants are generally required to inspect both residential and private commercial facilities (Gostin, 2000). For a public health agency or official to conduct a search, there must be a supporting legislative statute to provide for such activity. An inspection or search without a warrant can be conducted under three conditions: (a) legally valid consent justifies an administrative search; (b) public health officials can inspect a facility in an emergency to avert any immediate threats to the public's health or safety; and (c) under the "open fields" doctrine, a public health office may search a public place. Pervasively regulated businesses forfeit some rights of privacy and are subject to routine searches. Also, inspections are permitted without a warrant for licensed businesses with substantial public health significance. Additionally, the acceptance of some licenses by businesses waives their right to privacy and opens them to routine searches. To secure a search warrant, public health officials need only to demonstrate specific evidence of an existing violation in health or safety regulations or a reason that is in the public health's valid interest (Gostin, 2000). Most states require that the search warrant be signed by a judge or neutral magistrate (Grad, 1990). Evidence secured during an administrative inspection cannot be used in criminal investigations unless the evidence was in plain view during the inspection. The "plain view" doctrine provides for criminal evidence to be used when it is uncovered during an administrative search as long as the evidence was in plain view of the public health inspector during the search (Grad, 1990).

Public health officials should minimize the intrusiveness of inspections and administrative searches. Recommendations to minimize this intrusiveness include the following:

- Search during the daytime.
- Public health officials should identify themselves and present credentials, politely request admission to the facility, and clearly state the nature and purpose of the inspection.
- If entrance is refused, the public health officer should politely explain the legal consequences of such refusal, inspect the facility in an expeditious manner, inform the institutional representative when the inspection is complete, leave a receipt for any evidence secured, and avoid any verbal confrontation or physical contact (Grad, 1990).

Embargo and Seizure

Public health professionals can embargo articles by affixing a tag or marking the article with a statement such as "this article is in violation of the law" (Grad, 1990). An embargo prohibits the use or removal of the identified articles. These articles are usually suspected of posing a public health threat, as in the case of dangerous dissemination of contaminated or potentially infected goods. An embargo is considered a public health preventive measure. Sometimes the embargo is extended into condemnation proceedings by the public health official. Condemnation proceedings can order the destruction, denaturing, reexportation, or return of the goods. The cost of destroying embargoed goods is usually the responsibility of the owner of the goods (Grad, 1990).

Seizure means taking possession of goods that belong to another. Before potentially harmful goods are seized, the public health officer attempts to have the goods recalled or asks the owner to voluntarily destroy them. If the owner chooses not to comply, the goods are embargoed until a seizure order can be obtained (Grad, 1990).

Nuisances

A *private nuisance* means unreasonable interference with the use or enjoyment of private property (Gostin, 2000; Grad, 1990). Private nuisances are subject to tort law, and injunctions can be issued to stop the interference. A *public nuisance* means unreasonable interference with the community's use and enjoyment of a public place or interference with the right to pursue the normal conduct of life, without a threat to health, comfort, or repose (Gostin, 2000; Grad, 1990). Local ordinances or statutes provide the definition for a public nuisance. Public nuisances are subject to legal action by injunction or criminal prosecution. Some "nuisances" are licensed, such as garbage dumps, garbage disposal plants, or sewage treatment facilities.

Public health professionals are responsible for assisting the community with the elimination of public nuisances. The purpose of stopping a public nuisance is to maintain a healthy community environment. The following actions can be implemented to relieve the community of the public nuisance:

- *Summary abatement order.* This orders direct action to remove the offending condition prior to a hearing or court authorization. It is justified if there is significant and imminent risk or threat to the public's health.
- *Violations order.* This is an administrative order from a state or federal health officer or agency that informs the property owner of a legal violation.

- *Order to abate.* This is an order to stop the activity or condition for that time period detailed in the order (typically a "reasonable amount of time")
- *Order to cease and desist.* This is an order to end a prohibited condition.
- *Injunction.* This is an order by a court that directs a person to perform a specific activity or refrain from engaging in a specific activity (Grad, 1990).

Malpractice and Negligence

The acceptable and safe practice of public health nursing is determined through standards. Standards are created to provide public health nurses with guidelines that define acceptable levels of quality patient care and safety. These standards of care are the measure of average skills, care, and diligence exercised by other nurses under the same or similar situations (Aiken, 2002; Buppert, 1999). Standards of care provide the baseline to determine the existence of malpractice or negligent practice. Standards of care are derived from accreditation agencies, state statutes and regulations, professional associations, professional publications, and policies and procedures (Aiken, 2002).

Malpractice and negligence is covered under tort law. A tort is a wrongful act committed by one person against another person or against his or her property (Aiken, 2002). The intent of tort law is to make the injured person whole again through the appropriate level of compensation for the damages endured. Torts may be either unintentional or intentional.

Unintentional torts are unintended, wrongful acts against another person or property that produces injury or harm (Aiken, 2002). Both malpractice and negligence are unintentional torts. Malpractice is a type of negligence that occurs when the standard of care that should be expected from a reasonable and prudent professional is not met. This is also known as professional negligence. Only professional individuals can be sued for malpractice.

Negligence is based on the premise that every individual is responsible for behaving in a reasonable manner. Negligence is the omission of an act that could have prevented the injury or harm that occurred to another individual (Aiken, 2002; Buppert, 1999). Four elements must be present to determine that negligence has occurred: duty to care, breach of duty, causation, and loss or damage (Aiken, 2002; Gostin, 2000). Duty to care is a legal obligation to conform to a standard of conduct that protects others against unreasonable risk of injury or harm. Breach of duty is a failure to comply with legally recognized standards of care and safety. A determination of breach of duty is based on whether the action would have been undertaken by another "reasonable or prudent person," whether the person committing the breach was following the usual customs of the profession, and whether the action causing the breach met regulatory standards ("rule of law"; Gostin, 2000). Causation is determined based on a close causal association between the unreasonable conduct and the injury or harm. Loss or damage indicates that the plaintiff must have suffered actual loss or damage and not mere insult to his or her dignity.

An intentional tort is a willful or intentional act that violates another's rights (Aiken, 2002). Intentional torts include such acts as assault, battery, and false imprisonment. Some intentional torts are also criminal violations.

Public Health Laws

Appendix G provides a chronological, summarized list of public health laws. The list is not intended to be exhaustive.

Summary

Key issues in the scope of public health law are as follows.

- Public health law is an appropriate community-level intervention for public health nurses.
- Four types of law are constitutional, legislative, judicial or common, and administrative law.
- The Fourteenth Amendment to the U.S. Constitution provides individuals with dual citizenship in the nation and their state.
- Public health officers have statutory authority for compulsory examination if there is sufficient belief that a communicable disease exists. Compulsory examinations cannot be based on mere suspicion.
- Quarantine consists of complete restriction of the person or persons to an identified location.
- Isolation is the separation from the public of individuals who are known to be infected during the period of communicability for the disease.
- The acceptance of a license by an individual or institution implies consent to submit to the conditions of continued regulatory control by the agency.
- Registration is a process of identification of and record keeping on certain individuals.
- A search implies that the public health officer is looking for conditions that violate laws or for an instrument that may have been used in criminal activity.
- An inspection is generally conducted on a routine basis.
- Public health officials should minimize the intrusiveness of inspections and administrative searches.

- An embargo prohibits the use or removal of identified articles.
- Seizure means taking possession of goods that belong to another.
- A public nuisance is unreasonable interference with the community's use and enjoyment of a public place or interference with the right to pursue the normal conduct of life, without a threat to health, comfort, or repose.
- A tort is a wrongful act committed by one person against another person or against his or her property.
- Malpractice is a type of negligence that occurs when the standard of care that should be expected from a reasonable and prudent professional is not met.
- Negligence is the omission of an act that could have prevented the injury or harm that occurred to another individual.
- An intentional tort is a willful or intentional act that violates another's rights.

References

Aiken, T. (2002). *Legal, ethical, and political issues in nursing* (2nd ed.). Philadelphia, PA: F. A. Davis.

Buppert, C. (1999). *Nurse practitioner's business practice and legal guide.* Gaithersburg, MD: Aspen.

Gostin, L. (2000). *Public health law: Power, duty, restraint.* Los Angeles: University of California Press.

Grad, F. (1990). *The public health law manual* (2nd ed.). Washington, DC: American Public Health Association.

28 Public Health Ethics

Public health practice is concerned with protecting the nation's health and safety. Therefore, public health nurses must ensure that population-based, community-level interventions and individual-level interventions are implemented in an ethical manner. This chapter focuses on describing ethical theories and principles, presenting an ethical decision-making process and framework, and examining ethical codes and international networks.

Introduction

Public health practice is challenged with providing services at the individual level and at the same time meeting the population-based health-care needs of a community. Public health nurses are continually faced with making decisions regarding the best manner in which to allocate scarce public health resources and ensure the health and safety of the populations within communities, states, and the nation.

Public health nurses respond to infectious disease epidemics, threats of bioterrorism, increasing community violence, and unsafe environmental conditions; continue to provide direct health-care services and ensure the rights of individuals; and protect the health and safety of the greater good as well. All this requires the public health nurse to act in a strictly legal and ethical manner. Public health practice must be consistent with public health law, as outlined in chapter 27.

Ethics is defined as the study of the nature and justification of principles that guide individuals to act in a moral manner that is consistent with society's customs, values, and beliefs. Ethics is commonly described as the study of how we should behave in a situation or as the basis for determining correct action. The field of ethics continues to change with advancements in technology, public health needs, and services delivered. As public health practice becomes more predominant within the health-care delivery system, ethical issues surrounding public health practice continue to emerge.

Public health ethics encompasses ethics *in* public health and the ethics *of* public health (Callahan & Jennings, 2002). Public health ethics is considered to be a "search for those values, virtues, and principles necessary for people to live together in peace, mutual respect, and justice" (p. 170). Callahan and Jennings describe the scope of public health ethics as encompassing four general categories: health promotion and disease prevention, risk reduction, epidemiological and other forms of public health research, and socioeconomic disparities in health status. They propose four types of ethical analysis for public health: professional ethics, applied ethics, advocacy ethics, and critical ethics.

Professional ethics "seek out the values and standards that have been developed by practitioners and leaders of a given profession over a long period of time and . . . identify those values that seem most salient and inherent" to the professional discipline (Callahan & Jennings, 2002, p. 172). Applied ethics adopts a point of view outside the history and values of public health and focuses on principles that can be applied to real-world ethical issues. Applied ethics focuses more on professional behavior and conduct in specific situations than on the virtues of a profession (Callahan & Jennings, 2002). Advocacy ethics has an orientation toward equality and social justice. Advocacy ethics focuses on asserting a position on behalf of another individual, or on groups or communities. Critical ethics is historical in nature and oriented toward real-world ethical issues and real-time problems in public health. Critical ethics proposes discussions of ethics and public health policy that are genuinely public and civic endeavors that are more than just an attempt by the well-intentioned elite to advocate on behalf of underserved or needy clients of another status or class (Callahan & Jennings, 2002). Regardless of the type of ethical analysis chosen, there are basic theoretical frameworks that guide ethical decision-making (Beauchamp & Childress, 2001).

Ethical Theories

Ethical theories provide an ethical framework on which ethical principles may be articulated. Ethical theories assist public health nurses by providing paths by which to approach ethical decision making and actions. These ethical theories serve as a theoretical framework that can guide ethical decision-making processes. Two classical ethical theories are deontology and utilitarianism.

Deontology

Deontology is a theoretical framework based on a sense of moral obligation or duty. Deontology states that an action's moral rightness or wrongness depends on the action itself and the motivation for the action. From this perspective, the motivation for the action is seen as guiding the decision and justification to act more than the consequences of the action (Beauchamp & Childress, 2001). Deontology also recognizes the moral obligation that individuals feel. Moral obligation refers to an individual feeling a sense of duty that requires him or her to act in certain ways in response to the moral norms of society.

Utilitarianism

Teleology is an ethical theory that determines rightness or wrongness based solely on the expected outcomes or consequences of an action. Utilitarianism is a theoretical framework that is part of teleology theory. The utilitarian framework proposes that the most ethical action is that resulting in the greatest good for the greatest number of individuals (Beauchamp & Childress, 2001). Others refer to the utilitarian perspective as supporting those actions that cause the least harm to the fewest number of individuals. Utilitarianism is based on the utility of an action and the resultant consequences of the action in respect to the number of individuals affected, rather than on the action itself.

Ethical Principles

Most ethical theories, as well as the common moral tone of society, include ethical principles on which ethical behavior is based. Ethical principles are also foundational to professional codes of ethics. Ethical principles provide a perspective from which to critically reason through an ethical dilemma. The most common principles encountered in ethics are beneficence, non-maleficence, justice, and autonomy (Beauchamp & Childress, 2001).

Beneficence consists of norms for providing benefits to an individual, group, or community. Beneficence also consists of weighing the benefits of an action against the risks or costs to the parties involved. Public health nurses may encounter a dilemma when actions pose a benefit to one community but considerable individual-level risks or risks to another community (Beauchamp & Childress, 2001).

Nonmaleficence is the ethical principle that requires the public health nurse to "do no harm." With nonmaleficence, the public health nurse is challenged with not causing harm to individuals, groups, or communities. Public health nurses are frequently faced with allocating or reallocating scarce resources. In these cases, the public health nurse must ensure that allocating resources to one group and not providing another does not create harm to either group (Beauchamp & Childress, 2001).

Justice is the ethical principle that ensures the fair and equitable distribution of benefits, risks, and cost. Justice is frequently known as the ethical principle of fairness. The principle of justice must be considered in two dimensions. The two dimensions include (a) what is owed or due to an individual, group, or community and what is owed or due to society by the individual, group, or community (Beauchamp & Childress, 2001). Some community groups have an overwhelming sense of entitlement and feel that all public health services are due or owed to them at no cost or expense to them. This must be weighed against the basic public health services owed to all members of society and what services are beyond this basic level (if there is a predetermined "basic" level; Beauchamp & Childress, 2001).

Autonomy is the ethical principle known as "respect for persons." Autonomy provides individuals with the right to make autonomous decisions, also known as the right to self-determination. This principle provides individuals with the right to make free, uncoerced, and informed decisions. Autonomy is primarily ensured through the process of full disclosure and informed consent (Beauchamp & Childress, 2001).

In addition to the ethical principles of beneficence, nonmaleficence, justice, and autonomy, two other principles are considered essential in ethical behavior. These principles are fidelity and veracity. Fidelity and veracity are essential in ensuring that individuals, groups, and communities are sincere in filtering their actions through the four ethical principles. Fidelity is known as promise keeping. Fidelity ensures that public health nurses deliver those services that are considered promised to the community. Veracity is known as truth telling. Veracity consists of being honest in delivering information to community members. Both fidelity and veracity are essential in developing a trusting relationship with community members.

The Ethical Decision-Making Process

Ethical dilemmas encountered in public health nursing practice are complex, involving individuals, families, institutions, and communities. An ethical dilemma arises when there is a conflict in the principles, duties, rights, beliefs, and values of one individual, group, population, or community with another or with the greater society (Beauchamp & Childress, 2001). An understanding of ethical perspectives, principles, and codes assists public health nurses in exploring the best resolution to ethical dilemmas.

Ethical decision-making processes facilitate the selection of an ethical resolution by outlining the steps used to gain an understanding of the ethical dilemma and determining the best possible resolution. The following ethical decision-making process is recommended for public health nurses who encounter ethical dilemmas in public health situations. This process is designed to assist public health nurses with reasoning through an ethical dilemma.

1. Clearly define the ethical dilemma and outline the conflicting ethical issues and principles.

2. Identify the public health stakeholders at all levels: individual, family, group, and community.

3. Collect data relevant to both sides of the ethical dilemma.

4. List potential public health options to resolve the ethical dilemma.

5. Describe the public health consequences for each option listed.

6. Consider each ethical principle, review codes of ethics, and determine which option would be the best and most ethical resolution.

7. Implement the ethical resolution. Define what actions are to be taken by whom and when.

8. Evaluate the implementation and consequences of the ethical resolution, both positive and negative. Consider the impact of the ethical resolution on each stakeholder identified. Evaluate whether the ethical resolution and the community's reaction to the resolution has changed the moral attitude, values, or beliefs of the community or society.

Public Health Ethical Decision-Making Framework

A six-step public health ethical decision-making framework has been proposed by Gostin and Lazzarini (1997) as an analytical tool. This framework is designed to assist public health professionals in considering the ethical implications of proposed interventions, policy proposals, research projects, and programs (Gostin & Lazzarini, 1997; Kass, 2001). The process consists of proposing and examining the answers to the following questions:

- What are the public health goals of the proposed program?
- How effective is the program in achieving its stated goals?
- What are the known potential burdens of the program?
- Can the burdens be minimized? Are there alternative approaches that create less of a burden?
- Is the program implemented fairly?
- How can the benefits and burdens of the program be fairly balanced?

Codes of Ethics

Codes of ethics have been developed by several disciplines. Derived from normative ethics, these codes were developed to transmit moral guidelines

Table 28.1   Focuses of the APHA Principles of the Ethical Practice of Public Health

- Disease causation and prevention of adverse outcomes
- Respect for the individual community member's rights
- Need for community members to provide input into public health policies, programs, and priorities
- Advocacy and empowerment of disenfranchised community groups to ensure equitable access to resources
- Acquisition of information that will affect policies and programs
- Receipt of community consent for policies and programs
- Timely action
- Incorporation of diverse interventions that respect diverse values, beliefs, and cultures
- Enhancement of physical and social environments
- Protection of privacy and confidentiality of individuals and the community
- Competence of public health workers
- Engagement in collaborative partnerships to build trust and program effectiveness

SOURCE: American Public Health Association (2002).

of discipline and are a means by which to codify professional morality. Codes often represent the values inherent in a profession and specify its rules of etiquette and moral responsibilities. Ethical codes also are a means of fostering and reinforcing member identification with a profession (Beauchamp & Childress, 2001). Public health nurses have several codes of ethics that influence and guide their practice: the APHA Public Health Code of Ethics, the ANA Code for Nurses, and the International Council of Nursing (ICN) Code for Nurses.

American Public Health Association Public Health Code of Ethics

The APHA developed a professional code of ethics for public health practice that was intended for organizations in the United States that have public health as their explicit mission. The code is also considered to be relevant for individuals or institutions that are external to the traditional public health system but whose work has an impact on the health of communities. The APHA Public Health Code of Ethics states key ethical principles for the practice of public health (APHA, 2002). Table 28.1 presents these principles. This code is not considered to be an exhaustive code of health ethics. Public health professionals such as public health nurses can integrate the public health code of ethics with their own professional code of ethics (e.g., the ANA Code of Ethics).

The Public Health Code of Ethics is based on the key ethical principle of interdependence among all people. Interdependence is the essence of community: The Code of Ethics recognizes the status of communities but also recognizes that individuals are inexplicably tied to the life of their community. The individual affects the community, but the community also directly affects the individual, thus creating a cyclic interdependence of the people with their community (APHA, 2002). In addition to the key ethical principle

Table 28.2   APHA Public Health Code of Ethics: Focuses of Underlying Values and Beliefs

- The right to health resources
- The inherent social and environmental interdependence of individuals
- The public's trust
- Collaboration
- The reciprocal interdependence of individuals with their environment
- The opportunity of each individual to contribute to public discourse
- The identification and promotion of fundamental health requirements
- Knowledge is power
- Public health knowledge is based in science
- Individuals have a responsibility to act
- Information alone is not a basis for action

SOURCE: American Public Health Association (2002).

of interdependence, the code is based on key values and beliefs (outlined in Table 28.2) that are considered inherent to public health.

Nursing Codes

Public health nurses have their professional code of ethics, developed by the ANA. The ANA Code for Nurses (Table 28.3) provides guidelines for ethical conduct with clients and society at large, inclusive of communities. This code is not legally binding but provides broad ethical principles from which to determine nurses' level of professional ethical conduct. The ANA Code for Nurses also assists nurses in ethical decision-making processes (ANA, 1985).

In addition to the ANA Code for Nurses, public health nurses engaged in international public health practice must be familiar with the ICN Code for Nurses. The ICN Code for Nurses acknowledges that nurses provide care to individuals, families, and communities. The ICN Code for Nurses (Table 28.4) recognizes the fundamental responsibility of the nurse as four-fold: to promote health, to prevent illness, to restore health, and to alleviate suffering (ICN, 1973).

International Public Health Networks

International and European public health issues are being addressed through two networks. The European Public Health Ethics Network, also known as EuroPHEN, is intended to facilitate research on ethical issues that arise within public health and public health policy. The aim of EuroPHEN is to develop a framework for producing approaches to public health policy that will be common across the entire European Union. It is envisioned that this project will have three standards: ethical analysis, analysis of

Table 28.3 Focuses of the ANA Code for Nurses

- Respect for human dignity and uniqueness
- Safeguarding clients' right to privacy
- Safeguarding clients from incompetent, unethical, and illegal practices
- Assumption of responsibility and accountability for actions
- Maintaining competence
- Exercising informed judgment and competence in consultation and accepting responsibility and delegation
- Participating in ongoing development of nursing science and knowledge
- Improving standards of nursing
- Ensuring that employment environments are conducive to high-quality nursing care
- Protecting the public from misinformation and misrepresentation, thus maintaining the integrity of nursing
- Collaborating with other health professions

SOURCE: American Nurses Association (1985).

Table 28.4 Focuses of the ICN Code for Nurses

- Nurse is primarily response for individuals needing nursing care
- Promoting an environment that respects values, customs, and spiritual beliefs
- Maintaining personal information in confidence
- Assuming personal responsibility for practice and maintaining competence through continual learning
- Maintaining highest standards of nursing care possible
- Using judgment in acceptance of responsibility and with delegation
- Maintaining standards of personal conduct
- Sharing responsibility with citizens for health and social needs
- Sustaining cooperative coworker relationships
- Acting to safeguard individuals endangered by coworkers
- Determining and implementing desirable nursing standards of practice and education
- Actively developing nursing's professional knowledge
- Participating in professional organizations to establish and maintain equitable social and economic working conditions

SOURCE: International Council of Nurses (1973).

public policy and regulatory and legislative processes, and empirical qualitative and quantitative research on public attitudes and values (School of Health and Related Research, 2002a).

The EuroPHEN network will be associated with the International Public Health Ethics Network (InterPHEN). InterPHEN, a network developed by the International Association of Bioethics, is a forum in which to exchange information about public health policy in different countries and debate ethical issues that arise (School of Health and Related Research, 2002b). These two networks will build an international channel promoting the discussion of public health ethical issues, similar to the functions provided through the APHA.

Summary

Key issues in public health ethics are as follows.

- Ethics is defined as the study of the nature and justification of principles that guide individuals to act in a moral manner that is consistent with society's customs, values, and beliefs.
- Four types of ethical analysis for public health are professional ethics, applied ethics, advocacy ethics, and critical ethics.
- Deontology is a theoretical framework based on a sense of moral obligation or duty.
- The utilitarian framework is founded on the belief that the most ethical action is the action that results in the greatest good for the greatest number of individuals.
- Common principles encountered in ethics are beneficence, nonmaleficence, justice, and autonomy.
- An ethical dilemma arises when the principles, duties, rights, beliefs, and values of one individual, group, population, or community conflict with those of another or with the greater society.
- Codes of ethics are developed to transmit the moral guidelines of a discipline.
- The APHA Public Health Code of Ethics is based on the key ethical principle of the interdependence of people.
- The ANA Code for Nurses assists nurses in ethical decision-making processes.
- The ICN Code for Nurses recognizes the fundamental responsibility of the nurse as fourfold: to promote health, to prevent illness, to restore health, and to alleviate suffering.
- International and European public health issues are being addressed through two networks: EuroPHEN and InterPHEN

References

American Nurses Association. (1985). *Code for nurses, with imperative statements.* Kansas City, MO: Author.

American Public Health Association. (2002). *Public health code of ethics.* Retrieved June 29, 2003, from http://www.apha.org/codeofethics/ethics.htm

Beauchamp, T., & Childress, J. (2001). *Principles of biomedical ethics* (5th ed.). New York, New York: Oxford University Press.

Callahan, D., & Jennings, B. (2002). Ethics and public health: Forging a strong relationship. *American Journal of Public Health, 92*(2), 169-176.

Gostin, L., & Lazzarini, Z. (1997). *Human rights and public health in the AIDS pandemic.* New York: Oxford University Press.

International Council of Nurses. (1973). *ICN Code for nurses: Ethical concepts applied to nursing.* Geneva, Switzerland: Imprimeries Populaires.

Kass, N. (2001). An ethics framework for public health. *American Journal of Public Health, 91*(11), 1776-1782.

School of Health and Related Research. (2002a). *EuroPHEN (European Public Health Ethics Network)*. Retrieved June 29, 2003, from http://www.shef.ac.uk/~scharr/publich/research/ethics/europhen/index.html

School of Health and Related Research. (2002b). *InterPHEN: International Public Health Ethics Network*. Retrieved June 29, 2003, from http://www.shef.ac.uk/~scharr/publich/research/ethics/inter/index.html

Appendix A

Core Competencies for Public Health Professionals

Staff Descriptions

- Front-line staff: public health individuals who are involved in day-to-day public health activities
- Senior-level staff: public health individuals with specialized functions (does not include managers)
- Supervisory and management staff: public health individuals responsible for major programs or organizational functions with line authority for personnel

Competency Levels

1. Aware: basic mastery level; can identify the skill or concept but has limited ability to perform

2. Knowledgeable: intermediate mastery level; can apply and describe the skill

3. Proficient: advanced mastery level; can synthesize, critique, or teach the skill

Domain I. Analytic Assessment Skills

Specific Competencies	Front-Line Staff	Senior-Level Staff	Supervisory and Management Staff
Defines a problem	Knowledgeable to proficient	Proficient	Proficient
Determines appropriate uses and limitations of both quantitative and qualitative data	Aware to knowledgeable	Proficient	Proficient
Selects and defines variables relevant to problem	Aware to knowledgeable	Proficient	Proficient
Identifies relevant and appropriate data and information sources	Knowledgeable	Proficient	Proficient
Evaluates the integrity and comparability of data and identifies gaps in data sources	Aware	Proficient	Proficient
Applies ethical principles to the collection, maintenance, use, and dissemination of data and information	Knowledgeable to proficient	Proficient	Proficient
Partners with communities to attach meaning to collected quantitative and qualitative data	Aware to knowledgeable	Proficient	Proficient
Makes relevant inferences from quantitative and qualitative data	Aware to knowledgeable	Proficient	Proficient
Obtains and interprets information regarding risks and benefits to the community	Aware to knowledgeable	Proficient	Proficient
Applied data collection processes, information technology applications, and computer storage and retrieval strategies	Aware to knowledgeable	Knowledgeable to proficient	Knowledgeable to proficient
Recognizes how the data illuminate ethical, political, scientific, economic, and overall public health issues	Aware	Knowledgeable to proficient	Proficient

Domain 2. Policy Development and Program Planning Skills

Specific Competencies	Front-Line Staff	Senior-Level Staff	Supervisory and Management Staff
Collects, summarizes, and interprets information relevant to an issue	Knowledgeable	Proficient	Proficient
States policy options and writes clear and concise policy statements	Aware	Knowledgeable to proficient	Proficient
Identifies, interprets, and implements public health laws, regulations, and policies related to specific programs	Aware	Knowledgeable to proficient	Proficient
Articulates the health, fiscal, administrative, legal, social, and political implications of each policy option	Aware	Knowledgeable	Proficient
States the feasibility and expected outcomes of each policy option	Aware	Knowledgeable	Proficient
Uses current techniques in decision analysis and health planning	Aware	Knowledgeable to proficient	Proficient
Decides on the appropriate course of action	Aware	Knowledgeable to proficient	Proficient
Develops a plan to implement policy, including goals, outcome and process objectives, and implementation steps	Aware	Knowledgeable to proficient	Proficient
Translates policy into organizational plans, structures, and programs	Aware	Knowledgeable to proficient	Proficient
Prepares and implements emergency response plans	Aware to knowledgeable	Knowledgeable to proficient	Proficient
Develops mechanisms to monitor and evaluate programs for their effectiveness and quality	Aware to knowledgeable	Proficient	Proficient

Domain 3. Communication Skills

Specific Competencies	Front-Line Staff	Senior-Level Staff	Supervisory and Management Staff
Communicates effectively both in writing and orally, or in other ways	Proficient	Proficient	Proficient
Solicits input from individuals and organizations	Knowledgeable to proficient	Proficient	Proficient
Advocates for public health programs and resources	Knowledgeable	Proficient	Proficient
Leads and participates in groups to address specific issues	Knowledgeable	Proficient	Proficient
Uses the media, advanced technologies, and community networks to communicate information	Aware to knowledgeable	Proficient	Proficient
Effectively presents accurate demographic, statistical, programmatic, and scientific information for professional and lay audiences	Knowledgeable	Proficient	Proficient
Attitudes			
Listens to others in an unbiased manner, respects viewpoints of others, and promotes the expression of diverse opinions and perspectives	Proficient	Proficient	Proficient

Domain 4. Cultural Competency Skills

Specific Competencies	Front-Line Staff	Senior-Level Staff	Supervisory and Management Staff
Uses appropriate methods for interacting sensitively, effectively, and professionally with persons from diverse cultural, socioeconomic, educational, racial, ethnic and professional backgrounds and with persons of all ages and lifestyle preferences	Proficient	Proficient	Proficient
Identifies the role of cultural, social, and behavioral factors in determining the delivery of public health services	Knowledgeable	Proficient	Proficient
Develops and adapts approaches to problems that take into account cultural differences	Proficient	Proficient	Proficient
Attitudes			
Understands the dynamic forces contributing to cultural diversity	Knowledgeable	Knowledgeable to proficient	Proficient
Understands the importance of a diverse public health workforce	Knowledgeable	Proficient	Proficient

Domain 5. Community Dimensions of Practice Skills

Specific Competencies	Front-Line Staff	Senior-Level Staff	Supervisory and Management Staff
Establishes and maintains linkages with key stakeholders	Knowledgeable	Proficient	Proficient
Uses leadership, team building, negotiation, and conflict resolution skills to build community partnerships	Aware to proficient	Proficient	Proficient
Collaborates with community partners to promote the health of the population	Knowledgeable to proficient	Proficient	Proficient
Identifies how public and private organizations operate within a community	Knowledgeable	Proficient	Proficient
Accomplishes effective community engagements	Aware to knowledgeable	Proficient	Proficient
Identifies community assets and available resources	Knowledgeable to proficient	Proficient	Proficient
Develops, implements, and evaluates a community public health assessment	Knowledgeable	Proficient	Proficient
Describes the role of government in the delivery of community health services	Knowledgeable	Proficient	Proficient

Domain 6. Basic Public Health Sciences Skills

Specific Competencies	Front-Line Staff	Senior-Level Staff	Supervisory and Management Staff
Identifies the individual's and organization's responsibilities within the context of the essential public health services and core functions	Knowledgeable	Proficient	Proficient
Defines, assesses, and understands the health status of populations, determinants of health and illness, factors contributing to health promotion and disease prevention, and factors influencing the use of health services	Knowledgeable	Proficient	Proficient
Understands the historical development, structure, and interaction of public health and health-care systems	Aware	Knowledgeable	Proficient
Identifies and applies basic research methods used in public health	Aware	Proficient	Proficient
Applies the basic public health sciences, including behavioral and social sciences, biostatistics, epidemiology, environmental public health, and prevention of chronic and infectious diseases and injuries	Knowledgeable	Proficient	Proficient
Identifies and retrieves current relevant scientific evidence	Knowledgeable	Proficient	Proficient
Identifies the limitations of research and the importance of observations and interrelationships	Knowledgeable	Proficient	Proficient
Attitudes			
Develops a lifelong commitment to rigorous critical thinking	Knowledgeable to proficient	Proficient	Proficient

Domain 7.   Financial Planning and Management Skills

Specific Competencies	Front-Line Staff	Senior-Level Staff	Supervisory and Management Staff
Develops and presents a budget	Aware	Knowledgeable	Proficient
Manages programs within budget constraints	Aware	Knowledgeable to proficient	Proficient
Applies budget processes	Aware	Knowledgeable	Proficient
Develops strategies for determining budget priorities	Aware	Knowledgeable	Proficient
Monitors program performance	Aware to knowledgeable	Proficient	Proficient
Prepares proposals for funding from external sources	Aware	Proficient	Proficient
Applies basic human relations skills to the management of organizations, motivation of personnel, and resolution of conflicts	Aware to knowledgeable	Proficient	Proficient
Manages information systems for collection, retrieval, and use of data for decision making	Aware	Knowledgeable to proficient	Proficient
Negotiates and develops contracts and other documents for the provision of population-based services	Aware	Knowledgeable	Proficient
Conducts cost-effectiveness, cost:benefit, and cost utility analyses	Aware	Knowledgeable	Proficient

Domain 8. Leadership and Systems Thinking Skills

Specific Competencies	Front-Line Staff	Senior-Level Staff	Supervisory and Management Staff
Creates a culture of ethical standards within organizations and communities	Knowledgeable to proficient	Proficient	Proficient
Helps create key values and shared vision and uses these principles to guide action	Aware to knowledgeable	Knowledgeable to proficient	Proficient
Strategic planning: identifies internal and external issues that may affect delivery of essential public health services	Aware	Knowledgeable to proficient	Proficient
Facilitates collaboration with internal and external groups to ensure participation of key stakeholders	Aware	Knowledgeable to proficient	Proficient
Promotes team and organizational learning	Knowledgeable	Knowledgeable to proficient	Proficient
Contributes to development, implementation, and monitoring of organizational performance standards	Aware to knowledgeable	Knowledgeable to proficient	Proficient
Uses the legal and political system to effect change	Aware	Knowledgeable	Proficient
Applies theory of organizational structures to professional practice	Aware	Knowledgeable	Proficient

Appendix B

Healthy People 2010

Healthy People 2010 Goals

- Goal 1: Increase quality and years of healthy life
- Goal 2: Eliminate health disparities

Access to Quality Health Care

- Goal: Improve access to comprehensive, high-quality health-care services.

Clinical Preventive Care

1-1. Increase the proportion of persons with health insurance

1-2. (Developmental) Increase the proportion of insured persons with coverage for clinical preventive services

1-3. Increase the proportion of persons appropriately counseled about health behaviors

Primary Care

1-4. Increase the proportion of persons that has a specific source of ongoing care

1-5. Increase the proportion of persons with a usual primary care provider

1-6. Reduce the proportion of families that experiences difficulties or delays in obtaining health care or does not receive needed care for one or more family members

1-7. (Developmental) Increase the proportion of schools of medicine, schools of nursing, and other health professional training schools whose basic curriculum for health-care providers includes the core competencies in health promotion and disease prevention

1-8. In the health professions, allied and associated health profession fields, and the field of nursing, increase the proportion of all degrees awarded to members of underrepresented racial and ethnic groups

1-9. Reduce hospitalization rates for three ambulatory-care–sensitive conditions: pediatric asthma, uncontrolled diabetes, and immunization-preventable pneumonia and influenza

Emergency Services

1-10. (Developmental) Reduce the proportion of persons that delays or has difficulty in getting emergency medical care

1-11. (Developmental) Increase the proportion of persons that has access to rapid-response pre–hospital emergency medical services

1-12. Establish a single toll-free telephone number for access to poison control centers on a 24-hour basis throughout the United States

1-13. Increase the number of tribes and states (including the District of Columbia) with trauma care systems that maximize survival and functional outcomes of trauma patients and help prevent injuries from occurring

1-14. Increase the number of states (including the District of Columbia) that has implemented guidelines for prehospital and hospital pediatric care

Long-Term Care and Rehabilitative Services

1-15. (Developmental) Increase the proportion of persons with long-term care needs who have access to the continuum of long-term care services

1-16. Reduce the proportion of nursing home residents with a current diagnosis of pressure ulcers

Arthritis, Osteoporosis, and Chronic Back Conditions

Goal: Prevent illness and disability related to arthritis and other rheumatic conditions, osteoporosis, and chronic back conditions.

Arthritis and Other Rheumatic Conditions

2-1. (Developmental) Increase the mean number of days without severe pain among adults who have chronic joint symptoms

2-2. Reduce the proportion of adults with chronic joint symptoms who experience a limitation in activity due to arthritis

2-3. Preserve independence by reducing the proportion of all adults with chronic joint symptoms who have difficulty in performing two or more personal care activities

2-4. (Developmental) Increase the proportion of adults 18 years old and older with arthritis that seeks help in coping when experiencing personal and emotional problems

2-5. Increase the employment rate among adults with arthritis in the working-age population

2-6. (Developmental) Eliminate racial disparities in the rate of total knee replacements

2-7. (Developmental) Increase the proportion of adults that has seen a health-care provider for their chronic joint symptoms

2-8. (Developmental) Increase the proportion of persons with arthritis that has had effective, evidence-based arthritis education as an integral part of the management of the condition

Osteoporosis

2-9. Reduce the proportion of adults with osteoporosis

2-10. Reduce the proportion of adults that is hospitalized for vertebral fractures associated with osteoporosis

Chronic Back Conditions

2-11. Reduce activity limitation due to chronic back conditions.

Cancer

Goal: Reduce the number of new cancer cases, as well as the illness, disability, and death caused by cancer.

3-1. Reduce the overall cancer death rate

3-2. Reduce the lung cancer death rate

3-3. Reduce the breast cancer death rate

3-4. Reduce the death rate from cancer of the uterine cervix

3-5. Reduce the colorectal cancer death rate

3-6. Reduce the oropharyngeal cancer death rate

3-7. Reduce the prostate cancer death rate

3-8. Reduce the rate of deaths from melanoma

3-9. Increase the proportion of persons that uses at least one of the following protective measures that may reduce the risk of skin cancer: avoid the sun between 10 a.m. and 4 p.m., wear sun-protective clothing when exposed to sunlight, use sunscreen with a sun-protective factor of 15 or higher, and avoid artificial sources of ultraviolet light

3-10. Increase the proportion of physicians and dentists that counsels at-risk patients about tobacco use cessation, physical activity, and cancer screening

3-11. Increase the proportion of women that receives a Pap test

3-12. Increase the proportion of adults that receives a colorectal cancer screening examination

3-13. Increase the proportion of women 40 years old and older that has received a mammogram within the preceding 2 years

3-14. Increase the number of states that has a statewide population-based cancer registry that captures case information on at least 95% of the expected number of reportable cancers

3-15. Increase the proportion of cancer survivors that lives 5 years or longer after diagnosis

Chronic Kidney Disease

Goal: Reduce new cases of chronic kidney disease and its complications, disability, death, and economic costs.

4-1. Reduce the rate of new cases of end-stage renal disease

4-2. Reduce deaths from cardiovascular disease in persons with chronic kidney failure

4-3. Increase the proportion of treated chronic kidney failure patients that has received counseling on nutrition, treatment choices, and cardiovascular care 12 months before the start of kidney replacement therapy

4-4. Increase the proportion of new hemodialysis patients that uses arteriovenous fistulas as the primary mode of vascular access

4-5. Increase the proportion of dialysis patients registered on the waiting list for transplantation.

4-6. Increase the proportion of patients with treated chronic kidney failure who receive a transplant within 3 years of registration on the waiting list

4-7. Reduce kidney failure due to diabetes

4-8. (Developmental) Increase the proportion of persons with type 1 or type 2 diabetes and proteinuria that receives recommended medical therapy to reduce progression to chronic renal insufficiency

Diabetes

Goal: Through prevention programs, reduce the disease and economic burden of diabetes and improve the quality of life for all persons who have or are at risk for diabetes.

5-1. Increase the proportion of persons with diabetes that receives formal diabetes education

5-2. Prevent diabetes

5-3. Reduce the overall rate of diabetes that is clinically diagnosed

5-4. Increase the proportion of adults with diabetes whose condition has been diagnosed

5-5. Reduce the diabetes death rate

5-6. Reduce diabetes-related deaths among persons with diabetes

5-7. Reduce deaths from cardiovascular disease in persons with diabetes

5-8. (Developmental) Decrease the proportion of pregnant women with gestational diabetes

5-9. (Developmental) Reduce the frequency of foot ulcers in persons with diabetes

5-10. Reduce the rate of lower extremity amputations in persons with diabetes

5-11. (Developmental) Increase the proportion of persons with diabetes that obtains an annual urinary microalbumin measurement

5-12. Increase the proportion of adults with diabetes that has a glycosylated hemoglobin measurement at least once a year

5-13. Increase the proportion of adults with diabetes that has an annual dilated eye examination

5-14. Increase the proportion of adults with diabetes that has at least an annual foot examination

5-15. Increase the proportion of persons with diabetes that has at least an annual dental examination

5-16. Increase the proportion of adults with diabetes that takes aspirin at least 15 times per month

5-17. Increase the proportion of adults with diabetes that performs self-monitoring of blood glucose at least once daily

Disability and Secondary Conditions

Goal: Promote the health of people with disabilities, prevent secondary conditions, and eliminate disparities between people with and without disabilities in the U.S. population.

6-1. Include in the core of all relevant Healthy People 2010 surveillance instruments a standardized set of questions that identify "people with disabilities"

6-2. Reduce the proportion of children and adolescents with disabilities that is reported to be sad, unhappy, or depressed

6-3. Reduce the proportion of adults with disabilities that reports feelings such as sadness, unhappiness, or depression that prevent them from being active

6-4. Increase the proportion of adults with disabilities that participates in social activities

6-5. Increase the proportion of adults with disabilities reporting sufficient emotional support

6-6. Increase the proportion of adults with disabilities reporting satisfaction with life

6-7. Reduce the number of people with disabilities in congregate care facilities, consistent with permanency planning principles

6-8. Eliminate disparities in employment rates between working-age adults with and without disabilities

6-9. Increase the proportion of children and youth with disabilities that spends at least 80% of the time in regular education programs

6-10. (Developmental) Increase the proportion of health and wellness and treatment programs and facilities that provides full access for people with disabilities

6-11. (Developmental) Reduce the proportion of people with disabilities that reports not having the assistive devices and technology they need

6-12. (Developmental) Reduce the proportion of people with disabilities reporting environmental barriers to participation in home, school, work, or community activities

6-13. Increase the number of tribes and states (including the District of Columbia) that has public health surveillance and health promotion programs for people with disabilities and caregivers

Educational and Community-Based Programs

Goal: Increase the quality, availability, and effectiveness of educational and community-based programs designed to prevent disease and improve health and quality of life.

School Setting

7-1. Increase high school completion

7-2. Increase the proportion of middle, junior high, and senior high schools that provides school health education to prevent health problems in the following areas: unintentional injury; violence; suicide; tobacco use and addiction; alcohol and other drug use; unintended pregnancy, HIV/AIDS, and STD infections; unhealthy dietary patterns; inadequate physical activity; and environmental health

7-3. Increase the proportion of college and university students that receives information from their institution on each of the six priority health-risk behavior areas

7-4. Increase the proportion of the nation's elementary, middle, junior high, and senior high schools that has a nurse-to-student ratio of at least 1:750

Worksite Setting

7-5. Increase the proportion of worksites that offers a comprehensive employee health promotion program to their employees

7-6. Increase the proportion of employees that participates in employer-sponsored health promotion activities

Health-Care Setting

7-7. (Developmental) Increase the proportion of health-care organizations that provides patient and family education

7-8. (Developmental) Increase the proportion of patients that reports satisfaction with the patient education received from the health-care organization

7-9. (Developmental) Increase the proportion of hospitals and managed care organizations that provides community disease prevention and health promotion activities that address the priority health needs identified by the community

Community Setting and Select Populations

7-10. (Developmental) Increase the proportion of tribal and local health service areas or jurisdictions that has established a community health promotion program that addresses multiple Healthy People 2010 focus areas

7-11. Increase the proportion of local health departments that has established culturally appropriate and linguistically competent community health promotion and disease prevention programs

7-12. Increase the proportion of older adults that has participated during the preceding year in at least one organized health promotion activity

Environmental Health

Goal: Promote health for all through a healthy environment.

Outdoor Air Quality

8-1. Reduce the proportion of persons exposed to air that does not meet the U.S. Environmental Protection Agency's health-based standards for harmful air pollutants

8-2. Increase use of alternative modes of transportation to reduce motor vehicle emissions and improve the nation's air quality

8-3. Improve the nation's air quality by increasing the use of cleaner alternative fuels

8-4. Reduce air toxic emissions to decrease the risk of adverse health effects caused by airborne toxins

Water Quality

8-5. Increase the proportion of persons served by community water systems that receives a supply of drinking water that meets the regulations of the Safe Drinking Water Act

8-6. Reduce waterborne disease outbreaks arising from water intended for drinking among persons served by community water systems

8-7. Reduce per capita domestic water withdrawals

8-8. (Developmental) Increase the proportion of assessed rivers, lakes, and estuaries that is safe for fishing and recreational purposes

8-9. (Developmental) Reduce the number of beach closings that results from the presence of harmful bacteria

8-10. (Developmental) Reduce the potential human exposure to persistent chemicals by decreasing fish contaminant levels

Toxins and Waste

8-11. Eliminate elevated blood lead levels in children

8-12. Minimize the risks to human health and the environment posed by hazardous sites

8-13. Reduce pesticide exposures that result in visits to a health-care facility

8-14. (Developmental) Reduce the amount of toxic pollutants released, disposed of, treated, or used for energy recovery

8-15. Increase recycling of municipal solid waste

Healthy Homes and Healthy Communities

8-16. Reduce indoor allergen levels

8-17. (Developmental) Increase the number of office buildings that is managed using good indoor air quality practices

8-18. Increase the proportion of persons that lives in homes tested for radon concentrations

8-19. Increase the number of new homes constructed to be radon resistant

8-20. (Developmental) Increase the proportion of the nation's primary and secondary schools that has official school policies ensuring the safety of students and staff in relation to environmental hazards, such as chemicals in special classrooms, poor indoor air quality, asbestos, and exposure to pesticides

8-21. (Developmental) Ensure that state health departments establish training, plans, and protocols and conduct annual multiinstitutional exercises to prepare for response to natural and technological disasters

8-22. Increase the proportion of persons living in pre-1950s housing that has been tested for the presence of lead-based paint

8-23. Reduce the proportion of occupied housing units that is substandard

Infrastructure and Surveillance

8-24. Reduce exposure to pesticides as measured by urine concentration of metabolites

8-25. (Developmental) Reduce exposure of the population to pesticides, heavy metals, and other toxic chemicals, as measured by blood and urine concentrations of the substances or their metabolites

8-26. (Developmental) Improve the quality, utility, awareness, and use of existing information systems for environmental health

8-27. Increase or maintain the number of territories, tribes, and states (including the District of Columbia) that monitors diseases or conditions that can be caused by exposure to environmental hazards

8-28. (Developmental) Increase the number of local health departments or agencies that uses data from surveillance of environmental risk factors as part of their vector control programs

Global Environmental Health

8-29. Reduce the global burden of disease due to poor water quality, sanitation, and personal and domestic hygiene

8-30. Increase the proportion of the population in the U.S.-Mexico border region that has adequate drinking water and sanitation facilities

Family Planning

Goal: Improve pregnancy planning and spacing and prevent unintended pregnancy.

9-1. Increase the proportion of pregnancies that is intended

9-2. Reduce the proportion of births occurring within 24 months of a previous birth

9-3. Increase the proportion of females at risk of unintended pregnancy (and their partners) who use contraception

9-4. Reduce the proportion of females experiencing pregnancy despite use of a reversible contraceptive method

9-5. (Developmental) Increase the proportion of health-care providers that provides emergency contraception

9-6. (Developmental) Increase male involvement in pregnancy prevention and family planning efforts

9-7. Reduce pregnancies among adolescent females

9-8. Increase the proportion of adolescents that has never engaged in sexual intercourse before they are 15 years old

9-9. Increase the proportion of adolescents that has never engaged in sexual intercourse

9-10. Increase the proportion of sexually active, unmarried adolescents 15 to 17 years old that uses contraception that both effectively prevents pregnancy and provides barrier protection against disease

9-11. Increase the proportion of young adults that has received formal instruction before turning 18 years old on reproductive health issues, including all of the following topics: birth control methods, safer sex to prevent HIV, prevention of sexually transmitted diseases, and abstinence

9-12. Reduce the proportion of married couples whose ability to conceive or maintain a pregnancy is impaired

9-13. (Developmental) Increase the proportion of health insurance policies that covers contraceptive supplies and services

Food Safety

Goal: Reduce food-borne illnesses.

10-1. Reduce infections caused by key food-borne pathogens

10-2. Reduce outbreaks of infections caused by key food-borne bacteria

10-3. Prevent an increase in the proportion of isolates of *Salmonella* species from humans and from animals at slaughter that are resistant to antimicrobial drugs

10-4. (Developmental) Reduce deaths from anaphylaxis caused by food allergies

10-5. Increase the proportion of consumers that follows key food safety practices

10-6. (Developmental) Improve food employee behaviors and food preparation practices that directly relate to food-borne illnesses in retail food establishments

10-7. (Developmental) Reduce human exposure to organophosphate pesticides from food

Health Communication

Goal: Use communication strategically to improve health.

11-1. Increase the proportion of households with access to the Internet at home

11-2. (Developmental) Improve the health literacy of persons with inadequate or marginal literacy skills

11-3. (Developmental) Increase the proportion of health communication activities that includes research and evaluation

11-4. (Developmental) Increase the proportion of health-related World Wide Web sites that discloses information that can be used to assess the quality of the site

11-5. (Developmental) Increase the number of centers for excellence that seeks to advance the research and practice of health communication

11-6. (Developmental) Increase the proportion of persons that reports that health-care providers have satisfactory communication skills

Heart Disease and Stroke

Goal: Improve cardiovascular health and quality of life through the prevention, detection, and treatment of risk factors; early identification and treatment of heart attacks and strokes; and prevention of recurrent cardiovascular events.

Heart Disease

12-1. Reduce coronary heart disease deaths

12-2. (Developmental) Increase the proportion of adults 20 years old and older that is aware of the early warning symptoms and signs of a heart attack and the importance of accessing rapid emergency care by calling 911

12-3.   (Developmental) Increase the proportion of eligible patients with heart attacks that receives artery-opening therapy within an hour of symptom onset

12-4.   (Developmental) Increase the proportion of adults 20 years old and older that calls 911 and administer cardiopulmonary resuscitation when witnessing an out-of-hospital cardiac arrest

12-5.   (Developmental) Increase the proportion of eligible persons with witnessed out-of-hospital cardiac arrest that receives the first therapeutic electrical shock within 6 minutes after collapse recognition

12-6.   Reduce hospitalizations of older adults with congestive heart failure as the principal diagnosis

Stroke

12-7.   Reduce stroke deaths

12-8.   (Developmental) Increase the proportion of adults that is aware of the early warning symptoms and signs of a stroke

Blood Pressure

12-9.   Reduce the proportion of adults with high blood pressure

12-10. Increase the proportion of adults with high blood pressure whose blood pressure is under control

12-11. Increase the proportion of adults with high blood pressure that is taking action (for example, losing weight, increasing physical activity, or reducing sodium intake) to help control blood pressure

12-12. Increase the proportion of adults that has had blood pressure measured within the preceding 2 years and can state whether blood pressure was normal or high

Cholesterol

12-13. Reduce the mean total blood cholesterol levels among adults

12-14. Reduce the proportion of adults with high total blood cholesterol levels

12-15. Increase the proportion of adults that has had blood cholesterol checked within the preceding 5 years

12-16. (Developmental) Increase the proportion of persons with coronary heart disease that has LDL-cholesterol level treated, with the goal of reducing it to ≤100 mg/dL

HIV

Goal: Prevent human immunodeficiency virus (HIV) infection and its related illness and death.

13-1.   Reduce AIDS among adolescents and adults

13-2.   Reduce the number of new AIDS cases among adolescent and adult men who have sex with men

13-3.   Reduce the number of new AIDS cases among females and males who inject drugs

13-4.   Reduce the number of new AIDS cases among adolescent and adult men who have sex with men and inject drugs

13-5.   (Developmental) Reduce the number of cases of HIV infection among adolescents and adults

13-6.   Increase the proportion of sexually active persons that uses condoms

13-7.   (Developmental) Increase the number of HIV-positive persons that knows serostatus

13-8.   Increase the proportion of substance abuse treatment facilities that offers HIV/AIDS education, counseling, and support

13-9.   (Developmental) Increase the number of state prison systems that provides comprehensive HIV/AIDS, sexually transmitted disease, and tuberculosis education.

13-10. (Developmental) Increase the proportion of inmates in state prison systems that receives voluntary HIV counseling and testing during incarceration

13-11. Increase the proportion of adults with tuberculosis that has been tested for HIV

13-12. (Developmental) Increase the proportion of adults in publicly funded HIV counseling and testing sites that is screened for common bacterial sexually transmitted diseases (chlamydia, gonorrhea, and syphilis) and immunized against hepatitis B virus

13-13. Increase the proportion of HIV-infected adolescents and adults that receives testing, treatment, and prophylaxis consistent with current Public Health Service treatment guidelines

13-14. Reduce deaths from HIV infection

13-15. (Developmental) Extend the interval of time between an initial diagnosis of HIV infection and AIDS diagnosis to increase years of life in individuals infected with HIV

13-16. (Developmental) Increase years of life of HIV-infected persons by extending the interval of time between AIDS diagnosis and death.

13-17. (Developmental) Reduce new cases of perinatally acquired HIV infection

Immunization and Infectious Diseases

Goal: Prevent disease, disability, and death from infectious diseases, including vaccine-preventable diseases.

Diseases Preventable Through Universal Vaccination

14-1. Reduce or eliminate indigenous cases of vaccine-preventable diseases

14-2. Reduce chronic hepatitis B virus infections in infants and young children (perinatal infections)

14-3. Reduce hepatitis B

14-4. Reduce bacterial meningitis in young children

14-5. Reduce invasive pneumococcal infections

Diseases Preventable Through Targeted Vaccination

14-6. Reduce hepatitis A

14-7. Reduce meningococcal disease

14-8. Reduce Lyme disease

Infectious Diseases and Emerging Antimicrobial Resistance

14-9. Reduce hepatitis C

14-10. (Developmental) Increase the proportion of persons with chronic hepatitis C infection identified by state and local health departments

14-11. Reduce tuberculosis

14-12. Increase the proportion of all tuberculosis patients that completes curative therapy within 12 months

14-13. Increase the proportion of contacts and other high-risk persons with latent tuberculosis infection who complete a course of treatment

14-14. Reduce the average time for a laboratory to confirm and report tuberculosis cases

14-15. (Developmental) Increase the proportion of international travelers that receives recommended preventive services when traveling in areas of risk for select infectious diseases: hepatitis A, malaria, and typhoid

14-16. Reduce invasive early onset group B streptococcal disease

14-17. Reduce hospitalizations caused by peptic ulcer disease in the United States

14-18. Reduce the number of courses of antibiotics for ear infections for young children

14-19. Reduce the number of courses of antibiotics prescribed for the sole diagnosis of the common cold

14-20. Reduce hospital-acquired infections in intensive care unit patients

14-21. Reduce antimicrobial use among intensive care unit patients

Vaccination Coverage and Strategies

14-22. Achieve and maintain effective vaccination coverage levels for universally recommended vaccines among young children

14-23. Maintain vaccination coverage levels for children in licensed daycare facilities and children in kindergarten through the first grade

14-24. Increase the proportion of young children and adolescents that receives all vaccines that have been recommended for universal administration for at least 5 years

14-25. Increase the proportion of providers that has measured the vaccination coverage levels among children in the practice population within the past 2 years

14-26. Increase the proportion of children that participates in fully operational population-based immunization registries

14-27. Increase routine vaccination coverage levels for adolescents

14-28. Increase hepatitis B vaccine coverage among high-risk groups

14-29. Increase the proportion of adults that is vaccinated annually against influenza and ever vaccinated against pneumococcal disease

Vaccine Safety

14-30. Reduce vaccine-associated adverse events

14-31. Increase the number of persons under active surveillance for vaccine safety via large linked databases

Injury and Violence Prevention

Goal: Reduce injuries, disabilities, and deaths due to unintentional injuries and violence.

Injury Prevention

15-1.   Reduce hospitalization for nonfatal head injuries

15-2.   Reduce hospitalization for nonfatal spinal cord injuries

15-3.   Reduce firearm-related deaths

15-4.   Reduce the proportion of persons living in homes with firearms that are loaded and unlocked

15-5.   Reduce nonfatal firearm-related injuries

15-6.   (Developmental) Extend state-level child fatality review of deaths due to external causes for children 14 years old or younger

15-7.   Reduce nonfatal poisonings

15-8.   Reduce deaths caused by poisonings

15-9.   Reduce deaths caused by suffocation

15-10. Increase the number of states (including the District of Columbia) with statewide emergency department surveillance systems that collects data on external causes of injury

15-11. Increase the number of states (including the District of Columbia) that collects data on external causes of injury through hospital discharge data systems

15-12. Reduce hospital emergency department visits caused by injuries

Unintentional Injury Prevention

15-13. Reduce deaths caused by unintentional injuries

15-14. (Developmental) Reduce nonfatal unintentional injuries

15-15. Reduce deaths caused by motor vehicle crashes

15-16. Reduce pedestrian deaths on public roads

15-17. Reduce nonfatal injuries caused by motor vehicle crashes

15-18. Reduce nonfatal pedestrian injuries on public roads

15-19. Increase use of safety belts

15-20. Increase use of child restraints

15-21. Increase the proportion of motorcyclists using helmets

15-22. Increase the number of states (including the District of Columbia) that has adopted a model graduated driver licensing law

15-23. (Developmental) Increase use of helmets by bicyclists

15-24. Increase the number of states (including the District of Columbia) with laws requiring bicycle helmets for bicycle riders

15-25. Reduce residential fire deaths

15-26. Increase functioning residential smoke alarms

15-27. Reduce deaths from falls

15-28. Reduce hip fractures among older adults

15-29. Reduce drownings

15-30. Reduce hospital emergency department visits for nonfatal dog bite injuries

15-31. (Developmental) Increase the proportion of public and private schools that requires use of appropriate head, face, eye, and mouth protection for students participating in school-sponsored physical activities

Violence and Abuse Prevention

15-32. Reduce homicides

15-33. Reduce maltreatment and maltreatment fatalities of children

15-34. Reduce the rate of physical assault by current or former intimate partners

15-35. Reduce the annual rate of rape or attempted rape

15-36. Reduce sexual assault other than rape

15-37. Reduce physical assaults

15-38. Reduce physical fighting among adolescents

15-39. Reduce weapon carrying by adolescents on school property

Maternal, Infant, and Child Health

Goal: Improve the health and well-being of women, infants, children, and families.

Fetal, Infant, Child, and Adolescent Deaths

16-1.   Reduce fetal and infant deaths

16-2.   Reduce the rate of child deaths

16-3.   Reduce deaths of adolescents and young adults

Maternal Deaths and Illnesses

16-4.   Reduce maternal deaths

16-5.   Reduce maternal illness and complications due to pregnancy

Prenatal Care

16-6.   Increase the proportion of pregnant women that receives early and adequate prenatal care

16-7.   (Developmental) Increase the proportion of pregnant women that attends a series of prepared childbirth classes

Obstetrical Care

16-8.   Increase the proportion of very low birth weight infants born at level three hospitals or subspecialty perinatal centers

16-9.   Reduce cesarean births among low-risk (full-term, singleton, vertex presentation) women

Risk Factors

16-10. Reduce low birth weight and very low birth weight births

16-11. Reduce preterm births

16-12. (Developmental) Increase the proportion of mothers that achieves a recommended weight gain during their pregnancies

16-13. Increase the percentage of healthy, full-term infants that is put down to sleep on the back

Developmental Disabilities and Neural Tube Defects

16-14. Reduce the occurrence of developmental disabilities

16-15. Reduce the occurrence of spina bifida and other neural tube defects

16-16. Increase the proportion of pregnancies begun with an optimum folic acid level

Prenatal Substance Exposure

16-17. Increase abstinence from alcohol, cigarettes, and illicit drugs among pregnant women

16-18. (Developmental) Reduce the occurrence of fetal alcohol syndrome

Breastfeeding, Newborn Screening, and Service Systems

16-19. Increase the proportion of mothers that breastfeeds the baby

16-20. (Developmental) Ensure appropriate newborn bloodspot screening, follow-up testing, and referral to services

16-21. (Developmental) Reduce hospitalization for life-threatening sepsis among children 4 years old and younger with sickling hemoglobinopathies

16-22. (Developmental) Increase the proportion of children with special health-care needs that has access to a medical home

16-23. Increase the proportion of territories and states that has service systems for children with special health-care needs

Medical Product Safety

Goal: Ensure the safe and effective use of medical products.

17-1. (Developmental) Increase the proportion of health-care organizations that is linked in an integrated system that monitors and reports adverse events

17-2. (Developmental) Increase the use of linked, automated systems to share information

17-3. (Developmental) Increase the proportion of primary care providers, pharmacists, and other health-care professionals that routinely reviews with patients 65 years old and older and patients with chronic illnesses or disabilities all new prescribed and over-the-counter medicines

17-4   (Developmental) Increase the proportion of patients receiving information that meets guidelines for usefulness when new prescriptions are dispensed

17-5. Increase the proportion of patients that receives verbal counseling from prescribers and pharmacists on the appropriate use and potential risks of medications

17-6. Increase the proportion of persons that donates blood and thus ensure an adequate supply of safe blood

Mental Health and Mental Disorders

Goal: Improve mental health and ensure access to appropriate, quality mental health services.

Mental Health Status Improvement

18-1. Reduce the suicide rate

18-2. Reduce the rate of suicide attempts by adolescents

18-3. Reduce the proportion of homeless adults who have serious mental illness

18-4. Increase the proportion of persons with serious mental illness who are employed

18-5. (Developmental) Reduce the relapse rates for persons with eating disorders, including anorexia nervosa and bulimia nervosa

Treatment Expansion

18-6. (Developmental) Increase the number of persons seen in primary health care that receives mental health screening and assessment

18-7. (Developmental) Increase the proportion of children with mental health problems that receives treatment

18-8. (Developmental) Increase the proportion of juvenile justice facilities that screens new admissions for mental health problems

18-9. Increase the proportion of adults with mental disorders that receives treatment.

18-10. (Developmental) Increase the proportion of persons with cooccurring substance abuse and mental disorders that receives treatment for both disorders

18-11. (Developmental) Increase the proportion of local governments with community-based jail diversion programs for adults with serious mental illness

State Activities

18-12. Increase the number of states (including the District of Columbia) that tracks consumers' satisfaction with mental health services received

18-13. (Developmental) Increase the number of territories and states (including the District of Columbia) with an operational mental health plan that addresses cultural competence

18-14. Increase the number of territories and states (including the District of Columbia) with an operational mental health plan that addresses mental health crisis interventions, ongoing screening, and treatment services for elderly persons

Nutrition and Overweight

Goal: Promote health and reduce chronic disease associated with diet and weight.

Weight Status and Growth

19-1. Increase the proportion of adults who are at a healthy weight

19-2. Reduce the proportion of adults who are obese

19-3. Reduce the proportion of children and adolescents who are overweight or obese

19-4. Reduce growth retardation among low-income children under 5 years old

Food and Nutrient Consumption

19-5. Increase the proportion of persons 2 years old and older who consume at least two daily servings of fruit

19-6.   Increase the proportion of persons 2 years old and older who consume at least three daily servings of vegetables, with at least one third being dark green or orange vegetables

19-7.   Increase the proportion of persons 2 years old and older who consume at least six daily servings of grain products, with at least three being whole grains

19-8.   Increase the proportion of persons 2 years old and older who consume less than 10% of their total daily calories from saturated fat

19-9.   Increase the proportion of persons 2 years old and older who consume no more than 30% of their total daily calories from total fat

19-10.   Increase the proportion of persons 2 years old and older who consume 2400 mg or less of sodium daily

19-11.   Increase the proportion of persons 2 years old and older who meet dietary recommendations for calcium

Iron Deficiency and Anemia

19-12.   Reduce iron deficiency among young children and females of childbearing age

19-13.   Reduce anemia among low-income pregnant females in their third trimester

19-14.   (Developmental) Reduce iron deficiency among pregnant females

Schools, Worksites, and Nutrition Counseling

19-15.   (Developmental) Increase the proportion of children and adolescents 6 to 19 years old whose intake of meals and snacks at school contributes to good overall dietary quality

19-16.   Increase the proportion of worksites that offer nutrition or weight management classes or counseling

19-17.   Increase the proportion of physician office visits made by patients with a diagnosis of cardiovascular disease, diabetes, or hyperlipidemia that includes counseling or education related to diet and nutrition

Food Security

19-18.   Increase food security among U.S. households and thus reduce hunger

Occupational Safety and Health

Goal: Promote the health and safety of people at work through prevention and early intervention.

20-1. Reduce deaths from work-related injuries

20-2. Reduce work-related injuries resulting in medical treatment, lost time from work, or restricted work activity

20-3. Reduce the rate of injury and illness cases involving days away from work due to overexertion or repetitive motion

20-4. Reduce pneumoconiosis deaths

20-5. Reduce deaths from work-related homicides

20-6. Reduce work-related assaults

20-7. Reduce the number of persons who have elevated blood lead concentrations from work exposures

20-8. Reduce occupational skin diseases or disorders among full-time workers

20-9. Increase the proportion of worksites employing 50 or more persons that provide programs to prevent or reduce employee stress

20-10. Reduce occupational needlestick injuries among health-care workers

20-11. (Developmental) Reduce new cases of work-related, noise-induced hearing loss

Oral Health

Goal: Prevent and control oral and craniofacial diseases, conditions, and injuries and improve access to related services.

21-1. Reduce the proportion of children and adolescents who have experience of dental caries in their primary or permanent teeth

21-2. Reduce the proportion of children, adolescents, and adults with untreated dental decay

21-3. Increase the proportion of adults who have never had a permanent tooth extracted because of dental caries or periodontal disease

21-4. Reduce the proportion of older adults who have had all their natural teeth extracted

21-5.   Reduce periodontal disease

21-6.   Increase the proportion of oral and pharyngeal cancers detected at the earliest stage

21-7.   Increase the proportion of adults who, in the past 12 months, report having had an examination to detect oral and pharyngeal cancers

21-8.   Increase the proportion of children who have received dental sealants on their molar teeth

21-9.   Increase the proportion of the U.S. population served by community water systems with optimally fluoridated water

21-10. Increase the proportion of children and adults who use the oral health-care system each year

21-11. Increase the proportion of long-term care residents who use the oral health care system each year

21-12. Increase the proportion of low-income children and adolescents who received any preventive dental service during the past year

21-13. (Developmental) Increase the proportion of school-based health centers with an oral health component

21-14. Increase the proportion of local health departments and community-based health centers, including community, migrant, and homeless health centers, that has an oral health component

21-15. Increase the number of states (including the District of Columbia) that has a system for recording and referring infants and children with cleft lips, cleft palates, and other craniofacial anomalies to craniofacial anomaly rehabilitative teams

21-16. Increase the number of states (including the District of Columbia) that has an oral and craniofacial health surveillance system

21-17. (Developmental) Increase the number of tribal, state (including the District of Columbia), and local health agencies that serve jurisdictions of 250,000 or more persons that has in place an effective public dental health program directed by a dental professional with public health training

Physical Activity and Fitness

Goal: Improve health, fitness, and quality of life through daily physical activity.

Physical Activity in Adults

22-1.   Reduce the proportion of adults that engages in no leisure-time physical activity

22-2.   Increase the proportion of adults that engages regularly, preferably daily, in moderate physical activity for at least 30 minutes per day

22-3.   Increase the proportion of adults that engages in vigorous physical activity that promotes the development and maintenance of cardiorespiratory fitness 3 or more days per week for 20 or more minutes per occasion

Muscular Strength/Endurance and Flexibility

22-4.   Increase the proportion of adults that performs physical activities that enhance and maintain muscular strength and endurance

22-5.   Increase the proportion of adults that performs physical activities that enhance and maintain flexibility

Physical Activity in Children and Adolescents

22-6.   Increase the proportion of adolescents that engages in moderate physical activity for at least 30 minutes on 5 or more days out of 7

22-7.   Increase the proportion of adolescents that engages in vigorous physical activity that promotes cardiorespiratory fitness 3 or more days per week for 20 or more minutes per occasion

22-8.   Increase the proportion of the nation's public and private schools that requires daily physical education for all students

22-9.   Increase the proportion of adolescents that participates in daily school physical education

22-10. Increase the proportion of adolescents that spends at least 50% of school physical education class time being physically active

22-11. Increase the proportion of adolescents that views television 2 or fewer hours on a school day

Access

22-12. (Developmental) Increase the proportion of the nation's public and private schools that provides access to physical activity spaces and facilities for all persons outside of normal school hours (that is, before and after the school day, on weekends, and during summer and other vacations)

22-13. Increase the proportion of worksites offering employer-sponsored physical activity and fitness programs

22-14. Increase the proportion of trips made by walking

22-15. Increase the proportion of trips made by bicycling.

Public Health Infrastructure

Goal: Ensure that federal, tribal, state, and local health agencies have the infrastructure to provide essential public health services effectively.

Data and Information Systems

23-1. (Developmental) Increase the proportion of tribal, state, and local public health agencies that provide Internet and e-mail access for at least 75% of their employees and that teach employees to use the Internet and other electronic information systems to apply data and information to public health practice

23-2. (Developmental) Increase the proportion of federal, tribal, state, and local health agencies that have made information available to the public in the past year on the leading health indicators, health status indicators, and priority data needs

23-3. Increase the proportion of all major national, state, and local health data systems that use geocoding to promote nationwide use of geographic information systems at all levels

23-4. Increase the proportion of population-based Healthy People 2010 objectives for which national data are available for all population groups identified for the objective

23-5. (Developmental) Increase the proportion of leading health indicators, health status indicators, and priority data needs for which data—especially for select populations—are available at the tribal, state, and local levels

23-6. Increase the proportion of Healthy People 2010 objectives that is tracked regularly at the national level

23-7. Increase the proportion of Healthy People 2010 objectives for which national data are released within 1 year of the end of data collection

23-8.   (Developmental) Increase the proportion of federal, tribal, state, and local agencies that incorporates specific competencies in the essential public health services into personnel systems

23-9.   (Developmental) Increase the proportion of schools for public health workers that integrates into the curriculum specific content to develop competence in essential public health services

23-10. (Developmental) Increase the proportion of federal, tribal, state, and local public health agencies that provides continuing education to develop competence in essential public health services to employees

23-11. (Developmental) Increase the proportion of state and local public health agencies that meets national performance standards for essential public health services

23-12. Increase the proportion of tribes and states (including the District of Columbia) that has a health improvement plan and increase the proportion of local jurisdictions that has a health improvement plan linked with the state plan

23-13. (Developmental) Increase the proportion of tribal, state, and local health agencies that provides or ensures comprehensive laboratory services to support essential public health services

23-14. (Developmental) Increase the proportion of tribal, state, and local public health agencies that provides or ensures comprehensive epidemiology services to support essential public health services

23-15. (Developmental) Increase the proportion of federal, tribal, state, and local jurisdictions that reviews and evaluates the extent to which statutes, ordinances, and bylaws ensure the delivery of essential public health services

Resources

23-16. (Developmental) Increase the proportion of federal, tribal, state, and local public health agencies that gathers accurate data on public health expenditures, categorized by essential public health service

Prevention Research

23-17. (Developmental) Increase the proportion of federal, tribal, state, and local public health agencies that conducts or collaborates on population-based prevention research.

Respiratory Diseases

Goal: Promote respiratory health through better prevention, detection, treatment, and education efforts.

Asthma

24-1.   Reduce asthma deaths

24-2.   Reduce hospitalizations for asthma

24-3.   Reduce hospital emergency department visits for asthma

24-4.   Reduce activity limitations among persons with asthma

24-5.   (Developmental) Reduce the number of school or work days missed by persons with asthma due to asthma

24-6.   Increase the proportion of persons with asthma that receives formal patient education, including information about community and self-help resources, as an essential part of the management of the condition

24-7.   (Developmental) Increase the proportion of persons with asthma that receives appropriate asthma care according to the National Asthma Education and Prevention Program (NAEPP) guidelines

24-8.   (Developmental) Establish in at least 25 states a surveillance system for tracking asthma death, illness, disability, impact of occupational and environmental factors on asthma, access to medical care, and asthma management

Chronic Obstructive Pulmonary Disease

24-9.   Reduce the proportion of adults whose activity is limited due to chronic lung and breathing problems

24-10. Reduce deaths from chronic obstructive pulmonary disease among adults

Obstructive Sleep Apnea

24-11. (Developmental) Increase the proportion of persons with symptoms of obstructive sleep apnea whose condition is medically managed

24-12. (Developmental) Reduce the proportion of vehicular crashes caused by persons with excessive sleepiness

Sexually Transmitted Diseases (STDs)

Goal: Promote responsible sexual behaviors, strengthen community capacity, and increase access to quality services to prevent sexually transmitted diseases and their complications.

Bacterial STD Illness and Disability

25-1. Reduce the proportion of adolescents and young adults with *Chlamydia trachomatis* infections

25-2. Reduce gonorrhea

25-3. Eliminate sustained domestic transmission of primary and secondary syphilis

Viral STD Illness and Disability

25-4. Reduce the proportion of adults with genital herpes infection

25-5. (Developmental) Reduce the proportion of persons with human papillomavirus infection

STD Complications Affecting Females

25-6. Reduce the proportion of females who have ever required treatment for pelvic inflammatory disease

25-7. Reduce the proportion of childless females with fertility problems who have had a sexually transmitted disease or who have required treatment for pelvic inflammatory disease

25-8. (Developmental) Reduce HIV infections in adolescent and young adult females 13 to 24 years old that are associated with heterosexual contact

STD Complications Affecting the Fetus and Newborn

25-9. Reduce congenital syphilis

25-10. (Developmental) Reduce neonatal consequences from maternal sexually transmitted diseases, including chlamydial pneumonia, gonococcal and chlamydial *ophthalmia neonatorum*, laryngeal papillomatosis (from human papillomavirus infection), neonatal herpes, and preterm birth and low birth weight associated with bacterial vaginosis

Personal Behaviors

25-11. Increase the proportion of adolescents that abstains from sexual intercourse or uses condoms if currently sexually active

25-12. (Developmental) Increase the number of positive messages related to responsible sexual behavior during weekday and nightly prime-time television programming

Community Protection Infrastructure

25-13. Increase the proportion of tribal, state, and local sexually transmitted disease programs that routinely offers hepatitis B vaccines to all STD clients

25-14. (Developmental) Increase the proportion of youth detention facilities and adult city or county jails that screens for common bacterial sexually transmitted diseases within 24 hours of admission and treats STDs (when necessary) before persons are released

25-15. (Developmental) Increase the proportion of all local health departments that has contracts with managed care providers for the treatment of nonplan partners of patients with bacterial sexually transmitted diseases (gonorrhea, syphilis, and chlamy dia).

Personal Health Services

25-16. (Developmental) Increase the proportion of sexually active females 25 years old and younger that is screened annually for genital chlamydia infections

25-17. (Developmental) Increase the proportion of pregnant females screened for sexually transmitted diseases (including HIV infection and bacterial vaginosis) during prenatal health care visits, according to recognized standards

25-18. Increase the proportion of primary care providers that treats patients with sexually transmitted diseases and that manages cases according to recognized standards

25-19. (Developmental) Increase the proportion of all sexually transmitted disease clinic patients that is being treated for bacterial STDs (chlamydia, gonorrhea, and syphilis) and that is offered provider referral services for sex partners

Substance Abuse

Goal: Reduce substance abuse to protect the health, safety, and quality of life for all, especially children.

Adverse Consequences of Substance Use and Abuse

26-1. Reduce deaths and injuries caused by alcohol- and drug-related motor vehicle crashes

26-2. Reduce cirrhosis deaths

26-3. Reduce drug-induced deaths

26-4. Reduce drug-related hospital emergency department visits

26-5. (Developmental) Reduce alcohol-related hospital emergency department visits

26-6. Reduce the proportion of adolescents who report that they rode, during the previous 30 days, with a driver who had been drinking alcohol

26-7. (Developmental) Reduce intentional injuries resulting from alcohol- and illicit drug-related violence

26-8. (Developmental) Reduce the cost of lost productivity in the workplace due to alcohol and drug use

Substance Use and Abuse

26-9. Increase the age and proportion of adolescents who remain alcohol and drug free

26-10. Reduce past-month use of illicit substances

26-11. Reduce the proportion of persons engaging in binge drinking of alcoholic beverages

26-12. Reduce average annual alcohol consumption

26-13. Reduce the proportion of adults who exceed guidelines for low-risk drinking

26-14. Reduce steroid use among adolescents

26-15. Reduce the proportion of adolescents who use inhalants

Risk of Substance Use and Abuse

26-16. Increase the proportion of adolescents who disapprove of substance abuse

26-17. Increase the proportion of adolescents who perceive great risk associated with substance abuse

Treatment for Substance Abuse

26-18. (Developmental) Reduce the treatment gap for illicit drugs in the general population

26-19. (Developmental) Increase the proportion of inmates receiving substance abuse treatment in correctional institutions

26-20. Increase the number of admissions to substance abuse treatment centers for injection drug use

26-21. (Developmental) Reduce the treatment gap for alcohol problems

State and Local Efforts

26-22. (Developmental) Increase the proportion of persons who are referred for follow-up care for alcohol problems, drug problems, or suicide attempts after diagnosis or treatment for one of these conditions in a hospital emergency department

26-23. (Developmental) Increase the number of communities using partnerships or coalition models to conduct comprehensive substance abuse prevention efforts

26-24. Extend administrative license revocation laws, or programs of equal effectiveness, for persons who drive under the influence of intoxicants

26-25. Extend legal requirements for maximum blood alcohol concentration levels of 0.08% for motor vehicle drivers 21 years old and older

Tobacco Use

Goal: Reduce illness, disability, and death related to tobacco use and exposure to secondhand smoke.

Tobacco Use in Population Groups

27-1. Reduce tobacco use by adults

27-2. Reduce tobacco use by adolescents

27-3. (Developmental) Reduce the initiation of tobacco use among children and adolescents

27-4.   Increase the average age of first use of tobacco products by adolescents and young adults

Cessation and Treatment

27-5.   Increase smoking cessation attempts by adult smokers

27-6.   Increase smoking cessation during pregnancy

27-7.   Increase tobacco use cessation attempts by adolescent smokers

27-8.   Increase insurance coverage of evidence-based treatment for nicotine dependency

Exposure to Secondhand Smoke

27-9.   Reduce the proportion of children that is regularly exposed to tobacco smoke at home

27-10. Reduce the proportion of nonsmokers exposed to environmental tobacco smoke

27-11. Increase smoke-free and tobacco-free environments in schools, including all school facilities, property, vehicles, and school events

27-12. Increase the proportion of worksites with formal smoking policies that prohibit smoking or limit it to separately ventilated areas

27-13. Establish laws regarding smoke-free indoor air that prohibit smoking or limit it to separately ventilated areas in public places and worksites

Social and Environmental Changes

27-14. Reduce the rate of illegal sales to minors through enforcement of laws prohibiting the sale of tobacco products to minors

27-15. Increase the number of states (including the District of Columbia) that suspends or revokes state retail licenses for violations of laws prohibiting the sale of tobacco to minors

27-16. (Developmental) Eliminate tobacco advertising and promotions that influence adolescents and young adults

27-17. Increase adolescents' disapproval of smoking

27-18. (Developmental) Increase the number of tribes, territories, and states (including the District of Columbia) with comprehensive, evidence-based tobacco control programs

27-19. Eliminate laws that preempt stronger tobacco control laws

27-20. (Developmental) Reduce the toxicity of tobacco products by establishing a regulatory structure to monitor toxicity

27-21. Increase the average federal and state taxes on tobacco products

Vision and Hearing

Goal: Improve the visual and hearing health of the nation through prevention, early detection, treatment, and rehabilitation.

Vision

28-1. (Developmental) Increase the proportion of persons that has a dilated eye examination at appropriate intervals

28-2. (Developmental) Increase the proportion of preschool children 5 years old and younger that receives vision screening

28-3. (Developmental) Reduce uncorrected visual impairment due to refractive errors

28-4. Reduce blindness and visual impairment in children and adolescents 17 years old and younger

28-5. (Developmental) Reduce visual impairment due to diabetic retinopathy

28-6. (Developmental) Reduce visual impairment due to glaucoma

28-7. (Developmental) Reduce visual impairment due to cataract

28-8. (Developmental) Reduce occupational eye injuries

28-9. (Developmental) Increase the use of appropriate personal protective eyewear in recreational activities and hazardous situations around the home

28-10. (Developmental) Increase vision rehabilitation

Hearing

28-11. (Developmental) Increase the proportion of newborns that is screened for hearing loss by 1 month, has audiologic evaluation by 3 months, and is enrolled in appropriate intervention services by 6 months

28-12. Reduce otitis media in children and adolescents

28-13. (Developmental) Increase access by persons who have hearing impairments to hearing rehabilitation services and adaptive devices, including hearing aids, cochlear implants, or tactile or other assistive or augmentive devices

28-14. (Developmental) Increase the proportion of persons that has had a hearing examination on schedule

28-15. (Developmental) Increase the number of persons that is referred by a primary care physician for hearing evaluation and treatment

28-16. (Developmental) Increase the use of appropriate ear protection devices, equipment, and practices

28-17. (Developmental) Reduce noise-induced hearing loss in children and adolescents 17 years old and younger

28-18. (Developmental) Reduce adult hearing loss in the noise-exposed public

Reference

Department of Health and Human Services. (2000). *Healthy People 2010: Understanding and improving health* (2nd ed.). Washington, DC: U.S. Government Printing Office.

Appendix C

Epidemiological Glossary

Accuracy	The degree to which a measurement represents the true value of the attribute being measured.
Active immunity	The resistance developed in response to a stimulus by an antigen (agent or vaccine).
Agent	A factor whose presence, excessive presence, or relative absence is essential for the occurrence of a disease.
Analytic epidemiology	Use of epidemiological methods to test hypotheses about causality; the second phase of epidemiological investigations.
Antifactual association	Also known as a spurious association. A false association that occurs by chance or through bias due to confounding variables.
Association	A relationship between two factors or events, usually expressed as a degree of statistical dependence. Factors or events are said to be associated when they occur more frequently together than could be expected by chance alone.
Attack rate	A variant of an incidence rate in a narrowly defined population, usually expressed as a percent.
Attributable risk	The rate of disease in those with the characteristic minus the rate of disease in those without the characteristic.
Behavioral risk factor	A characteristic or behavior that is associated with increased probability of a specified outcome.
Bias	That which influences the outcome of a study, often to a degree sufficient to render questions regarding the validity of the results.
Biological plausibility	A reasonable physiological mechanism that explains how a causal factor could operate to bring about a particular disease
Biomodal epidemiologic curve	The distribution patterns have two peaks (which are part of the curve).
Blinding	An attempt to limit bias in a study by preventing the participant and/or investigator from knowing to which group the participant belongs.
Case	A person identified as having a particular disease, based on the presence of defined criteria
Case definition	Set of standard criteria established for deciding whether a person has a specific disease or other health-related condition.

Case fatality rate | The number of people dying during a specific period of time after disease onset or diagnosis, divided by the number of individuals with the specific disease, multiplied by 100.

Case finding | A concerted effort to search for previously unidentified cases of a disease.

Causality | The relating of causes to the effects they produce.

Cause | A stimulus that brings about an effect; usually defined operationally by determining that changing the amount or frequency of a suspected cause changes the amount or frequency of the related effect.

Clinical epidemiology | The application of epidemiological principles and methods to problems encountered in clinical medicine.

Cluster | An aggregation of cases within a specified period of time in a specific place.

Coherence | A biologically plausible phenomenon for an association between two factors.

Cohort | A subsection of a population with a common feature, usually age. The component of the population born during a particular period and identified by period of birth so that its characteristics can be ascertained as it enters successive time and age periods. The term has been broadened to describe any designated group of persons who are followed or traced over a period of time.

Cohort study | A study in which subsets of a defined population can be identified as exposed, not exposed, or exposed in varying degrees to a factor or factors hypothesized to cause a disease or other outcome.

Common source epidemic | An epidemic caused by exposure of a group of persons to the same source of an agent (the "point source").

Communicable disease | A disease in which the causative agent may be transmitted from one person to another person through direct or indirect contact.

Confounding variable | A factor that causes change in the frequency of a disease and also varies systematically with a third, potentially causal factor being studied.

Consistency | A criterion for inferring causality that requires similar findings from multiple studies of the relationships between two variables.

Control group | A group of subjects that receives no treatment.

Cross sectional study | A study that determines for each member of a study population or a representative sample of a population the presence or absence of hypothetical causal factors and disease at a single point in time.

Crude birth rate | The number of total live births in a year divided by the population size for that year.

Crude death rate | The number of total deaths in a year divided by the population size in that year.

Cumulative incidence | The proportion of persons who experience onset of a health-related event during a specified time interval.

Dependent variable | A variable which is dependent on the effect of other variables.

Descriptive epidemiology	Study of the occurrence of a disease or other health-related characteristics in human populations according to characteristics of person, place, and time. The first phase of epidemiological investigation.
Direct transmission	The transfer of an infectious agent from the reservoir to a receptive portal of entry through which human infection can take place.
Dose effect	An increase in disease incidence related to the level or dose of exposure.
Double-blind study	A study in which neither the participant nor the investigator knows which group any subject belongs to.
Ecological fallacy	Two populations differ in many factors other than the observed relationship, and one or more of those factors may be the underlying reason for the differences in the observed experience. An error in inference caused by failure to distinguish between different levels of organization, assuming that relationships between factors and diseases observed for groups can be equally applied to individuals.
Ecological study	A study that looks for relationships between factors or events and disease frequency or level, based on aggregate data for entire populations. The joint presence or absence of disease and the etiological factor for individuals is not established.
Endemic	A situation in which the occurrence of a disease is at a persistent level (usually low to moderate) for a defined area.
Environmental factors	Extrinsic factors that affect the host's potential for exposure to an agent. Physical, biological, and socioeconomic factors, such as crowding and sanitation.
Epidemic	A situation in which the occurrence of a disease within a defined area is clearly in excess of the expected level in that area for a defined period of time.
Epidemic curve	The distribution of the times of onset of a disease. A graphic plotting of the distribution of causes by time of onset.
Epidemiological triad	The interaction of agent, host, and environment.
Epidemiology	The study of the distribution and determinants of diseases or conditions in populations.
Etiologic agent	An agent that causes a specific disease state.
Etiology	Postulated causes that initiate the pathogenic process.
Experimental epidemiology	The use of experimental studies to establish disease causality.
Experimental group	A group that receives the treatment under investigation.
False negative	A negative test result in an individual who actually possesses the attribute for which the test was conducted.
False positive	A positive test result in an individual who actually does not possess the attribute for which the test was conducted.
Health risk appraisal	A method of estimating an individual's risk of developing a disease or other outcome.

Herd immunity	The immunity of a group or community. Resistance of a group to invasion and spread of an infectious agent, based on the resistance to infection of a high proportion of individual members of the group.
Horizontal transmission	A term used to describe transmission that generally occurs within a population.
Host factors	Intrinsic factors that influence a person's exposure, susceptibility, or response to an agent.
Hyperendemic	A persistently high level of occurrence. A persistently high endemic.
Incidence	The number of new cases of a disease in a population during a defined period of time. Also, the number of new cases of a disease occurring in a population during a specific time period divided by the number of persons at risk of developing the disease during the period of time multiplied by 1000 and expressed as a rate per 1000 persons.
Incubation period	The period of time from the development of an illness or infection to the onset of the illness (presentation of symptoms). The period of time from the causal event to the initiation of disease.
Independent variable	The exposure of a characteristic being observed or measured that is hypothesized to influence the outcome of interest.
Index case	The first case in a defined population unit to come to the attention of the investigator.
Indirect transmission	Transport of an organism by means of air, vehicles, or vectors from a reservoir to a receptive portal of entry through which human infection can take place.
Interrater reliability	Test consistency of value obtained by two individuals rating the same phenomenon using the same method.
Intrarater reliability	Test consistency of values produced by an individual rater.
Life expectancy	The average number of years an individual is expected to live.
Life-time incidence	A cumulative incidence rate in which the time interval is a person's lifespan.
Mass screening	Application of screening test unselectively to entire populations or selectively to high-risk groups.
Multiphasic screening	Simultaneous application of screening tests for a variety of diseases or conditions. Multiple tests on single sample of blood.
Natural history	Stages in the process of development and progression of a disease without intervention by man.
Natural immunity	Species-determined inherent resistance to a disease or agent.
Necessary cause	A factor that must be present before an event occurs.
Odds	Ratio of occurrence of an event to that of a nonoccurrence.
Odds ratio	A comparison of the presence of a risk factor for a disease in a sample of diseased subjects and nondiseased controls.
Outbreak	An epidemic in the defined area.

Pandemic	An epidemic that spreads over several countries or continents, affecting a large number of people.
Parallel testing	The simultaneous application of multiple diagnostic tests.
Pathogen	An organism capable of causing disease.
Period prevalence	The prevalence of a disease at any time during a specified time interval.
Person-year	Statistical measure representing the risk over one year of one person developing a disease.
Point prevalence	The prevalence of the disease at a specific point in time.
Population at risk	All the people who are identified as vulnerable to a condition.
Potential years of life lost	A measure of the loss to society due to youthful or early deaths, calculated as the sum, over all persons dying from that cause, of the years these individuals would have lived had they fulfilled a normal life expectancy.
Predictive value negative	The probability that an individual with a negative test is a true negative; that is, that the individual with the negative test actually does not have the disease for which the test was conducted.
Predictive value positive	The probability that an individual with a positive test is a true positive; that is, that the individual with the positive test actually does have the disease for which the test was conducted.
Prepathogenesis	First period in the natural history of disease, before initiation of any changes at the cellular level in the host.
Presymptomatic disease	Early stage in the natural history of disease, before initiation of any changes at the cellular level in the host and before the development of symptoms.
Prevalence	The number of existing cases in a population during a defined period of time. This includes the number of new and old cases. Also, the number of cases of a disease present in a population during a specific time divided by the number of persons in the population at that specific time, multiplied by 1000, and expressed as a rate per 1000 persons.
Primary prevention	Actions taken to prevent the development of a disease in a person who is well and does not have the disease. It occurs at the prepathological level.
Propagated epidemic	An epidemic caused by person-to-person transmission of a disease agent.
Proportion	Specific type of ratio in which the numerator is included in the denominator and the resultant value is expressed as a percentage.
Rates	Fractions derived from a numerator and a denominator. The numerator counts the number of times that a particular event occurs. The denominator counts the population at risk during the time interval in question.
Ratio	The relationship between two numbers expressed as a fraction; the value obtained by dividing the numerator of the fraction by the denominator.

Relative risk	The ratio of the risk of disease or death among those exposed to the risk as compared to those not exposed.
Reliability	The extent to which repeated measurements of a relatively stable phenomenon provide consistent results.
Reportable disease	Also known as a notifiable disease. A disease, usually infectious in nature, that is required by law to be reported to the appropriate health officer or authority.
Reservoir	The habitat in which an agent lives, grows, or multiplies.
Risk	Probability that an unfavorable event will occur.
Risk appraisal	An estimation of an individual's risk for developing an outcome.
Risk factor	An attribute or exposure associated with increased probability of a specified outcome (a risk marker). An attribute or exposure that increases the probability of occurrence of disease (a determinant). A determinant that can be modified by intervention, thus reducing the risk (a modifiable risk factor).
Secondary attack rate	The number of new cases of a disease among the contacts of the index case. Expressed as a percentage.
Secondary prevention	The screening, testing, and treatment of a disease that is at the pathological level.
Sensitivity	The ability of a screening test to identify correctly those cases that truly have the disease.
Serial testing	Application of diagnostic test consecutively to one subject at a time.
Single-blind study	A study in which only participants do not know to which group they belong.
Specificity	The ability of a screening test to identify correctly those cases that do not have the disease.
Standard metropolitan statistical area	A county or group of counties containing at least one city with a population of 50,000 people or more.
Standardization	Technique used to remove the effects of differences in age, sex, race, or other confounding variables when comparing two rates for two or more populations.
Standardized mortality ratio	The observed number of deaths per year divided by the expected number of deaths per year multiplied by 100.
Statistical power	The relative frequency with which a true difference of specified size between populations would be detected by the proposed experiment or test.
Substantive epidemiology	The collection of epidemiological knowledge about disease.
Surveillance of disease	System of monitoring all aspects of occurrence and spread of a disease that are relevant to disease control.
Temporality	Evidence that exposure to a causal factor occurred before initiation of the disease process.
Tertiary prevention	Actions taken to limit the disability of a disease state.

Test-retest reliability	Test consistency of values across time with repeated testing.
Triple-blind study	A study in which the subject and investigator are ignorant of the group to which the subject belongs and the data analysis is done without information about which group individual subjects belong to.
Type I error	The error of rejecting a true null hypothesis. Alpha error.
Type II error	The error of failing to reject a false null hypothesis. Beta error.
Unimodal epidemiologic curve	The distribution pattern has only one peak.
Validity	The degree to which the results of a measurement correspond to the true state of the phenomenon being measured. The degree to which the instrument measures what it is expected to measure.
Vector	The insect or other living thing that transports an infectious agent from an infected individual or its wastes to a susceptible individual or its food or immediate surroundings.
Vehicle	An inanimate substance that transports an infectious agent to a susceptible host.
Vertical transmission	Transmission that occurs when a mother conveys an infection to her unborn offspring.
Vital statistics	Data relating to births (natality), deaths (mortality), marriage, divorce, and illness (morbidity).

References

Gordis, L. (2000). *Epidemiology* (2nd ed.). Philadelphia, PA: W. B. Saunders.

Last, J. (1988). *Dictionary of epidemiology* (2nd ed.). New York: Oxford University Press.

Valanis, B. (1999). *Epidemiology in health care* (3rd ed.). Stamford, CT: Appleton & Lange.

Appendix D

Community-Based Organization Assessment

This assessment tool provides a sample of the areas questioned but is not intended to be comprehensive.

Organizational Infrastructure

- The organization has established a recruitment and relationship-building committee charged with developing, evaluating, and monitoring resource development policies, practices, and goals.
- The organization has the resources it needs to accomplish its strategic objectives on its own.
- Staff employed include
  - Full-time staff
  - Part-time staff
  - Volunteers
  - Interns
  - Board
  - Other
- Chapters and offices
  - Members
  - Staff
- Committees have
  - a clear statement of purpose
  - clear written goals and objectives
  - function
  - specific roles and responsibilities
- The committee structure and membership are reviewed annually for relevance.
- The organization's by-laws are up to date.
- The roles of the board and the executive director are defined and respected. The executive director is the manager of the organization's operations. The board is focused on policy and planning.

- The executive director is recruited, selected, and employed by the board of directors. The board provides clearly written expectations and qualifications for the position, as well as reasonable compensation.
- Board organization is documented, with a description of the board and board committee responsibilities.
- The bylaws include
  - how and when notices for board meetings are made
  - how members are elected or appointed by the board
  - what the terms of office are for officers and members
  - how board members are rotated
  - how ineffective board members are removed from the board
  - how many board members makes up the quorum required for all policy decisions
- The organization has a written personnel handbook or policy that is regularly reviewed and updated.
- The organization has job descriptions, including qualifications, duties, reporting relationships, and key indicators.

Strategic Development

- The organization has a written, updated, strategic plan.
- The written strategic plan has been developed by researching the internal and external environment.
- The strategic plan identifies changing community needs, including the agency's strengths, weaknesses, opportunities, and threats.
- The organization has a clear, meaningful, written mission statement that reflects its fundamental purpose, values, and people served.
- The organization has developed a vision statement that communicates the organization's future direction and desired results.
- The mission statement is widely understood, agreed on, and communicated by the board, staff, volunteers, constituents, and community.
- The strategic plan sets goals and measurable objectives that address identified critical issues for the next 3 to 5 years.
- The plan establishes an evaluation process and performance indicators to measure progress toward the achievement of goals and objectives.
- Through work plans, human and financial resources are allocated to ensure the accomplishment of the goals in a timely fashion.

Board Functions

- The organization has completed a formal review of its current board profile and has identified deficiencies.
- Board members serve without payment unless the agency has a policy identifying reimbursable out-of-pocket expenses.

- Board members are accessible to stakeholders and to staff (volunteer and paid).
- The board members receive orientation, regular training, and information about their responsibilities. Orientation includes information on the organization's mission, bylaws, policies, practices, and programs, as well as board members' governance roles and responsibilities as board members.
- Each board has a board operations manual that summarizes responsibilities (including job descriptions for officers) and operation procedures. This manual includes a copy of the organization's bylaws.
- The number of current board members is consistent with what is required in the bylaws or state statutes.
- The board reviews the bylaws on at least an annual basis. Bylaws should clearly state the organization's purpose, service area, defined members, defined board of directors, specific meeting guidelines, defined officers, defined committees, guidelines for amending bylaws, guidelines for dissolution of the organization, and guidelines for financial and legal procedures.
- The board has developed an annual meeting calendar with tasks that routinely need to be done at specific board meetings.
- All board meetings have written agendas and materials that are given to the board in advance of the meetings. Board reports and minutes are recorded and action taken on the minutes of all meetings.
- The board takes the leadership role in fundraising and financial management.
- The board oversees the annual audit and uses it to strengthen the organization's financial policies.
- The board prepares a budget (based on a recommendation from the executive director, if one exists) that allocates funds to the major priorities identified in the strategic plan of the organization.
- The board reviews monthly reports of expenditures and revenues.

Financial Management

- A financial plan has been developed to ensure financial stability for 3 to 4 years and is consistent with the organization's strategic plan.
- The current budget information is used as a base for future budgeting and board meetings.
- The organization has a cash operating reserve of at least 90 days.
- The organization follows accounting practices that conform to accepted standards and fulfill Internal Revenue Service requirements.
- The organization has an ongoing training program for staff and board members that addresses how to read, interpret, and use the organization's financial statements.

- The organization has documented a set of internal controls, including the handling of cash and deposits and approval of spending and disbursements.
- The organization develops an annual comprehensive operating budget that includes all expenses and revenue sources for all programs. The budget is reviewed and approved by the board of directors.
- The board of directors reviews assets and liabilities every 12 months to determine if the organization has enough liquidity.
- There is a 5-year capital expenditures plan that is updated annually.
- There are written policies stating who can authorize debt.
- The organization monitors unit costs of programs and services through the documentation of staff time and direct expenses and use of a process for allocation of management and general fund-raising expenses.
- The organization reconciles all cash accounts monthly.

Human Resources

- The board has a nominating process that ensures that the board remains appropriately diverse with respect to ethnicity, gender, economic status, culture, disabilities, age, skills and expertise.
- Volunteers are viewed as nonsalaried personnel.
- Job descriptions have been developed for volunteer positions.
- There are written policies for and about volunteers.
- Written job descriptions have been developed for each volunteer work assignment.
- The organization follows nondiscriminatory hiring practices.
- The organization has a timely process for filling vacant positions to prevent an interruption of program services or disruption to organization operations.

Leadership and Management Effectiveness

- The executive director regularly meets with staff to discuss both financial and nonfinancial information.
- The organization is guided by sound business principles.
- Leadership has the courage to embrace change.
- The organization uses its resources efficiently.
- Key management possess leadership and management skills.
- Patterns of organizational communication promote effectiveness.

Physical and Technological Resources

- List physical assets.
- Describe office space.
- Describe computer and telecommunication capabilities.

Outcome Measurement and Evaluation

- Stakeholders are involved in the evaluation process.
- The evaluation includes a review of the organizational programs and systems to ensure that they comply with the organization's mission, values, and goals.
- Periodically the organization conducts a comprehensive evaluation of its programs.
- A plan has been developed to clearly communicate the importance of outcome measurement to all important members of the public, including staff (volunteers and paid staff).
- The organization has selected the outcomes that are important to measure.
- Data sources for the outcome indicators have been identified.
- Data collection methods have been designed.
- Data collection instruments and procedures have been pretested and are valid and reliable.
- The outcome measurement process has been monitored.
- The data have been analyzed.
- Findings are used to guide budgets and resource allocations.
- Findings are presented regularly to the board to help board members focus on programmatic issues.
- Findings are used to communicate program results to stakeholders.

Program Planning, Development, and Implementation

- The organization has a program planning process in place that includes stakeholders.
- Each program has a program plan written that includes program goals, objectives, specific activities, timeline for each activity, responsible individuals, and outcome and evaluation measures.
- The organization has developed programs that inform, educate, and involve the public.
- The organization has developed a formal process to identify and expand its most effective and needed programs.
- A timeline for major implementation steps has been completed.
- The planning process identifies the critical issues facing the organization.

Reference

Lewis, A. (2000). *Nonprofit organizational assessment tool*. Retrieved July 2, 2003, from http://www.uwex.edu/li/learner/assessment.htm

Appendix E

Hazardous Environmental Agents, Routes of Entry, and Symptoms

Metals

Arsenic

Routes of entry: Ingestion, inhalation, and permeation of skin or mucous membranes.

Symptoms: Burning lips, throat constriction, and dysphagia, followed by excruciating abdominal pain, hemorrhagic gastritis, gastroenteritis, severe nausea, projectile vomiting, profuse "rice-water–like" diarrhea, with hypovolemia, resulting in hypotension and an irregular pulse. Muscle cramps, facial edema, bronchitis, dyspnea, chest pain, dehydration, intense thirst, and fluid-electrolyte disturbances are also common. A garlic-like odor of the breath and feces may occur. Hypotension and tachycardia are common early signs. Fever and tachypnea may occur.

Arsine

Routes of entry: Inhalation or through cuts and breaks in the skin.

Symptoms: Acute poisoning causes severe vomiting and diarrhea, muscular cramps, facial edema, and cardiac abnormalities. Shock is also possible. Chronic arsine exposure can affect the skin, respiratory tract, heart, liver, kidneys, blood and blood-producing organs, and the nervous system. Death may occur quickly following a massive or concentrated exposure.

Beryllium

Routes of entry: Inhalation, ingestion, or skin contact.

Symptoms: Pulmonary and systemic granulomatous disease. Nodular skin lesions in patients with chronic beryllium disease. Acute chemical pneumonitis, tracheobronchitis, conjunctivitis, dermatitis, and chronic granulomatous pulmonary disease with systemic manifestations. Acute beryllium disease consists of respiratory tract irritation and dermatitis, sometimes with conjunctivitis. Respiratory tract symptoms range from mild nasopharyngitis to a severe chemical pulmonitis that may be fatal.

Cadmium

Routes of entry: Ingestion or inhalation of dust or fumes.

Symptoms: Acute poisoning after inhalation results in chest pain, cough (with bloody sputum), difficulty breathing, sore throat, "metal fume fever" (shivering, sweating, body pains, headache), dizziness, irritability, weakness, nausea, vomiting, diarrhea, tracheobronchitis, pneumonitis, and pulmonary edema. After acute ingestion, symptoms include abdominal pain, burning sensation, nausea, vomiting, salivation, muscle cramps, vertigo, shock, unconsciousness and convulsions. Chronic exposure (by inhalation or ingestion) results in kidney damage, gastrointestinal symptoms, loss of sense of smell, nasal discharge, nose and throat irritation, lack of appetite, weight loss, nausea, tooth discoloration, bone defects, liver damage, anemia, pulmonary emphysema, chronic bronchitis, bronchopneumonia, and death.

Chromium

Routes of entry: Inhalation, ingestion, or skin absorption.

Symptoms: Irritation to the upper respiratory tract, severe nasal irritation. Ingestion of hexavalent chromium may cause intense gastrointestinal irritation or ulceration and corrosion, epigastric pain, nausea, vomiting, diarrhea, vertigo, fever, muscle cramps, hemorrhagic diathesis, toxic nephritis, renal failure, intravascular hemolysis, circulatory collapse, peripheral vascular collapse, liver damage, acute multisystem shock, coma, and even death, depending on the dose.

Lead

Routes of entry: Inhalation or ingestion of dust.

Symptoms: Acute exposure produces symptoms in the nervous, hematologic, renal, gastrointestinal, and cardiovascular systems. Symptoms include anorexia, vomiting, malaise, and convulsions; may cause permanent brain damage and reversible renal injury.

Mercury

Routes of entry: Vapor inhalation or skin absorption.

Symptoms: Weakness, chills, metallic taste, nausea, vomiting, abdominal pain, diarrhea, headache, visual disturbances, dyspnea, cough, and chest tightness. Chronic mercury exposure may cause rashes and corneal and lens changes with visual impairment.

Nickel

Route of entry: Inhalation of dust or fumes.
Symptoms: Asthma, urticaria, erythema multiforme, contact dermatitis, and hand eczema. Acute toxicity from nickel inhalation includes sore throat and hoarseness.

Zinc Oxide

Route of entry: Inhalation of dust or fumes.
Symptoms: Metal fume fever (zinc chills, brass founder's ague, etc.) from the inhalation of zinc oxide fumes. Fever, chills, muscular pain, nausea, and vomiting. Tachycardia and/or dyspnea may be present.

Hydrocarbons

Benzene

Routes of entry: Vapor inhalation or skin absorption.
Symptoms: The major toxic effect is on the CNS. Symptoms include dizziness, weakness, euphoria, headache, nausea, vomiting, tightness in chest, and staggering. With severe exposure, symptoms include blurred vision, tremors, shallow and rapid respiration, ventricular dyrhythmia, paralysis, and unconsciousness. Toxicities from inhalation of benzene include irritation of conjunctiva and visual blurring, irritation of mucous membranes, dizziness, headache, unconsciousness, convulsions, tremors, ataxia, delirium, tightness in chest, irreversible brain damage with cerebral atrophy, fatigue, vertigo, dyspnea, respiratory arrest, cardiac failure and ventricular arrhythmias, leukopenia, anemia, thrombocytopenia, petechiae, blood dyscrasia, leukemia, bone marrow aplasia, death, and fatty degeneration and necrosis of heart, liver, and adrenal glands.

Toluene

Routes of entry: Vapor inhalation or skin absorption.
Symptoms: Irritation of eyes and upper respiratory tract, dizziness, headache, anesthesia, and respiratory arrest. Liquid also irritates eyes; if aspirated, causes coughing, gagging, distress, and rapidly developing

pulmonary edema. If ingested, causes vomiting, griping, diarrhea, and depressed respiration. Kidney and liver damage may follow ingestion. Toluene embryopathy is characterized by microcephaly, central nervous system dysfunction, attention deficits and hyperactivity, developmental delay with greater language deficits, minor craniofacial and limb anomalies, and variable growth deficiency.

Xylene

Routes of entry: Vapor inhalation or skin absorption.

Symptoms: Vapor irritates eyes and mucous membranes and may cause dizziness, headache, nausea, and mental confusion. Liquid irritates eyes and mucous membranes. Swallowing or absorption through skin causes poisoning. Prolonged exposure to skin contact may result in dermatitis. Repeated, prolonged exposure to fumes may produce conjunctivitis of the eye and dryness of the nose, throat, and skin. Direct liquid contact may result in flaky or moderate dermatitis. Inhalation of vapors may cause CNS excitation, then depression, characterized by paresthesia, tremors, apprehension, impaired memory, weakness, nervous irritation, vertigo, headache, anorexia, nausea, and flatulence, and can lead to anemia and mucosal hemorrhage.

Formaldehyde

Route of entry: Inhalation.

Symptoms: Conjunctivitis, corneal burns, brownish discoloration of skin, dermatitis, urticaria (hives), pustulovesicular eruption. Inhalation results in rhinitis and anosmia (loss of sense of smell), pharyngitis, laryngospasm; tracheitis and bronchitis, pulmonary edema, cough, chest tightness, dypsnea (difficult breathing), headache, weakness, palpitation (rapid heart beat), gastroenteritis (inflammation of the stomach and intestines), burning in mouth and esophagus, nausea and vomiting, abdominal pain, diarrhea, vertigo (dizziness), unconsciousness, jaundice, albuminuria, hematuria, anuria, acidosis, convulsions.

Trichloroethylene

Routes of entry: Ingestion, inhalation, or skin exposure.

Symptoms: Acute inhalation produces rapid coma and may result in death.

Carbon Disulfide

Routes of entry: Vapor inhalation or skin absorption.

Symptoms: Conjunctivitis, epithelial hyperplasia of cornea, and eczematous inflammation of eyelids.

Ethylene Oxide

Route of entry: Inhalation.
Symptoms: Nausea, vomiting, neurological disorders, and death.

Polychlorinated Diphenyls

Routes of entry: Inhalation, ingestion, or skin absorption.
Symptoms: Abdominal pain, anorexia, nausea, vomiting, jaundice, rare cases of coma and death. Neurological symptoms, such as headache, dizziness, depression, nervousness. Other symptoms, such as fatigue, loss of weight, loss of libido, and muscle and joint pains.

Gases

Ammonia

Route of entry: Inhalation.
Symptoms: Vapors cause irritation of eyes and respiratory tract. Contact with skin can cause burns and vesication. If systemic absorption becomes extensive, coma may occur, preceded by hypertonic contractions and convulsions.

Hydrochloric Acid

Routes of entry: Inhalation or skin absorption.
Symptoms: Inhalation of hydrochloric acid fumes produces nose, throat, and laryngeal burning and irritation; pain and inflammation; coughing; sneezing; choking; hoarseness; dyspnea; bronchitis; chest pain; laryngeal spasms and upper respiratory tract edema; headache; and palpitations. Contact with fumes or liquid can produce corrosive burns. Dermal exposure also results in irritation, pain, dermatitis, and ulceration. Contact with refrigerated liquid can produce frostbite. Eye contact with fumes is extremely irritating. Contact with liquid produces pain, swelling, conjunctivitis, corneal erosion, and necrosis of conjunctiva and corneal epithelium, with perforation or scarring.

Hydrofluoric Acid

Routes of entry: Inhalation, ingestion, or contact (skin, eyes) with vapors or dusts.

Symptoms: Irritation of eyes, nose, and throat; pulmonary edema; skin and eye burns; nasal congestion; and bronchitis.

Sulfur Dioxide

Routes of entry: Inhalation or direct contact with skin or mucous membrane.

Symptoms: Acute symptoms include respiratory tract irritation, cough, burning, lacrimation, conjunctival injection, difficulty in swallowing, and oropharyngeal erythema after substantial exposure. Vomiting, diarrhea, abdominal pain, fever, headache, vertigo, agitation, tremor, convulsions, and peripheral neuritis may also be experienced.

Chlorine

Route of entry: Inhalation.

Symptoms: Burning of eyes, nose, and mouth; lacrimation; rhinorrhea; coughing; choking and substernal pain; nausea; vomiting; headache; dizziness; syncope; pulmonary edema; pneumonia; hypoxemia; dermatitis; eye and skin burns.

Ozone

Route of entry: Inhalation.
Symptoms: Irritation of eye, nose, throat, and skin.

Nitrogen Oxides

Route of entry: Inhalation.
Symptoms: Usually no symptoms occur at the time of exposure, with the exception of a slight cough, fatigue, and nausea. Fatigue, uneasiness, restlessness, cough, hyperpnea, and dyspnea appear insidiously, with adult respiratory distress syndrome developing gradually.

Asphyxiants

Carbon Monoxide

Route of entry: Inhalation.
Symptoms: Rapidly fatal cases of carbon monoxide poisoning are characterized by congestion and hemorrhages in all organs. Headache, dizziness, and blurred vision.

Hydrogen Sulfide

Route of entry: Inhalation.

Symptoms: Eye irritation, painful conjunctivitis, photophobia, tearing, and corneal opacity. Respiratory symptoms include rhinitis with anosmia, tracheobronchitis, pulmonary edema. Death from rapid respiratory paralysis.

Cyanide

Routes of entry: Inhalation of vapor or aerosol, skin absorption.

Symptoms: Massive doses can produce a sudden loss of consciousness and prompt death from respiratory arrest without warning. Ingestion can produce a bitter, acrid, burning taste, followed by a feeling of constriction or numbness in the throat. Salivation, nausea, and vomiting are common. Anxiety, confusion, vertigo, giddiness, and often a sensation of stiffness in the lower jaw. Hyperpnea and dyspnea. Odor of bitter almonds may be noted on the breath or vomitus. A bright pink coloration of the skin due to high concentrations of oxyhemoglobin in the venous return may be confused with that of carbon monoxide poisoning. The skin color appears red. Death from respiratory arrest.

Pesticides

Organophosphates (e.g., parathion)

Routes of entry: Inhalation, ingestion, or skin absorption.

Symptoms: Headache, giddiness, nervousness, blurred vision, weakness, nausea, cramps, diarrhea, and discomfort in the chest. Sweating, miosis, tearing, salivation, and other excessive respiratory tract secretion, vomiting, cyanosis, papilledema, uncontrollable muscle twitches followed by muscular weakness, convulsions, coma, loss of reflexes, and loss of sphincter control. Cardiac arrhythmias, various degrees of heart block, and cardiac arrest may occur. Acute emphysema, pulmonary edema, pink froth in the trachea and bronchi, and considerable congestion of the organs are found at autopsy.

References

Environmental Defense. (2003). *Scorecard: About the chemicals.* Retrieved July 2, 2003, from http://www.scorecard.org/chemical-profiles/

Environmental Protection Agency. (2003). *Green book: Nonattainment areas for critical pollutants.* Retrieved July 2, 2003, at http://www.epa.gov/air/oaqps/greenbk/

Helvie, C. (1998). *Advanced practice nursing in the community.* Thousand Oaks, CA: Sage.

Appendix F

Integrated Community Assessment Process and Tool

The Integrated Community Assessment Process

Phase I: Data Collection. Primary and secondary data collection are used to identify community assets and needs. Data are collected for each component's area of inquiry. Behavioral assessment, public health agency, and environmental assessment data sources are tapped.

Phase II: Data Analysis. A comprehensive review, critique, and analysis of all data are completed to develop a list of assets, deficits, or needs.

Phase III: Community Diagnosis. Health-care assets, deficits, and needs, as identified through data collection and analysis, are listed.

Phase IV: Proposed Multilevel Community Interventions. Recommendations based on community assets and deficits are made for identified concerns.

Phase V: Report. An oral and written report on the community assessment is disseminated to key community stakeholders.

Phase VI: Evaluation. The community assessment process is evaluated.

The Integrated Community Assessment Tool

Phase I: Data Collection

Part I. Community Description

Instructions: Provide a general, broad-based description of the community that includes what you know about the geographical area, population demographics, political factors, community resources and institutions, and environment. From this information, describe what population group constitutes the defining characteristics of the community. This description should provide clear, defining boundaries of the population and the community being assessed.

Part II. Windshield Survey (Primary Data Collection)

Conduct the windshield survey at various times of the day and night. List community assets and deficits noted during the windshield survey. Secondary data can cover areas of inquiry unanswered during the windshield survey.

Components	Areas of Inquiry	Assets	Deficits
Housing	What is age, type of architecture, material of construction for the homes? How are houses spaced? What is the condition of housing? Do housing conditions vary in certain areas of the community? If so, how?		
Zoning	What is the political district? What is the parish or county seat? What are the zip codes? What is the police or fire district?		
Use of space	How is the land used (open space, residential, agricultural, commercial or industrial)? What is the quality of the land space (flowers, road condition, condition of lawns)? Is open space public or private? Who is using the open space? Are there any national geographical boundaries (rivers, mountains)? Are any landfills or waste management centers present? Is there any evidence of pollution (air, water, rodents)?		
Boundaries	Do signs indicate the community boundaries? How are the boundaries determined—natural or political, economic, cultural, or ethnic? What is the official and unofficial name of the community? Are there any clear boundaries identified according to race or ethnicity or urban, suburban, or rural boundaries? Is there evidence of different subgroups within the community, cultural or racial?		
Common areas	Where are people gathering? Do the gathering places differ by age, sex, socioeconomic status, or other factors? Are common areas territorial or open to strangers? What is the distribution of the common areas in the community?		

(Continued)

453

Components	Areas of Inquiry	Assets	Deficits
Transportation	What are the major sources of transportation, public and private? What is the condition of the transportation system and roads? Do street names reveal history or other community characteristics? Are appropriate safety precautions evident for the respective modes of transportation?		
Service centers	What types of service centers exist? Are there social agencies, health facilities, recreation centers, and school activity evident?		
Stores	What types of shopping centers exist? Where do residents shop? Is there a difference in the types of stores available in different neighborhoods in the community? What kinds of goods and services are available to local residents?		
Street scene	Who do you see on the streets, what types of people? What is the street activity like? Are the people typical of people you would expect to see on the streets at the time you see them? Are the people clothed as you would expect? If not, how do they differ from what you expected? Do you see animals, such as stray cats or dogs? What warning signage is present?		
Community growth and dynamics	Do you see signs of community growth, such as real estate signs, new construction (home and industrial), remodeling, or street repair? Do you see signs of community decline such as trash, abandoned cars, blighted housing, real estate signs? If so, are these signs concentrated in certain areas? Is there evidence of graffiti? If so, what is the meaning and significance of the graffiti?		

(Continued)

Components	Areas of Inquiry	Assets	Deficits
Race and ethnicity	What do you feel are the racial characteristics of the people (genetic characteristics, skin color, hair type)? What evidence do you see of the ethnic characteristics of the people (food stores, churches, private schools, information in a language other than English)?		
Religion	What are the major religious churches? Where are they located in the community? Do you see evidence of religious homogeneity or heterogeneity? Do you see religious institutions associated with other agencies (schools, community centers)?		
Politics	Do you see any political campaign posters? What are the political party affiliations? Which seems predominant?		
Media	Do you see TV antennas or TV station advertisements? What local magazines or newspapers are available to the residents? Which media seem most important to residents (radio, TV, print)?		
Community personality	How does the community affect your senses (sight, hearing, smell, feeling)? Does the community create a good feeling or uncomfortable feeling? Why? Did the local residents interact with you? If so, how? What is the local dialect? What languages are spoken? Which is predominant?		

Part III. Community Data Collection (Primary and Secondary Data Collection)

Collect existing data for each of the areas of inquiry. Potential data sources are identified.

Components	Areas of Inquiry	Data Source	Assets	Deficits
History of the community	What was the settlement date of the community? What were the nationalities of the initial settlers? Who were they? What important events or factors affect the development of the community? Who were the important persons in the growth of the community?	Chamber of Commerce Library Maps Government documents Local historical societies Museums Interviews and focus groups		
Population profile	What is the population density? What are the community demographics? What is the population of the community? How does it vary by census area? What is the age, gender, and racial distribution? What social classes are represented in the community? What are the demographic shifts occurring in the community (in-migration and out-migration)? To and from where? What family types (single parent, nuclear, extended, nontraditional, same sex) exist? Which type predominates? How do family types differ throughout the area? Average family size? Number of children in foster care? What child rearing practices are predominant? What ethnic or cultural groups exist within the community? Does the community have refugee or migrant populations? What are housing and utility costs? What are the marriage and divorce rates? What are the birth rates?	U.S. Census Local library Real estate office Chamber of commerce City government Local ethnic and cultural centers State office of public health		
Transportation system	What are the major highways that make the community accessible? How do people travel within the community (taxi, bus, train, airplane, private car, volunteer transportation, bicycle)? Does the cost of transportation affect community members?	Chamber of commerce Library Regional transportation authority Bus and train stations Social service agencies Interviews and focus groups		

(Continued)

Components	Areas of Inquiry	Data Source	Assets	Deficits
Economic system	What occupations (retail, industrial, farming, service, government, tourism, unemployed) are represented in the community? Which ones predominate? What is the relationship between occupations and lifestyles? Do people work within or commute out of the community for employment? Is unemployment a current, past, continuing, or occasional problem for the community? How do industries influence local life? What is the industrial or economic base that supports the growth of the community? Is the economic base remaining stable or decreasing? What is the tax base of the community? What are typical (median, average) income levels of persons living within the community?	Chamber of commerce Local businesses Industries Unemployment office Social service agencies Department of Labor		
Protective systems (police)	What are the crime statistics? What are the predominant types of crimes? What is the geographic distribution of crimes? What are the full-time and part-time police workforce statistics? Are these numbers adequate? What is the police response time? Do the police have adequate equipment and training? Does the community support the department financially? Does the police department sponsor crime prevention programs? What are they? Are there security systems in the houses? Are there bars on the windows? Are there private police control programs in certain neighborhoods? Do neighborhood watch programs exist? How are they coordinated and managed? What is the relationship between the police department and the emergency medical system? Is there universal police signage in the community?	Police department Legal or court system Neighborhood associations Emergency medical system Interviews and focus groups		

(Continued)

Components	Areas of Inquiry	Data Source	Assets	Deficits
Protective systems (fire)	What are the fire statistics in the community? What are the predominant types of fires and their causes in the community? What is the geographic distribution of fires? What is the composition of the fire department workforce: full-time, part-time, volunteer firemen? Are these numbers adequate? What is the fire department response time? Does the department have adequate equipment and training? Does the community support the department financially? Is there a central water supply for fire fighting? Does the department offer fire prevention education? What methods or programs are used? Are there any universal signals used for fire and rescue (e.g., children's bedrooms have special signs)?	Fire department Neighborhood associations Emergency medical system Interviews and focus groups		
Protective systems (emergency health)	What are the predominant situations to which emergency medical systems (EMS) respond in the community? How many full-time, part-time, and volunteer personnel does the EMS department have? Is there a communitywide EMS system (911)? What is the response time? Does the department have adequate equipment and training to do the job? Are the ambulances up to date? How is the EMS system activated? Does the community support the department financially? Does EMS sponsor education and safety programs? Does the community have an emergency disaster plan? Who is responsible for it? What types of emergencies does it address? Has it been used? If so, how did it work?	Police department Fire department Emergency medical system departments Hospital emergency departments Interviews and focus groups		
Food supply systems	What types of restaurants are within the community? What are the menu selections (ethnic, healthy)? How often do people in the community tend to eat out?	Local stores Social service agencies Volunteer groups		

(Continued)

Components	Areas of Inquiry	Data Source	Assets	Deficits
	What grocery stores (chain or locally owned), specialty food stores, and fresh or locally grown sources are available in the community? Does the cost of food affect the availability of food or certain types of food? Are there food supply programs for persons unable to afford, purchase, or prepare their own food? Do you see evidence of differences in diet preferences among community subgroups? What are these differences? What is the typical diet regimen?	Churches Interviews and focus groups		
Religious and ethnic groups	What religious groups exist? What belief systems are represented? What are the ethnic groups' influences? How significant is the role of religion or ethnicity in the community? How many people in the community have church or religious affiliations? What is the average size of congregations for these religious affiliations? What are the churches' associations with national affiliations? What is the relationship between religion and health beliefs? How is death typically managed? What rituals, burial rites, or resources are used to manage the care of deceased persons? Are there subgroups within the community in which death is handled in a different manner than the methods used by the majority of the community? What are these?	Local clergy Religious representatives Telephone book Church directories Local funeral home directors Religious groups and organizations Census data Interviews and focus groups		
Community culture	What are predominant cultural beliefs? Are these representative of the entire community? What cultural groupings are there in the community? How significant is the role of culture in the community? What are the intercultural and intracultural variations? What are the cultural values and beliefs	Clergy Ethnic leaders Religious organizations Census data Interviews and focus groups Local newspaper		

(Continued)

Components	Areas of Inquiry	Data Source	Assets	Deficits
	about health, wellness, health care, research, family, and parenting? Does the community have planned cultural events such as blessings of boats, crops, fairs, festivals?			
Educational systems	How many schools (public or private) exist for each grade level? If education beyond high school is not available in the community, what schools are accessible within the region? How many students (adults and children) attend the schools? What are the average daily attendance, graduation rates, and drop-out rates? Are particular populations at risk? What are the standardized national examination test scores? What are the average class size and student-teacher ratio? What types of programs do schools offer, curricular and extracurricular? What is the utilization of these programs? How are the programs paid for? Are there special programs for adults? What recreational activities are there? Do schools offer advanced placement or programs for gifted children? What percentage of students pursues a college education? What types of vocational options are available? How do schools address special education needs of children (e.g., learning disabled, hearing impaired, visually impaired, children needing to learn English as a second language)? Is there a comprehensive school health program? Is there a school nurse? What are the responsibilities of the school nurse? What is the school or student-to-school-nurse ratio? Who pays the school nurse's salary? What are the significant health needs, concerns, or issues of students in the school system? What community agencies are involved in meeting the	Board of education office Local school principal School nurse and health curriculum Telephone directory Census data School records School reports Interviews and focus groups		

(Continued)

Components	Areas of Inquiry	Data Source	Assets	Deficits
	needs of students in the school or school-age population of the community? What state and federally funded programs based on economic needs are the schools in your community eligible to receive? What are the eligibility requirements for these programs? What is the prevailing educational level of adults in the community? How valued is education by members of the community?			
Health-care systems	What western-type (allopathic) health-care facilities, programs, and personnel are available? Who is available within the community to provide western-type health care (physicians, nurses, dentists, psychologists, physical therapists, other)? What hospitals are used by community members? Which is the closest? What kinds of inpatient care are available? What kinds of outpatient services are available? What emergency and urgent-care facilities are included within or easily accessible to the community? What extended-care facilities are included within or easily accessible to the community? What residential care facilities are included within or easily accessible to the community? Is there a hospice program? What agency(s) provides these services? Who is eligible to use these services? Are respite and adult day-care services available? Who provides them? What official health department services and programs are conducted within the community? What is the relationship between the public health department and other health-care services? How is prevention and monitoring of communicable disease managed within the community? How are environmental and	Telephone book Local physicians' offices Local care providers Public health officials Census data Community resource book		

(Continued)

461

Components	Areas of Inquiry	Data Source	Assets	Deficits
	sanitation problems addressed? What services to mothers and children are provided through official agency programs? What programs are available for people with special problems such as AIDS and other chronic diseases? What traditional health-care facilities, programs, and personnel exist within the community (e.g., folk healers or practitioners, spiritual healers)? Is there evidence that eastern-type medicine, such as acupuncture, acupressure, and meditation, is used by community members? Do members of the community rely on folk or home remedies? What are they? Are there veterinarians for animal care? What kinds of animals play a role in community life? How do animals affect the well-being of community members? What are the primary health-care payment sources? What resources are available for indigent health care? What are the uninsured and underinsured rates? Do those who live in the community perceive barriers to health care? What health education programs are available? Who provides the programs? What health-care issues have been addressed recently? Who pays for these programs? What self-help or mutual assistance programs exist?			
Communication systems	What newspapers (local or regional) are read by community members? What radio stations are available for entertainment or information? What TV stations (local, regional, national, cable) are used as a source of entertainment or information? Are community bulletin boards used to share information or buy and sell goods and services? Where are they located? Do you see displays and posters in stores	Local radio stations Local newspaper office TV stations Library Interviews and focus groups		

(Continued)

Components	Areas of Inquiry	Data Source	Assets	Deficits
	that provide information about life in the community? What libraries (general use or specialty type) are available? How many people use library services, and what kinds of services does the library provide? What informal communication systems (gossip centers) do you identify in the community? What are the patterns of communication (horizontal and vertical communication)? Who are the major advertisers within the community?			
Governmental and political systems	What are the political parties in the community? What political parties dominate decision making in the community? How politically organized and active is the community? What are the political processes used? What issues have most affected the community in recent years (housing, transportation, health, water and sewage, police and fire, group homes, other)? What government structure exists in the community? What are the major public health policies that have been developed that are specific to this community? Evaluate the community budget to determine governmental priorities.	Library Local campaign information Local political headquarters City or town hall Newspapers Billboards Interviews and focus groups		
Recreational systems	Does the community have any recreational programs? Are there any recreational parks nearby? What recreational activities do community members take part in? Are there any movie theaters in the community? Are there any health and fitness clubs in the community? Are there any senior citizen recreational programs available for members of the community? What are the primary hobbies of the citizens? What is the number of walking tracts or	Local health department Parks and recreational services Telephone book Community resource book Interviews and focus groups		

(Continued)

Components	Areas of Inquiry	Data Source	Assets	Deficits
	neighborhood fitness trails? Are there community pools, baseball fields, and basketball courts? What is the percentage of people who exercise? Are there bars or local clubs? How many? What types? Where are they located?			
Environmental systems	What environmental issues (personal or industrial) affect community life? What agencies, policies, or programs affect environmental issues in the community? What is the source of the water supply? Are sources adequate for current and future use? How is the water supply tested and maintained free from contamination? What are the waste management systems (sanitation systems, trash removal, recycling programs and facilities, landfills, cost, industrial, hazardous waste)? Does the disposal of waste constitute an economic or environmental concern for the community? What is the air quality? Are there contaminants (natural, industrial, energy-production related, or transportation related) that affect the community? How is air quality monitored? What energy sources are used by the community (gas, electric, nuclear, or other)? Does the cost or availability of energy affect individual consumers or industrial growth? How does the community provide for low-income persons who cannot pay for adequate energy supplies? Does the community have or need vector control programs (insects, rodents, mosquitoes, other)? What is the topography of the land? Are there potential environmental hazards such as rivers that may flood, hills with potential for rock slides? What is the climate (average temperature, precipitation)?	National weather service Local newspaper TV stations Environmental Protection Agency Local health department Sanitation or environmental engineer Interviews and focus groups		

(Continued)

Components	Areas of Inquiry	Data Source	Assets	Deficits
Health status and wellness	What are the major causes of morbidity and mortality, by age, race, and gender? What is the infant mortality rate? What is the perinatal mortality rate? What is the maternal mortality rate? What are the common communicable diseases and their rates? What is the percentage of low-birth-weight infants? How adequate is prenatal care? What are the types of disability? What is the level of tobacco, alcohol, and drug use? Types of drugs used? What are the major biological and psychological health problems and concerns that exist? What is the average life expectancy for males and females? What is the teen pregnancy rate? What is the level of domestic violence (child abuse, elder abuse, intimate partner abuse)? What are the major acute illnesses? Are they seasonal? What are the major chronic illnesses?	State health report card *Morbidity and Mortality Weekly Report* Local health department Census data Local hospital data		
Community-based associations	What are the trade and labor, professional, neighborhood, religious, and special interest associations within the community? What is the mission of these associations? What services are provided by each association?	Community resource book Local health department Telephone directory Interviews and focus groups		
Community-based institutions	What are the community-based institutions within the community (institutions immersed within the community to meet the community's needs), such as community-based AIDS service organizations? What is the mission of these institutions? What services are provided by these institutions? What is the power base of the institutions?	Community resource book Telephone directory Interviews and focus groups		

Phase II: Data Analysis

Analysis of Windshield Survey

Assets	Deficits	Potential Interventions
1.	1.	1.
2.	2.	2.
3.	3.	3.

Focus Group Thematic Analysis (Community Constituents, Community Leaders)

Assets	Deficits	Potential Interventions
1.	1.	1.
2.	2.	2.
3.	3.	3.

Interview Thematic Analysis (Community Constituents, Community Leaders)

Assets	Deficits	Possible Interventions
1.	1.	1.
2.	2.	2.
3.	3.	3.

Analysis of Community Assessment Data Components (Data from Phase I, Part II)

Assets	Deficits	Possible Interventions
1.	1.	1.
2.	2.	2.
3.	3.	3.

Phase III: Community Diagnosis

List community asset and diagnosis statements. These statements provide direction for the evaluation of community interventions.

Community Diagnosis Statement

[Community deficit or problem] related to [potential causes or associated factors] as evidenced by [community assessment data].

Community Assets Statement

[Community asset] promotes a healthy community, as evidenced by [outcomes of community asset].

Phase IV: Proposed Multilevel Community-Level Interventions

Interventions should be proposed that relate to community diagnosis and community asset statements.

Assets	Interventions for Expansion of Assets
1.	1.
2.	2.
3.	3.

Assets	Interventions for Expansion of Assets
1.	1.
2.	2.
3.	3.

Phase V: Report

Narrative community action plan is developed with appropriate objectives, interventions, and methods of evaluation identified and a timeline provided.

Community Diagnosis or Asset Statement	Oojective	Interventions	Timeline	Evaluation Method

Phase VI: Evaluation

Evaluate each community assessment process.

Reference

Krieger, N., & Harton, M. (1992). Community health assessment tool: A pattern approach to data collection and diagnosis. *Journal of Community Health Nursing, 9*, 229-234.

Appendix G

Chronological List of Public Health Laws

1902: P.L. 57-244, Biologics Control Act
1906: P.L. 59-384, Pure Food and Drug Act (also known as Wiley Act)
1920: P.L. 66-141, Snyder Act
1921: P.L. 67-97, Maternity and Infancy Act (also known as Sheppard-Towner Act)
1935: P.L. 74-271, Social Security Act
1936: P.L. 74-846, Walsh-Healy Act
1937: P.L. 75-244, National Cancer Institute Act
1938: P.L. 75-540, LaFollette-Bulwinkle Act; P.L. 75-717, Food, Drug and Cosmetic Act
1939: P.L. 76-19, Reorganization Act
1941: P.L. 77-146, Nurse Training Act
1944: P.L. 78-410, Public Health Service Act
1945: P.L. 79-15, McCarran-Ferguson Act
1946: P.L. 79-487, National Mental Health Act; P.L. 79-725, Hospital Survey and Construction Act (also known as Hill-Burton Act)
1948: P.L. 80-655, National Health Act; P.L. 80-845, Water Pollution Control Act
1952: P.L. 82-414, Immigration and Nationality Act (also known as McCarran-Walter Act)
1954: P.L. 83-482, Medical Facilities Survey and Construction Act; P.L. 83-703, Atomic Energy Act
1955: P.L. 84-159, Air Pollution Control Act; P.L. 84-377, Polio Vaccination Assistance Act
1956: P.L. 84-569, Dependents Medical Care Act; P.L. 84-652, National Health Survey Act; P.L. 84-660, Water Pollution Control Act Amendments of 1956; P.L. 84-911, Health Amendments Act
1958: P.L. 85-544, Grants-in-aid to Schools of Public Health; P.L. 85-929, Food Additive Amendment
1959: P.L. 86-121, Indian Sanitation Facilities Act; P.L. 86-352, Federal Employees Health Benefits Act
1960: P.L. 86-778, Social Security Amendments (also known as Kerr-Mills Act)

1962: P.L. 87-692, Health Services for Agricultural Migratory Workers Act; P.L. 87-781, Drug Amendments (also known as Kefauver-Harris amendments)

1963: P.L. 88-129, Health Professions Educational Assistance Act; P.L. 88-156, Maternal and Child Health and Mental Retardation Planning Amendments; P.L. 88-164, Mental Retardation Facilities and Community Mental Health Centers Construction Act; P.L. 88-206, Clean Air Act

1964: P.L. 88-443, Hospital and Medical Facilities Amendments (amended the Hill-Burton Act); P.L. 88-452, Economic Opportunity Act; P.L. 88-581, Nurse Training Act

1965: P.L. 89-4, Appalachian Redevelopment Act; P.L. 89-73, Older Americans Act; P.L. 89-92, Federal Cigarette Labeling and Advertising Act; P.L. 89-97, Social Security Amendments; P.L. 89-239, Heart Disease, Cancer and Stroke Amendments; P.L. 89-272, Clean Air Act Amendments; P.L. 89-290, Health Professions Educational Assistance Amendments

1966: P.L. 89-564, Highway Safety Act; P.L. 89-642, Child Nutrition Act; P.L. 89-749, Comprehensive Health Planning Act (also known as Partnership for Health Act); P.L. 89-751, Allied Health Professions Personnel Training Act; P.L. 89-794, Economic Opportunity Act Amendments

1967: P.L. 90-31, Mental Health Amendments; P.L. 90-148, Air Quality Act; P.L. 90-170, Mental Retardation Amendments; P.L. 90-174, Clinical Laboratory Improvement Act; P.L. 90-189, Flammable Fabrics Act; P.L. 90-248, Social Security Amendments

1968: P.L. 90-490, Health Manpower Act

1969: P.L. 91-173, Federal Coal Mine Health and Safety Act; P.L. 91-190, National Environmental Policy Act

1970: P.L. 91-222, Public Health Cigarette Smoking Act; P.L. 91-224, Water Quality Improvement Act; P.L. 91-296, Medical Facilities Construction and Modernization Amendments (amended Hill-Burton Act); P.L. 91-464, Communicable Disease Control Amendments; P.L. 91-513, Comprehensive Drug Abuse Prevention and Control Act; P.L. 91-572, Family Planning Services and Population Research Act; P.L. 91-596, Occupational Safety and Health Act; P.L. 91-601, Poison Prevention Packaging Act; P.L. 91-604, Clean Air Amendments; P.L. 91-616, Comprehensive Alcohol Abuse and Alcoholism Prevention, Treatment, and Rehabilitation Act; P.L. 91-623, Emergency Health Personnel Act; P.L. 91-695, Lead-Based Paint Poisoning Prevention Act

1971: P.L. 92-157, Comprehensive Health Manpower Training Act

1972: P.L. 92-294, National Sickle Cell Anemia Control Act; P.L. 92-303, Federal Coal Mine Health and Safety Amendments; P.L. 92-426, Uniformed Services Health Professions Revitalization Act;

P.L. 92-433, National School Lunch and Child Nutrition Amendments (amended Child Nutrition Act); P.L. 92-573, Consumer Product Safety Act; P.L. 92-574, Noise Control Act; P.L. 92-603, Social Security Amendments; P.L. 92-714, National Cooley's Anemia Control Act

1973: P.L. 93-29, Older Americans Act; P.L. 93-154, Emergency Medical Services Systems Act; P.L. 93-222, Health Maintenance Organization Act

1974: P.L. 93-247, Child Abuse Prevention and Treatment Act; P.L. 93-270, Sudden Infant Death Syndrome Act; P.L. 93-296, Research in Aging Act; P.L. 93-344, Congressional Budget and Impoundment Control Act; P.L. 93-360, Nonprofit Hospital Amendments; P.L. 93-406, Employee Retirement Income Security Act (also known as ERISA); P.L. 93-523, Safe Drinking Water Act; P.L. 93-641, National Health Planning and Resources Development Act; P.L. 93-647, Social Security Amendments (also known as Social Services Amendments)

1976: P.L. 94-295, Medical Devices Amendments; P.L. 94-317, National Consumer Health Information and Health Promotion Act; P.L. 94-437, Indian Health Care Improvement Act; P.L. 94-460, Health Maintenance Organization Amendments; P.L. 94-469, Toxic Substances Control Act (TSCA); P.L. 94-484, Health Professions Educational Assistance Act

1977: P.L. 95-142, Medicare-Medicaid Antifraud and Abuse Amendments; P.L. 95-210, Rural Health Clinic Services Amendments

1978: P.L. 95-292, Medicare End-Stage Renal Disease Amendments; P.L. 95-559, Health Maintenance Organization Amendments

1979: P.L. 96-79, Health Planning and Resources Development Amendments

1980: P.L. 96-398, Mental Health Systems Act; P.L. 96-499, Omnibus Budget Reconciliation Act (OBRA '80); P.L. 96-510, Comprehensive Environmental Response, Compensation and Liability Act (CERCLA)

1981: P.L. 97-35, Omnibus Budget Reconciliation Act (OBRA '81)

1982: P.L. 97-248, Tax Equity and Fiscal Responsibility Act (TEFRA); P.L. 97-414, Orphan Drug Act (ODA)

1983: P.L. 98-21, Social Security Amendments

1984: P.L. 98-369, Deficit Reduction Act (DEFRA); P.L. 98-417, Drug Price Competition and Patent Term Restoration Act; P.L. 98-457, Child Abuse Amendments; P.L. 98-507, National Organ Transplant Act

1985: P.L. 99-177, Emergency Deficit Reduction and Balanced Budget Act (also known as Gramm-Rudman-Hollins Act); P.L. 99-272, Consolidated Omnibus Budget Reconciliation Act (COBRA '85)

1986: P.L. 99-509, Omnibus Budget Reconciliation Act (OBRA '86); P.L. 99-660, Omnibus Health Act

1987: P.L. 100-177, National Health Service Corps Amendments; P.L. 100-203, Omnibus Budget Reconciliation Act (OBRA '87)

1988: P.L. 100-360, Medicare Catastrophic Coverage Act; P.L. 100-578, Clinical Laboratory Improvement Amendments; P.L. 100-582, Medical Waste Tracking Act; P.L. 100-607, National Organ Transplant Amendments; P.L. 100-647, Technical and Miscellaneous Revenue Act

1989: P.L. 101-239, Omnibus Budget Reconciliation Act (OBRA '89)

1990: P.L. 101-336, Americans with Disabilities Act (ADA); P.L. 101-381, Ryan White Comprehensive AIDS Resources Emergency Act (CARE); P.L. 101-508, Omnibus Budget Reconciliation Act (OBRA '90); P.L. 101-629, Safe Medical Devices Act; P.L. 101-649, Immigration and Nationality Act of 1990

1992: P.L. 102-585, Veterans Health Care Act

1993: P.L. 103-43, National Institutes of Health Revitalization Act; P.L. 103-66, Omnibus Budget Reconciliation Act (OBRA '93)

1995: P.L. 104-65, Lobbying Disclosure Act

1996: P.L. 104-134, Departments of Veterans Affairs, Housing and Urban Development, and Independent Agencies Appropriations Act; P.L. 104-191, Health Insurance Portability and Accountability Act (also known as Kassebaum-Kennedy Act); P.L. 104-193, Personal Responsibility and Work Opportunity Reconciliation Act (also known as Welfare Reform Act)

1997: P.L. 105-33, Balanced Budget Act of 1997; P.L. 105-115, Food and Drug Administration Modernization and Accountability Act

1998: P.L. 105-357, Controlled Substances Trafficking Prohibition Act; P.L. 105-369, Ricky Ray Hemophilia Relief Fund Act

1999: P.L. 106-113, Medicare, Medicaid, and SCHIP Balanced Budget Refinement Act of 1999 (BBRA); P.L. 106-117, Veterans Millennium Health Care and Benefits Act

2000: P.L. 106-354, Breast and Cervical Cancer Prevention and Treatment Act; P.L. 106-430, Needlestick and Safety Prevention Act; P.L. 106-525, Minority Health and Health Disparities Research and Education Act; P.L. 106-554, Medicare, Medicaid, and SCHIP Benefits Improvement and Protection Act of 2000 (BIPA); P.L. 106-580, National Institute of Biomedical Imaging and Bioengineering Establishment Act

2001: P.L. 107-9, Animal Disease Risk Assessment, Prevention and Control Act; P.L. 107-38, Emergency Supplemental Appropriations Act for Recovery from and Response to Terrorist Attacks on the United States

Note: Public health laws can be accessed at http://www.firstgov.gov or http://www.access.gpo.gov. P.L. = public law. The first number before the hyphen refers to the Congress that enacted the legislation. The number after the hyphen refers to the sequence in which the law was enacted. For example, P.L. 107-38 is the 38th public law enacted by the 107th Congress.

Reference

Longest, B. (2002). *Health policymaking in the United States* (3rd ed.). Washington, DC: Association of University Programs in Health Administration.

Appendix H

Institutions Concerned With Public Health

Agency for Health Care Research and Quality
2101 E. Jefferson St., Suite 501
Rockville, MD 20852
Phone: 301-594-1364
http://www.ahcpr.gov

American Medical Association
1101 Vermont Ave. NW, 12th Floor
Washington, DC 20005
Phone: 202-789-7400
http://www.ama-assn.org

American Nurses Association
600 Maryland Ave. SW, #100W
Washington, DC 20024-2571
Phone: 202-651-7000
http://www.nursingworld.org

American Public Health Association
800 I St., NW
Washington, DC 20001-3710
Phone: 202-777-2742
http://www.apha.org

Association of State and Territorial Health Officials
1275 K St., N.W., Suite 800
Washington, DC 20005
Phone: 202-371-9090
http://www.astho.org

Association of Clinicians for the Underserved
501 Darby Creek Rd., Suite 20
Lexington, KY 40509-1606
Phone: 606-263-0046
http://www.clinicians.org

Brookings Institution
1775 Massachusetts Ave. NW
Washington, DC 20036
Phone: 202-797-6302
http://www.brook.edu/

Center for the Advancement of Health
2000 Florida Ave., NW, Suite 210
Washington, DC 20009
Phone: 202-387-2829
http://www.cfah.org

Centers for Medicare and Medicaid Services (CMS)
7500 Security Boulevard
Baltimore, MD 21244
Phone: 410-786-3000
http://www.cms.hhs.gov

Center for Patient Advocacy
1350 Beverly Rd., #108
McLean, VA 22101
Phone: 800-846-7444
http://www.patientadvocacy.org

Environmental Protection Agency
Headquarters Information
Resources Center
401 M St., SW
Mailcode 3404
Washington, DC 20460
Phone: 202-260-5922
http://www.epa.gov

Food and Drug Administration
5600 Fishers Lane
Rockville, MD 20857
Phone: 888-463-6332
http://www.fda.gov/

**Health Resources and Services
Administration (HRSA)**
Information Center
P.O. Box 2910
Merrifield, VA 22116
Phone: 888-275-4772
http://www.ask.hrsa.gov

**Immunization Action
Coalition**
1573 Selby Ave.
Suite 234
St. Paul, MN 55104
Phone: 651-647-9009
http://www.immunize.org

Institute of Medicine
2101 Constitution Ave., NW
Washington, DC 20418
Phone: 202-334-2169
http://www.iom.edu

Migrant Clinicians Network
P. O. Box 164285
Austin, TX 78716
Phone: 512-327-2017
http://www.migrantclinician.org

National Alliance for Hispanic Health
1501 16th St., NW
Washington, DC 20036
Phone: 202-387-5000
http://www.hispanichealth.org

**National Association for the
Advancement of Colored People
(NAACP)**
4805 Mount Hope Dr.
Baltimore, MD 21215
Phone: 410-358-8900
http://www.naacp.org

**National Association of Community
Health Centers**
1330 New Hampshire Ave., NW
Suite 122
Washington, DC 20036
Phone: 202-659-8008
http://www.nachc.com

**National Association of County and City
Health Officials**
1100 17th St., N.W., Second Floor
Washington, DC 20036
Phone: 202-783-5550
http://www.naccho.org

National Association of Home Care
228 7th St. SE
Washington, DC 20003
Phone: 202-547-6586

**National Association of Local Boards of
Health**
1840 East Gypsy Lane Rd.
Bowling Green, OH 43402
Phone: 419-353-7714
http://www.nalboh.org

**National Black Nurses'
Association, Inc.**
8630 Fenton St., Suite 330

Silver Spring, MD 20910
Phone: 301-589-3200
http://www.nbna.org/

**National Black Women's Health Project
(NBWHP)**
Public Education/Policy Office
1211 Connecticut Ave., NW, Suite 310
Washington, DC 20036
Phone: 202-835-0117
http://www.blackwomenshealth.org/
site/PageServer

**National Center for
Health Statistics**
3311 Toledo Rd.
Hyattsville, MD 20782
Phone: 301-458-4636
http://www.cdc.gov/nchs/

**National Center for Injury Prevention
and Control (NCIPC)**
Mailstop K65
4770 Buford Highway, NE
Atlanta, GA 30341-3724
Phone: 770-488-1506
http://www.cdc.gov/ncipc

**National Coalition Building Institute
(NCBI)**
1835 K St. N.W., Suite 715
Washington, DC 20006
Phone: 202-785-9400
http://www.ncbi.org

**National Health Resource Center on
Domestic Violence**
6400 Flank Dr.
Suite 1300
Harrisburg, PA 17112
Phone: 800-537-2238
http://endabuse.org/programs/display.php
3?DocID=41

**National Hospice and Palliative Care
Organization**
1901 North Moore St., #901
Arlington, VA 22209
Phone: 800-658-8898
http://www.nho.org/templates/1/home-
page.cfm

**National Immunization
Program (NIP)**
Centers for Disease Control and
Prevention
1600 Clifton Road, NE
Mailstop E52
Atlanta, GA 30333
Phone: 800-232-2522
http://www.cdc.gov/nip

National Indian Health Board
1385 South Colorado Blvd.,
Suite A-707
Denver, CO 80222
Phone: 303-759-3075
http://www.nihb.org

**National Institute for Occupational
Safety and Health (NIOSH)**
4676 Columbia Parkway
Cincinnati, OH 45226
Phone: 800-356-4674
http://www.cdc.gov/niosh

National Lead Information Center
8601 Georgia Ave.
Suite 503
Silver Spring, MD 20910
Phone: 800-424-5323
http://www.epa.gov/lead/nlic.htm

National Medical Association
1012 10th St., NW
Washington, DC 20001
Phone: 202-347-1895
http://nmanet.org

**Office of Minority Health Resource
Center, Public Health Service, US
Department of Health and Human
Services**
P.O. Box 37337
Washington, DC 20013-7337
Phone: 301-230-7199
http://www.omhrc.gov/omhrc/index.htm

Office of Population Affairs
1101 Wootton Parkway, Suite 700
Rockville, MD 20852
Phone: 301-654-6190
http://opa.osophs.dhhs.gov/

Public Health Foundation
1220 L St., N.W., Suite 350
Washington, DC 20005
Phone: 202-898-5600
http://www.phf.org

**Resources for Cross Cultural
Health Care**
27 Aspen Circle
Albany, NY 12208
Phone: 518-435-1972
http://www.diversityrx.org/HTML/
WERCCH.htm

Robert Wood Johnson Foundation
Route One and College Road East
P.O. Box 2316
Princeton, NJ 08543-2316
http://www.rwjf.org

**Sexuality Information and Education
Council of the U.S. (SIECUS)**
130 W. 42nd Street, Suite 350
New York, NY 10036-7802
Phone: 212-819-9770
http://www.siecus.org

The Center for Mental Health Services
P.O. Box 42490
Washington, DC 20015
Phone: 800-789-2647
http://www.mentalhealth.org

**Office on Violence Against Women
Office**
U.S. Department of Justice
810 7th St., NW
Washington, DC 20531
Phone: 202-307-6026
http://www.ojp.usdoj.gov/vawo/
welcome.html

Author Index

Subject Index

About the Author

Demetrius James Porche, Ph.D., is Professor of Nursing and Associate Dean for Nursing Research and Evaluation at the Louisiana State University Health Sciences Center in New Orleans, Louisiana, and Adjunct, Associate Professor at Tulane University School of Public Health and Tropical Medicine in the Community Health Sciences Department. He received his Bachelor of Science in Nursing degree from Nicholls State University and his Master of Nursing and Doctor of Nursing Science degrees from Louisiana State University Medical Center. A certified clinical specialist in community health nursing and family nurse practitioner, his clinical experience includes critical care nursing, home health nursing, hospice nursing, infection control and epidemiological surveillance, and clinical specialization in HIV and other blood-borne illnesses. His community health experience is concentrated in comprehensive school health program management, the homeless population, HIV prevention, community capacity building, and program planning. His research interests include health promotion and disease prevention, men's health, behavior change and modification, and community-level evaluation. He is currently a research and evaluation consultant to several community-based organizations. His professional leadership roles include Vice President of the New Orleans District Nurses Association, Louisiana State Nurses Association Consultant to the Louisiana Association of Student Nurses, President of Xi Zeta Sigma (Theta Tau Chapter), and HIV/AIDS Expert Panel Member for the International Council for Nurses. He currently serves as associate editor of the *Journal of the Association of Nurses in AIDS Care* and associate editor of the *Journal of Multicultural Nursing and Health Care.*